CLINICAL APPLICATION OF BLOOD GASES
Fourth Edition

Clinical Application of Blood Gases
Fourth Edition

Barry A. Shapiro, M.D.
Professor of Clinical Anesthesia
Director of Respiratory/Critical Care Medicine
Department of Anesthesiology
Northwestern University Medical School
Medical Director of Respiratory Care Services
Northwestern Memorial Hospital
Chicago, Illinois

Ronald A. Harrison, M.D.
Associate Professor of Clinical Anesthesia
Northwestern Medical School
Chicago, Illinois

Roy D. Cane, M.D.
Professor of Clinical Anesthesia
Associate Director of Respiratory/Critical Care Medicine
Department of Anesthesiology
Northwestern University Medical School
Associate Medical Director of Respiratory Care Services
Northwestern Memorial Hospital
Chicago, Illinois

Rozanna Kozlowski-Templin, B.A., C.C.P.T.
Director of Blood Gas Laboratories
Department of Respiratory Care
Northwestern Memorial Hospital
Chicago, Illinois

YEAR BOOK MEDICAL PUBLISHERS, INC.
CHICAGO • LONDON • BOCA RATON

1   2   3   4   5   6   7   8   9   0   K   R   93   92   91   90   89

Library of Congress Cataloging-in-Publication Data
Clinical application of blood gases / Barry A. Shapiro ... [et al.]. -
  - 4th ed.
     p. cm.
   Rev. ed. of: Clinical application of blood gases / Barry A.
Shapiro, Ronald A. Harrison, John R. Walton, 3rd ed. 1982.
   Includes bibliographies and index.
   ISBN 0-8151-7657-0
   1. Blood gases—Analysis.   I. Shapiro, Barry A., 1937-
II. Shapiro, Barry A., 1937-   Clinical application of blood gases.
   [DNLM: 1. Blood Gas Analysis.   QY 450 C641]
RB45.2.C55 1989   88-26184
616.07'561—dc19   CIP
DNLM/DLC
for Library of Congress

Sponsoring Editor: Richard H. Lampert
Assistant Director, Manuscript Services: Fran Perveiler
Production Project Manager: Nancy Baker
Proofroom Manager: Shirley E. Taylor

To David, Leslie and Pat

FOREWORD TO THE FIRST EDITION

In the early 1950s many clinicians assumed that an arbitrary "normal" blood pressure was necessary to sustain life. With little concern for maintaining blood flow to vital organs, an attempt was usually made to keep systolic blood pressure, measured by indirect and imprecise methods, above 100 mm Hg. As a result, for a decade few patients died in shock or from an acute illness without having received an infusion of the pressor substance norepinephrine, sometimes in extraordinary concentration. At autopsy, pathologic evidence of excessive vasoconstriction was often apparent, raising questions as to whether the disease or the treatment was responsible for death. Today, this practice has waned and less attention is paid to an arbitrary blood pressure level; more thought is given to the basic principles of cardiovascular regulation, vasopressors are used less frequently, more fluid is given to expand the vascular space, and therapy is directed at specific components of the cardiovascular system.

We appear to be in the middle of another, similar cycle, also concerning clinical physiologic measurements, namely, blood gas determinations. These values, like blood pressure, are subject to errors in measurement as well as errors in sampling and handling. As with blood pressure, blood gases are valid only at the instant the measurement is made and do not reveal anything about the status of tissue perfusion.

The periodic measurement of blood gases in sick patients was not common until the mid-1960s. Even today, the analyses are usually not available in small hospitals, and in many teaching hospitals blood gases can be obtained readily only from 8 A.M. to 5 P.M. These determinations have been accorded great importance in diagnosis and monitoring patient care, especially in acute medicine—so much so that there are those who appear to believe that if blood gases were measured, then the patient obviously had received the best possible care. If the findings were within normal limits and the patient died, nothing more could have been done; if the results were abnormal and the patient died, then the cause of death was apparent.

Measurement of blood oxygen or carbon dioxide tension and hydrogen ion concentration yields information otherwise unobtainable, but such analyses cannot be considered independently of other laboratory tests or clinical observations any more than can a high specific gravity of urine, a low hematocrit or a high body temperature. This is only one of a series of tests and it must be placed in perspective. Doctor Shapiro proposes to do this in his monograph—and I think he does it well!

James E. Eckenhoff, M.D.
Professor of Anesthesia and Dean
Northwestern University Medical School
Chicago, Illinois

PREFACE

Since the original publication of *Clinical Application of Blood Gases* in 1973, it has been updated twice and translated into four languages. Like its predecessors, this fourth edition is devoted to a single purpose—to aid and promote the appropriate interpretation of blood gas measurements in the acute clinical setting. For more than 15 years both praise and criticism have been offered as to how well or poorly that goal is accomplished. The task is especially difficult because numerous educational and professional levels of health care providers (physicians, critical care nurses, respiratory therapists) are involved in acute respiratory care. In this fourth addition I have attempted to retain those elements well received in the past while adding relevant discussion of new information and technology. The result is five Sections composed of 14 new chapters and 14 chapters containing updated material from previous editions.

Section I contains six updated chapters reviewing the physics, chemistry, and respiratory physiology fundamental to pH and blood gas interpretation. This presentation is intended as an overview for the student and others requiring introductory information. Since these chapters serve only as review for most clinicians, appropriate references to this background information are included throughout the text. Section V is composed of two chapters presenting basic and advanced case studies keyed to text chapters. These are intended to aid the student and relatively inexperienced clinician.

Section II presents eight chapters devoted to the body of knowledge upon which pH and blood gas measurements can be appropriately applied to monitor respiratory homeostasis and guide therapy in the acutely ill patient. This section includes information that was not available at the time the third edition was written, e.g., the effects of metabolic abnormalities, low flow cardiac output states, and temperature variation. These complex factors are common in critically ill patients, yet only recently understood as to their potential impact on interpretation of blood gases.

Section III addresses the utilization and limitations of continuous in-vivo measurements that potentially reflect the blood gases, i.e., pulse oximetry, transcutaneous electrodes, capnography, pulmonary artery oximetry, and fluorescent optode technology. Most of this information has accumulated since the third edition was published and is presented in five new chapters.

Section IV is composed of seven chapters. The first three chapters coalesce and update technical information presented in previous editions. Four new chapters discuss technology that has become important since the last edition. These chapters are not intended to be laboratory manuals but rather to serve as a resource for clinically relevant information pertaining to the technical aspects of blood gas measurement.

This fourth edition is in large part the product of my co-authors. Dr. Ronald Harrison's significant contributions to the second and third editions continue to stand the test of time. Dr. Roy Cane contributes his significant clinical knowledge and experience to this edition, as does Rozanna Kozlowski-Templin in the technical areas. I am indebted to their consistent support, patience and dedication. I wish to acknowledge Dr. Hak Yui Wong for his contribution to the information pertaining to temperature correction, Judith Stutz for manuscript preparation and E. Kelly Quinn for secretarial coordination.

Although the medical scientific community has decided to gradually adopt the use of System Internationale (S.I.) Units, I have chosen to not utilize S.I. units for purposes of clarity and readability. The S.I. system calls for pressure to be expressed as kilopascals (kPa) rather than millimeters of mercury (mm Hg). The conversion factor for mm Hg to kPa is 0.133. Bicarbonate is expressed in mmol/L rather than mEq/L with a conversion factor of 1. I leave it to each reader to make the transition as deemed appropriate.

The physiologic data provided by blood gas analysis remains the cornerstone of monitoring respiratory homeostasis. Appropriate interpretation and clinical application of these measurements demands an in-depth knowledge of the associated physics, chemistry, pathophysiology, and technology. It is my hope that this fourth edition of *Clinical Application of Blood Gases* will provide a useful resource for all health care providers involved in acute respiratory care.

Barry A. Shapiro, M.D.

CONTENTS

PART ONE

Fundamentals of Blood Gas Interpretation

1

Physics and Chemistry

THE PHYSICS OF GAS

The exchange of gas molecules across permeable membranes (respiration) is a physical phenomenon essential to the maintenance of life. Gas molecules are constantly in motion and randomly colliding with each other and with various surfaces. The nature of these gas molecules dictates three intuitive truths:

1. The gas occupies a volume. The nature of that volume and the number of gas molecules affect the behavior of the gas.
2. The gas exerts a pressure within the volume. The frequency of the random collisions of the molecules against the sides of the container determines the pressure.
3. The gas has a temperature because molecular movement is a process of heat expenditure. This temperature determines how fast the molecules move.

Intuitive understanding may be a helpful beginning, but the pertinent physics and chemistry must be understood before extending these generalities to the clinical setting.

Matter is defined as the material from which physical substances are formed. Matter exists in three primary forms on the earth's surface: solid, liquid, and gas. Gases are distinguished from other states of matter by their ability to expand without limit to fill the available space and to exert pressure uniformly on all surfaces. Knowledge of certain physical properties of gases (e.g., volume, temperature, pressure) is essential for understanding their behavior.

1. *Volume* refers to the space that a gas occupies and is measured in terms of cubic centimeters (cc) or milliliters (ml).

2. *Pressure* is defined mathematically as force per unit area. In practice, the measurement is obtained by noting the height to which the force can support a column of mercury. This is most often expressed as millimeters of mercury (mm Hg).*

On the earth's surface, gas molecules are in constant motion (kinetic movement). Such molecular movement produces heat. Quantitation of the heat is called *temperature.*

3. *Temperature* is classically measured with a thermometer—an instrument that registers a change in volume in response to a change in heat.

Volume changes due to heat variability are carefully calibrated at reproducible points in various liquids—e.g., the boiling point and freezing point of water. With standard substances such as mercury or alcohol, these incremental changes in volume are measured and so-called temperature scales are derived. There are three temperature scales commonly used today: the Fahrenheit, centigrade, and Kelvin scales.

The Fahrenheit scale is seldom used in medicine although it is the most commonly used temperature scale in the United States. On this scale, the freezing point of water is set at 32° and the boiling point of water at 212°.

The centigrade (Celsius) scale is so designed that the total change in volume from the freezing point of water (0°) to the boiling point of water (100°) is divided into 100 equal increments. This is the most common temperature scale used in medicine and is considered the metric temperature scale.

The Kelvin (absolute) temperature scale uses the same incremental volume changes per degree as does the centigrade scale. However, 0° Kelvin is equal to −273° centigrade—a temperature that theoretically represents the point where all molecular movement ceases; this is called absolute zero.

When comparing the behavior of different gases (or different amounts of the same gas), it is necessary to quantitate the amount of gas (i.e., the number of molecules) in the sample. Although gas particles are small, they do have a mass. When mass is measured in relation to the earth's gravitational force, it is called *weight.* The mass or weight of a defined amount of gas is quantitated by *Avogadro's number*; that is, 6.023×10^{23} molecules of any gas equal 1 gm molecular weight (gram atomic weight).

*The classic mercury scale is known as the *Torricelli scale*; often the units of the Torricelli scale (mm Hg) are referred to as *Torr.*

When gases in physical chemistry are described, n stands for the number of molecules in a gas sample.* This allows for the comparison of different gases by knowing both their atomic weight and the weight of the respective sample.

The Gas Laws

From physical chemistry it is known that all gases behave in an "ideally" predictable fashion at exceedingly low pressures—commonly referred to as the behavior of an "ideal gas." Real gases behave in extremely complicated ways at great extremes of pressure; however, in the range of pressures found at the earth's surface, the behavior of these real gases closely approximates that of the ideal gas. A mathematical relationship known as the *ideal gas law* has been developed to describe the behavior of these real gases under conditions found at the earth's surface:

$$P \times V = nR \times T$$

P is pressure in atmospheres—1 atm equals 760 mm Hg; V is volume in liters (L)—1 ml equals 0.001 L; T is temperature on the Kelvin scale; n equals the amount of gas present; and R is the gas constant—a fixed value of 0.082 expressed in liter atmospheres per mole degree. Mathematically, R is referred to as a constant of proportionality and allows for the interrelationship of the various properties of the gas, such as pressure, volume, and temperature.

From the ideal gas law, if the amount of gas remains constant (i.e., n remains constant), the interrelationships of temperature, pressure, and volume under differing sets of conditions may be predicted. In other words, assuming nR is constant:

$$\frac{P_1 \times V_1}{T_1} = \frac{P_2 \times V_2}{T_2}$$

When one of the three terms (P, V, T) remains unchanged while another changes its value, the third term must change in a predictable manner. When any one value remains unchanged, the three possible relationships are as follows:

1. Boyle's law: $P_1 \times V_1 = P_2 \times V_2$

*When $n = 1$, it means that the measured weight of that gaseous substance in grams is numerically equal to its gram atomic weight.

Boyle's law states that if temperature remains constant, pressure will vary inversely with volume. The disease tuberculosis (TB) is a useful mnemonic: T = temperature constant, B = Boyle's law.

2. Charles' law: $\dfrac{V_1}{T_1} = \dfrac{V_2}{T_2}$

Charles' law states that if pressure is held constant, volume and temperature will vary directly. The disease cerebral palsy (CP) is a useful mnemonic: C = Charles' law; P = pressure constant.

3. Gay-Lussac's law: $\dfrac{P_1}{T_1} = \dfrac{P_2}{T_2}$

Gay-Lussac's law states that if volume is held constant, pressure and temperature will vary directly. Vitamin G is a useful mnemonic: V = volume constant; G = Gay-Lussac's law.

Partial Pressure of Gases

The earth's atmosphere is composed primarily of gas molecules. These molecules have mass and are attracted toward the earth's center by the force of gravity. At the earth's surface, this atmospheric weight exerts a pressure sufficient to support a column of mercury 760 mm high. This *atmospheric pressure* affects everything on the earth's surface; life forms are no exception.

The earth's atmosphere is composed of varying amounts of several different gases; therefore, understanding the behavior of gases when they are mixed together is imperative. *Dalton's law* summarizes a very important physical principle pertaining to the mixture of gases: *In a mixture of gases, the total pressure is equal to the sum of the partial pressures of the separate components* (Fig 1–1). It is sometimes easier to think of a partial pressure of a component gas as the pressure that gas would exert if it were present alone in the system. In other words, since each of the individual gases may be considered as acting independently, its contribution to the total pressure is dependent on what fraction or percent of the total gases it occupies (Table 1–1).

Water Vapor Pressure

Some substances exist in more than one state of matter under certain environmental conditions. Within a given range of temperatures and

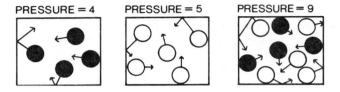

FIG 1–1.
A simplified illustration of the principle of partial pressures according to Dalton's law. The three *squares* represent containers of equal volumes and constant temperatures. The *circles* represent gas molecules in motion. The pressure within the container is the result of gas molecules colliding with the sides of the container.

If four molecules of gas A *(black circles)* are present, the total pressure may be theoretically expressed as 4; if five molecules of gas B *(white circles)* are present, the total pressure may be theoretically expressed as 5; if a mixture of gases A and B is present, the total pressure may be theoretically expressed as 9.

Since the total pressure of 9 is the sum of the partial pressures (i.e., partial pressure of gas A is 4, partial pressure of gas B is 5), the pressure exerted by each individual gas is the same whether it occupies the space by itself or is present in a mixture of other gases.

pressures, water can exist as a liquid, a gas, or a solid.* Water in the gaseous form is called *water vapor* or molecular water and is referred to as *humidity*. When water vapor exists in a mixture of gases, it follows the gas laws and exerts a partial pressure. Alveolar gas is 100% humidified at body temperature; therefore, "ideal" alveolar gas has a water vapor pressure (PH_2O) of 47 mm Hg.

Clinical measurements are usually accomplished under "standard" conditions. In blood gas measurements, the standard conditions are body temperature and pressure fully saturated (BTPS). Body temperature is 37°C; the pressure is the atmospheric pressure to which the body is exposed; saturated refers to maximum water vapor at 37°C, which is 47 mm Hg.

Diffusion and Blood Gas Solubility

The constant random movement of gas molecules results in those molecules moving from an area of relatively high concentration toward an area of lower concentration. This net passive movement of gas molecules is called *diffusion*.[†] All life is dependent on the ability of gas

---

*When a substance such as H_2O exists simultaneously in both the liquid and gaseous phases, the partial pressure it exerts as a gas is directly related to the existing temperature. In general, the partial pressure of the gas increases as the temperature increases until it equals the ambient pressure, at which point the liquid (H_2O) boils.

†The presence of a semipermeable membrane, such as the alveolar capillary membrane of the lung, can be visualized as a limiting factor allowing for only selective diffusion of certain substances.

TABLE 1–1.

Partial Pressures of Component Gases Comprising Air Under Various Conditions

Component Gas	Percent of Total Gas	Partial Pressure (mm Hg)
Air at sea level (760 mm Hg)		
Oxygen (O_2)	20.9	159
Nitrogen (N_2)	79.0	600
Others	0.1	1
Ideal *alveolar gas* at sea level (760 mm Hg) (air sample)		
Oxygen (O_2)	13.3	101
Nitrogen (N_2)	75.2	572
Carbon dioxide (CO_2)	5.3	40
Water vapor (H_2O)	6.2	47
Air at 18,000 ft above sea level (380 mm Hg)		
Oxygen (O_2)	20.9	79.4
Nitrogen (N_2)	79.0	300.2
Others	0.1	0.4
Ideal *alveolar gas* at 18,000 ft above sea level (380 mm Hg) (air sample)		
Oxygen (O_2)	5.9	22
Nitrogen (N_2)	73.9	271
Carbon dioxide (CO_2)	10.6	40
Water vapor (H_2O)	12.4	47

molecules to cross cell membranes. This process of *gas diffusion* across a semipermeable membrane occurs primarily in response to a pressure gradient; that is, the pressure on one side of the membrane must be greater than the pressure on the other side. In general, the greater the pressure difference, the faster will be the net movement of molecules. *Each gas moves according to its own pressure gradient without regard to what other gases in the mixture may be doing.* Net movement stops when the partial pressures are equal on both sides, a situation referred to as a state of *dynamic equilibrium*.

If a membrane separates a gas mixture from a liquid, the degree to which the gases can dissolve in the liquid will affect the diffusion process. In general, when a gas is exposed to a liquid, the gas molecules move into the liquid and become dissolved unless they combine chemically with constituents of the liquid. Eventually the number of gas molecules leaving the liquid equals the number of gas molecules entering the liquid, and a state of dynamic equilibrium is established. In other words, the pressure of the gases in the liquid will then be equal to the pressure of the gases in the atmosphere or, more exactly, the *partial pressures in solution* will be equal to the atmospheric partial pressures. *Henry's law* states that the amount of gas that can be dissolved in a liquid is proportional to the partial pressure of the gas to which the liquid is exposed.

There are several other factors that determine how effectively gas will diffuse across the alveolar capillary membrane. One factor is the weight of the gas and is expressed in *Graham's law*. This states that the diffusibility of a gas is inversely proportional to the square root of its molecular weight; in other words, the heavier the molecule, the less its diffusibility.

CHEMISTRY OF ACID-BASE BALANCE

Solutions

An element is a simple substance that cannot be decomposed by ordinary chemical means. An *atom* is the smallest quantity of an element that can exist and still retain the chemical properties of the element. An atom is composed of negatively charged electrons orbiting around a nucleus containing positively charged *protons* and uncharged *neutrons*. The majority of the mass (weight) of an atom exists in its nucleus.

Most elements in their natural state have an equal number of positively and negatively charged particles.* An atom is in the *ionized state* when one or more electrons are either removed from or added to the outermost orbit.

A *solution* is a liquid consisting of a mixture of two or more substances that are molecularly dispersed throughout one another in a homogeneous manner. A solution consists of a *solvent* (the major component) and one or more *solutes* (minor components). In biologic solutions, water may be considered the major component (solvent); all other substances in solution are considered solutes.

In biologic solutions, solutes exist in both un-ionized (undissociated) and ionized (dissociated) states. That portion of the substance existing in the dissociated state is referred to as an *ion*. It should be obvious that ions have an excess or a deficit of electrons in their outer orbits; that is, ions have net electric charges. Ions with net positive charges are *cations*; ions with net negative charges are *anions*.

The equilibrium between two states of a substance in solution depends on several factors, including the chemical interrelationships of the substance and the numbers and types of other substances in the

---

*The *atomic number* is based on the number of protons in the nucleus. The number of protons plus the number of neutrons equals the *atomic weight* of the atom.

solution (Table 1–2). Certain substances such as strong acids, strong bases, and salts exist in solution primarily in the ionized state. Weak acids and bases exist in solution in varying degrees of ionization. It is important to realize that a small number of water molecules exist in the ionized state.

Hydrogen Ion Activity

The maintenance of cellular function is dependent on cellular metabolism (biochemical and enzymatic processes). This metabolic process demands an exacting environment. There are many factors, such as temperature, osmolarity, electrolytes, nutrients, and oxygen, that must be maintained within narrow limits if the cell is to preserve its normal metabolic function. One of the most important factors in this cellular environment is the *hydrogen ion activity*—often referred to as the "free hydrogen ion in solution." This is most commonly expressed as *hydrogen ion concentration* ($[H^+]$).

Substances that tend to donate hydrogen ions to the solution are called *acids*; substances that tend to remove hydrogen ions from the solution are *bases*. Thus, strong acids are capable of donating many free hydrogen ions to the solution, and strong bases can accept many free hydrogen ions from the solution. This situation may be visualized as two points of a spectrum, one end representing a strong acid and the other end representing a strong base. In between these two extremes substances can act as weak acids or weak bases.

Weak acids or weak bases accept or donate hydrogen ions in response to the availability of free hydrogen ions in solution. This phenomenon is extremely important in minimizing changes in the free hydrogen ion concentration and thus stabilizing the free hydrogen ion concentration in the cells of biologic systems. A substance that prevents extreme changes in the free hydrogen ion concentration within a solution

TABLE 1–2.

Substances in Solution

Example	Undissociated	Dissociated
Strong acid: hydrochloric acid	$HCl \rightleftharpoons$	$H^+ + Cl^-$
Strong base: sodium hydroxide	$NaOH \rightleftharpoons$	$Na^+ + OH^-$
Salt: sodium chloride	$NaCl \rightleftharpoons$	$Na^+ + Cl^-$
Weak acid: carbonic acid	$H_2CO_3 \rightleftharpoons$	$H^+ + HCO_3^-$
Water	$H_2O \rightleftharpoons$	$H^+ + OH^-$

is defined as a *buffer* substance. These buffers allow cellular metabolism to continue unimpeded when the cells are subjected to significant increases or decreases in the number of hydrogen ions. There are four major buffer systems in the body: hemoglobin, bicarbonate, phosphate and serum protein.

The importance of hydrogen activity in cellular function necessitates its quantitative measurement. The most widely accepted method uses the pH scale. This scale is derived from and dependent on the fact that water dissociates very weakly to form some hydrogen (H^+) and hydroxyl (OH^-) ions. The relationship can be expressed as an *ionization constant of water* known as a K_w.

$$H_2O \leftrightharpoons H^+ + OH^-$$

$$K_w = \frac{[H^+][OH^-]}{H_2O}$$

Since the concentration of hydrogen and hydroxyl ions is so small, the concentration of undissociated water $[H_2O]$ remains essentially unchanged. Therefore, the K_w of water can be written as follows:

$$K_w = [H^+][OH^-]$$
$$= [1 \times 10^{-7}][1 \times 10^{-7}]$$
$$= 1 \times 10^{-14}$$

Note that there are equal numbers of hydrogen and hydroxyl ions; thus, the solution is referred to as a *neutral* solution.

Since humans are composed of 50% to 60% water, it is appropriate to use water as the biologic reference solvent. The ionization constant of water (1×10^{-14}) is equal to the product of the concentrations of hydrogen ions and hydroxyl ions; the product of these two concentrations must remain numerically unchanged. Therefore, as hydrogen ions increase in number (an acid solution), there must be a corresponding decrease in the number of hydroxyl ions. Conversely, as hydrogen ions decrease in number (a basic solution), there must be a corresponding increase in the number of hydroxyl ions.

In clinical medicine, emphasis is placed on the hydrogen ion concentration. Because of the small concentrations of hydrogen ion, their expression in the customary fraction or decimal form would be extremely unwieldy. Therefore, an *exponential* form is used to denote the value (Table 1–3). In the exponential form, the power to which 10 must be

TABLE 1–3.

Comparison of Fraction, Decimal, and
Exponential Forms

Fraction	Decimal	Exponent
$\frac{1}{10}$	0.1	10^{-1}
$\frac{1}{1,000}$	0.001	10^{-3}
$\frac{1}{10,000,000}$	0.0000001	10^{-7}
$\frac{1}{100,000,000}$	0.00000001	10^{-8}

multiplied is the exponent; for example, in (10^{-3}) the minus three (-3) is the exponent. When a number is written in a logarithmic form, it can be thought of as a simplified expression of a routine exponential form; 10^{-3} is logarithmically expressed as -3.

At the turn of the century, a Scandinavian scientist, S. P. L. Sorenson, who was studying hydrogen ion activity, referred to the concentration 10^{-7} as "7 puissance hydrogen." This is French for describing the hydrogen ion exponent of the base 10 on the logarithmic scale.

The Danish biochemist and physician, Karl Hasselbalch, embraced Sorenson's concept and expressed 10^{-7} mole/L as "the negative logarithm of the hydrogen ion activity." This he called the pH (puissance hydrogen). The mathematical definition of pH is as follows:

$$pH = -\log[H^+]$$

The introduction of a second minus multiplied by the log value allows *all pH values to be expressed as positive numbers* (Table 1–4).

In clinical medicine, most blood levels of hydrogen ion concentration are between 1×10^{-7} mole/L (pH 7) and 1×10^{-8} mole/L (pH 8). The

TABLE 1–4.

Comparison of
Exponential and
Logarithmic Forms

Exponent	pH $(-)$ Log
10^{-1}	1
10^{-3}	3
10^{-7}	7
10^{-8}	8

average value for hydrogen ion concentration in blood is 0.4×10^{-8} mole/L (pH 7.4).

Henderson-Hasselbalch Equation

The Henderson-Hasselbalch equation expresses the biologic acid-base relationship by looking at one specific component of the system—namely, the carbonic acid (H_2CO_3) to bicarbonate ion (HCO_3^-) relationship:

$$H_2CO_3 \rightleftharpoons H^+ + HCO_3^- \tag{1}$$

The amount of hydrogen ion activity secondary to the dissociation of carbonic acid is in turn governed by the interrelationship of all the blood acids, bases, and buffers. It is this vital interrelationship that allows for a complete analysis of acid-base balance by looking at only one component of the system.

The *law of mass action* states that in equation (1), the product of the concentrations of the substances on the right divided by the concentration of the substance on the left is equal to a constant written as a value K_A:

$$K_A = \frac{[H^+][HCO_3^-]}{[H_2CO_3]} \tag{2}$$

To express the hydrogen ion concentration in pH form, the log of both sides of equation (2) must be taken. This will not change the value of the equation.

$$\log K_A = \log \frac{[H^+][HCO_3^-]}{[H_2CO_3]} \tag{3}$$

$$\log K_A = \log[H^+] + \log \frac{[HCO_3^-]}{[H_2CO_3]} \tag{4}$$

The transposition of the log of the hydrogen ion concentration ($\log[H^+]$) to the left side of equation (4) and the log of K_A to the right side of the equation produces:

$$-\log[H^+] = -\log K_A + \log \frac{[HCO_3^-]}{[H_2CO_3]} \tag{5}$$

The term for minus the log of hydrogen ion concentration ($-\log[H^+]$) has already been defined as pH; the term for minus the log of $K_A (-\log K_A)$ is pK.

$$pH = pK + \log \frac{[HCO_3^-]}{[H_2CO_3]} \qquad (6)$$

The pK represents the pH value at which the solute is 50% dissociated. In equation (6), if the pH equaled the pK, there would be equal amounts of bicarbonate ion and carbonic acid. The importance of the pK is that it represents the pH at which maximum buffering capacity can be achieved for that particular reaction.

In equation (6), the carbonic acid concentration is dependent on the amount of dissolved carbon dioxide. The amount of carbon dioxide dissolved is in turn dependent on its solubility (expressed as a solubility coefficient s) and the partial pressure of carbon dioxide measured in the blood (P_{CO_2}). Therefore, in most clinical forms of equation (6), the carbonic acid concentration (H_2CO_3) is replaced by the solubility coefficient times the partial pressure of carbon dioxide (s $\times$ P_{CO_2}):

$$pH = pK + \log \frac{[HCO_3^-]}{s \times P_{CO_2}} \qquad (7)$$

The pK is 6.1; s is 0.0301.

Carbon Dioxide Chemistry

When carbon dioxide (CO_2) is dissolved in water (dCO_2) the formation of carbonic acid (H_2CO_3) takes place very slowly (Table 1–5). In plasma, the concentration of dissolved carbon dioxide (dCO_2) is approximately 1,000 times greater than the concentration of carbonic acid.

An enzyme is a substance that alters the speed at which a chemical reaction takes place but is not consumed or altered in the process. *Car-*

TABLE 1–5.

Formation of Carbonic Acid

Plasma
$$H_2O + dCO_2 \rightarrow H_2CO_3 \rightleftarrows H^+ + HCO_3^-$$
$$\qquad\qquad 1,000 \quad : \quad 1$$
Red blood cells
$$H_2O + dCO_2 \rightleftarrows H_2CO_3 \rightleftarrows H^+ + HCO_3^-$$

---

bonic anhydrase is an enzyme that exists in red blood cells and kidney tubular cells. This enzyme speeds the reaction forming carbonic acid (see Table 1–5). Remember, this enzyme does *not* exist in plasma.

Total Dissolved Carbon Dioxide

It is difficult to distinguish between dissolved carbon dioxide (dCO_2) and carbonic acid (H_2CO_3); therefore, it is convenient to add the respective concentrations and refer to this sum as the *total* dissolved carbon dioxide in plasma:

$$\text{Total } dCO_{2\text{Plasma}} = [dCO_2 + H_2CO_3]_{\text{Plasma}}$$

At BTPS the relationship of this total carbon dioxide dissolved to carbon dioxide partial pressure (PCO_2) can be written as follows:

$$\text{Total carbon dioxide dissolved} = (0.0301)(PCO_2)$$

In other words, the carbon dioxide partial pressure (PCO_2) times its solubility coefficient ($s = 0.0301$) gives the value of the total carbon dioxide dissolved. In essence, a measurement of blood PCO_2 can be considered equivalent to a measurement of the plasma carbonic acid plus the dissolved carbon dioxide.

Figure 1–2 illustrates the plasma relationship of dissolved carbon dioxide (dCO_2) and carbonic acid. Most of the carbon dioxide enters the red blood cell, while a small portion remains dissolved in plasma. This

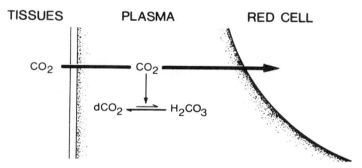

FIG 1–2.
The plasma relationship of dissolved carbon dioxide (dCO_2) and carbonic acid (H_2CO_3). Note that only a small amount (approximately 5%) of the CO_2 that enters the blood remains in the plasma. Virtually 99.9% of this plasma CO_2 remains in the dissolved state, while approximately 0.1% reacts with water to form H_2CO_3: i.e., by volume, the relationship dCO_2/H_2CO_3 is 1,000/1. The dissolved CO_2 exerts a pressure (Henry's law) and is measured clinically as the PCO_2 (partial pressure of carbon dioxide).

small portion is a critical factor that determines carbon dioxide movement into or out of the blood. As the carbon dioxide tension in cells and extracellular fluid is increased by metabolism, the rate and amount of carbon dioxide movement into the blood are increased. Since carbon dioxide can be dissolved in plasma to only a limited degree, most of the carbon dioxide enters the red blood cells. The red blood cells transport carbon dioxide much more efficiently because of carbonic anhydrase and hemoglobin.

In general, the greater the total amount of carbon dioxide in the blood, the greater is the amount in the plasma (as either dissolved carbon dioxide or carbonic acid). This total dissolved carbon dioxide, although an extremely small portion of the total carbon dioxide content, is extremely critical because it exerts the pressure in the blood that determines the gradient by which carbon dioxide enters or leaves the blood.

2

Physiology of Respiration

Homeostasis . . . the tendency of a system, esp. the physiological system of higher animals, to maintain internal stability, owing to the coordinated response of its parts to any situation or stimulus tending to disturb its normal condition or function.—*The Random House Dictionary of the English Language*

CARDIOPULMONARY HOMEOSTASIS

The single-celled animal directly acquires oxygen from the environment and expels the carbon dioxide metabolite; the entire process requires nothing more than simple diffusion across the cell membrane. In man, the homeostatic necessity of gas exchange (respiration) involves the cardiopulmonary system—two distinct sets of capillary beds plus the pulmonary and cardiovascular systems.

Cardiopulmonary homeostasis may be conceived as the resultant of the mechanisms acting on the cardiovascular and pulmonary systems to maintain adequate respiration. Figure 2–1 illustrates many of the components of this delicate balance. One must comprehend the primary factors that determine cardiopulmonary homeostasis because *it is this homeostasis that the blood gases reflect.*

Systemic Capillary System

At the distal end of the systemic arterial system is the *systemic capillary bed*, which pervades nearly all tissues. This is where gas exchange between blood and tissue takes place—the exchange known as *internal respiration*. It is traditionally measured by the *respiratory quotient*, which is the ratio of the carbon dioxide produced to the oxygen consumed.

EXTERNAL RESPIRATION

PULMONARY CAPILLARY BED

$\dot{V}_A/\dot{Q}$

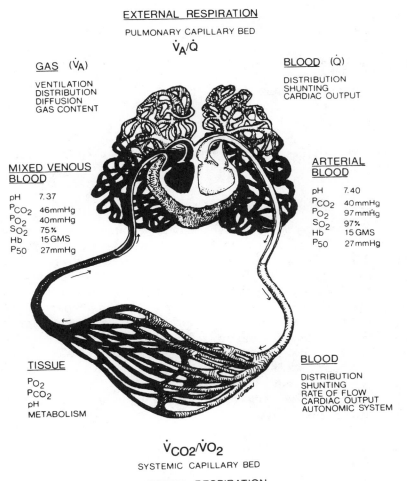

GAS ($\dot{V}_A$)

VENTILATION
DISTRIBUTION
DIFFUSION
GAS CONTENT

BLOOD ($\dot{Q}$)

DISTRIBUTION
SHUNTING
CARDIAC OUTPUT

MIXED VENOUS
BLOOD

pH	7.37
P_{CO_2}	46mmHg
P_{O_2}	40mmHg
S_{O_2}	75%
Hb	15 GMS
P_{50}	27mmHg

ARTERIAL
BLOOD

pH	7.40
P_{CO_2}	40mmHg
P_{O_2}	97mmHg
S_{O_2}	97%
Hb	15 GMS
P_{50}	27mmHg

TISSUE

P_{O_2}
P_{CO_2}
pH
METABOLISM

BLOOD

DISTRIBUTION
SHUNTING
RATE OF FLOW
CARDIAC OUTPUT
AUTONOMIC SYSTEM

$\dot{V}_{CO_2}/\dot{V}_{O_2}$

SYSTEMIC CAPILLARY BED

INTERNAL RESPIRATION

FIG 2–1.
The cardiopulmonary homeostatic schema (see text).

The normal value of the respiratory quotient is 0.8.

Gas exchange in the systemic capillary bed depends on many factors, including but not limited to:

1. Values of arterial blood gases entering the capillary bed.
2. Blood distribution throughout the capillary bed.
3. Arterial–to–venous shunting—i.e., the bypassing of the capillaries.

4. Rate of blood flow through the capillary bed.
5. Cardiac output—i.e., the total amount of blood circulated per minute.
6. Autonomic nervous system effects on the capillaries.
7. Tissue oxygen tension.
8. Tissue carbon dioxide tension.
9. Tissue pH.
10. Metabolic rate.

If one or more of these factors are abnormal, the homeostatic cycle will be affected.

Pulmonary Capillary System

Blood entering a portion of the systemic venous system reflects only the gas exchange of that particular tissue and may have inconsistent relationships with the total body homeostasis; total body homeostatic reflection is possible only after venous blood mixes in the right ventricle. The mixed venous blood (pulmonary artery blood) enters the *pulmonary capillary bed*, where gas exchange between blood and atmosphere takes place. This exchange of oxygen and carbon dioxide, known as *external respiration*, is traditionally measured by the respiratory exchange ratio (RR). This ratio (approximately 0.8) is numerically very close to the respiratory quotient (RQ), since external and internal respiration are equal in the steady state.

The factors involved in gas exchange in the pulmonary capillary bed include but are not limited to:

1. Distribution of the blood flow.
2. Intrapulmonary shunting.
3. Cardiac output.
4. Total ventilation (air movement into and out of the airway).
5. Distribution of inspired gases throughout the tracheobronchial tree and the alveoli.
6. Diffusion across the alveolar-capillary membrane.
7. Content of the inspired air.

Homeostatic Balance and Blood Gases

Venous blood collected from the systemic and pulmonary capillary beds is mixed together in the corresponding ventricles. Thus, blood leaving those ventricles must be measured if reflection of total body gas exchange is desired. Since respiration does not occur in the arteries, any arterial blood sample should be representative of blood leaving the corresponding ventricle. The easy availability of systemic arteries has made them the universal standard for obtaining clinical blood gas samples.

A change of any factor in the cardiopulmonary homeostatic schema (see Fig 2–1) results in (1) the arterial blood gas values changing, (2) an organ system increasing its work to maintain the homeostatic balance—the blood gas values remain relatively unchanged, or (3) various combinations of these two alternatives.

The degree of abnormality in arterial blood gas measurement is determined by the balance between the severity of disease and the degree of compensation (increased work) by the cardiopulmonary system. *Normal arterial blood gases do not mean there is an absence of cardiopulmonary disease*; there may be disease present but totally compensated. *Abnormal arterial blood gases mean that uncompensated disease is present*, which may be life-threatening.

INTERNAL RESPIRATION

The primary biologic purpose of respiration is to provide oxygen to the cells; the secondary purpose is to remove carbon dioxide from the cells.

Cellular Oxygen

As the earth's atmosphere developed from containing primarily hydrogen (a reducing atmosphere) to containing primarily oxygen (an oxidizing atmosphere), oxygen became available as an energy source for the development of cellular life because it was abundant and accessible and possessed a high energy potential. Thus, life forms developed using oxygen as the primary biomedical storage type of energy; in fact, complex forms of life evolved only after mechanisms for maintaining the cellular oxygen environment were developed.

The transition to an oxygen atmosphere forced complex biologic systems to develop defenses against the toxic effects of oxygen. In 1785, Lavoisier noted that oxygen must be considered a biomedical double-edged sword—it not only promotes life but also destroys life.[1] He noted that when there is an excess of oxygen, an animal undergoes a severe illness; when oxygen is lacking, death is almost instantaneous.

We now understand that increasing the oxygen tension in tissues will increase the energy available for biologic processes. However, more cellular constituents will be destroyed as oxygen tension increases. These two effects occur at all concentrations of oxygen and, thus, *there must be an oxygen pressure at which biologic activity is optimal.*[2, 3] If the oxygen tension is significantly above or below this optimal pressure, there are dire biologic consequences.

Cellular energy is necessary for chemical reactions. Many essential biochemical reactions for sustaining life require a considerable amount of energy—in fact, so much energy that they have been referred to as "thermodynamically improbable." This means that the energy required for many necessary biochemical cellular functions is so great that it is almost impossible for the cell to manufacture such energy. The cell obtains this great amount of energy from substances called *high-energy phosphate bonds*, primarily the high-energy phosphate bonds contained in adenosine triphosphate (ATP). Most cellular energy is used, transported, and stored in the form of these high-energy phosphate bonds. Breakdown of these bonds is accompanied by a tremendous energy release.

Oxidative metabolism is the normal mechanism by which energy is stored and released from high-energy phosphate bonds. The *mitochondria* are cellular constituents that contain all the components necessary to form and break down ATP. Molecular oxygen must be available in the cell for the biochemical process within the mitochondria (Krebs cycle) to produce high-energy phosphate bonds and allow the release of energy for biochemical processes.

When the delivery of oxygen to the mitochondria is impaired, the energy contained within the Krebs cycle is no longer available. The cellular oxygen tension at which the mitochondrial respiratory rate begins to decrease is called the *critical oxygen tension.*[4] Various studies show that as long as other factors are normal, the mitochondria can function adequately when cellular oxygen tension is as low as 5 mm Hg. At the present time, however, it is not possible to delineate critical oxygen tensions for vital organ systems under various conditions.

Tissue Hypoxia

Tissue hypoxia exists when cellular critical oxygen tensions are inadequate. This statement seems clinically appropriate since the importance of tissue hypoxia is that mechanisms other than oxidative ones must be used to provide metabolic energy. These *anaerobic* mechanisms are homeostatically undesirable because they are far less efficient than aerobic pathways and they produce metabolites other than carbon dioxide.

Classically, hypoxia is subdivided into four types: (1) hypoxemic hypoxia, (2) anemic hypoxia, (3) circulatory hypoxia, and (4) histotoxic hypoxia.

Hypoxemic Hypoxia

This is deficient tissue oxygenation due to inadequate arterial oxygenation. The hemoglobin available is insufficiently oxygenated and the resulting oxygen content is inadequate to maintain an adequate blood to tissue oxygen tension gradient. *In essence, this is hypoxia due to hypoxemia!* However, the presence of arterial hypoxemia does not automatically indicate the presence of tissue hypoxia. The cardiovascular system may adequately compensate by increasing cardiac output so that less oxygen is removed from each quantity of blood presented to the tissues. This mechanism frequently allows tissue oxygen requirements to be met. It should be emphasized that although hypoxemia does not necessarily indicate that tissue hypoxia is present, it must strongly *suggest* tissue hypoxia and necessitates complete clinical evaluation.

Anemic Hypoxia

This represents deficient tissue oxygenation because of a reduction in the oxygen-carrying capacity of the blood—that is, a deficiency either in the amount of hemoglobin (anemia) or in the ability of the hemoglobin to carry oxygen (methemoglobinemia, carbon monoxide poisoning, and others). *The arterial blood may have a perfectly normal arterial oxygen tension.* This is one of the circumstances that stress the importance for the clinician to realize the difference between arterial oxygen tension and arterial oxygen content. The main compensatory mechanism for anemic hypoxia is an increase in cardiac output. Generally, it can be said that anemic hypoxia is rarely accompanied by hypoxemia.

Circulatory Hypoxia

Capillary circulation may become inadequate to meet the cellular requirement of oxygen. This can be thought of as either capillary stagnation (pooling) of the blood or failure of the capillaries to allow a flow of blood to the tissues (arterial-venous shunting).

Stagnant hypoxia is a result of sluggish peripheral capillary blood flow, which may be caused by decreased cardiac output, vascular insufficiency, or neurochemical abnormalities. The slow transit time of the blood through the capillaries results in prolonged oxygen exchange between a given amount of capillary blood and tissues. This exchange is eventually limited by a blood to tissue oxygen pressure gradient that is insufficient for oxygen movement from hemoglobin to tissue. Since tissue metabolism continues, a decrease in tissue oxygen tension (hypoxia) results. Stagnant hypoxia is primarily a cardiovascular phenomenon and commonly occurs unassociated with arterial hypoxemia; however, it is almost always associated with a severe reduction in venous oxygen content and venous oxygen tension.

Certain clinical conditions lead to *arterial-venous shunting* in the systemic capillaries. Where this occurs, capillary blood flow is absent and therefore oxygen is unavailable to the tissues. Often this type of tissue hypoxia is associated with above-normal cardiac outputs and is not associated with decreased arterial and venous oxygen tensions.

Histotoxic Hypoxia

This represents tissue oxygen deficiency due to failure of oxygen utilization at the cellular level. It is rarely accompanied by hypoxemia. The classic example is cyanide poisoning.

In summary, *tissue hypoxia is the condition in which inadequate oxygen is available at the cellular level.* Its direct measurement is not available and therefore it remains a purely clinical diagnosis. The condition is presumed from various clinical and laboratory findings.

Metabolic Rate

The basilar oxygen consumption of an average-size adult is approximately 250 ml/minute. Aerobic metabolism produces 80 ml carbon dioxide for each 100 ml oxygen consumed; this respiratory quotient (RQ) of 0.8 means that the normal adult produces 200 ml carbon dioxide for each 250 ml oxygen consumed. Increases in the metabolic rate can occur suddenly (such as in exercise) or they can gradually increase over periods of minutes to hours (such as a slow rise in a patient's temperature). An *increase* in body temperature is the most common reason for a change in the metabolic rate. Fever is responsible for a 10% increase in oxygen consumption for each degree Celsius (centigrade) rise in temperature (7% increase per degree Fahrenheit). Sudden increases in metabolic rate can be seen in patients who have had a grand mal seizure or a sudden increase in the work of breathing, such as would occur secondary to a partial upper airway obstruction. However, *under normal clinical circumstances the moment-to-moment demand for oxygen at the tissue level is fairly constant.*

EXTERNAL RESPIRATION

Gas exchange between blood and the external environment occurs in the pulmonary capillary bed—a process called *external respiration.* The quantities of carbon dioxide and oxygen exchanged must logically equal the exchange in the systemic capillaries, with oxygen being added to the blood while carbon dioxide is being removed. This relationship of volumes of carbon dioxide and oxygen exchanged per minute by the lungs is the *respiratory exchange ratio (RR)*. The respiratory exchange ratio represents the *overall* exchange capability of the lung, not individual variances within different parts of the lung.

An alternative method of expressing the effectiveness of pulmonary gas exchange is to consider the "matching" of ventilation and perfusion or, more precisely, the relationship between the volume of gas moving into an alveolus and the blood flow through the adjacent capillary. The advantage of this approach is that it takes into account the *efficiency* of molecular gas exchange in all areas of the lung. It is difficult to comprehend fully the complex ventilation to perfusion relationship; however, a basic understanding of the concept is necessary for the clinical application of blood gas measurements.

Distribution of Pulmonary Perfusion

The normal distribution of blood flow throughout the pulmonary vasculature is dependent on three major factors: (1) gravity, (2) cardiac output, and (3) pulmonary vascular resistance.

Gravity

In normal man standing erect, there is a distance of approximately 30 cm from the *apex* (top) to the *base* (bottom) of the lung. Assuming the pulmonary artery enters the lung halfway between top and bottom, the pulmonary artery pressure would have to be great enough to overcome a gravitational force of 15 cm of water to supply flow to the apex; a similar gradient would aid flow to the lung base. A column of blood (essentially H_2O) 15 cm high exerts a pressure of approximately 11 mm Hg. *This gravitational effect on blood flow results in a lateral wall pulmonary artery pressure at the lung base of greater magnitude than the pulmonary artery pressure at the apex.* Thus, blood will preferentially flow through the gravity-dependent areas of the lung (Fig 2–2).

Under normal circumstances, *alveolar* pressures are equal throughout the lung. Theoretically, the least gravity-dependent areas of the lung (the apex in the upright subject) may have alveolar pressures higher than the pulmonary arterial pressures at that level. This would result in the virtual absence of blood flow to these areas. It should be noted that the total absence of pulmonary blood flow to these areas does *not* exist to any significant extent in the normally perfused lung.[6] However, if

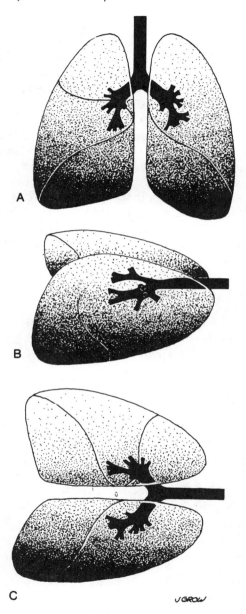

FIG 2–2.
The preponderance of pulmonary blood flow will normally occur in the gravity-dependent areas of the lung. Thus, body position has a significant effect on the distribution of pulmonary blood flow, as shown in the erect (**A**), supine (lying on the back) (**B**), and lateral (lying on the side) (**C**) positions.

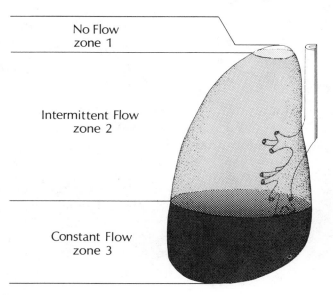

No Flow
zone 1

Intermittent Flow
zone 2

Constant Flow
zone 3

FIG 2–3.
The three-zone model illustrating the effects of gravity on pulmonary perfusion (see text).

pulmonary artery pressure is significantly decreased (e.g., shock) or alveolar pressures are significantly increased (e.g., intermittent positive-pressure breathing or positive end-expiratory pressure), the absence of perfusion to the least gravity-dependent areas of the lung may become significant.

The Three-Zone Model.—It has become well accepted to refer to the gravity effects of pulmonary perfusion in terms of the three-zone model (Fig 2–3). Zone 3 is the gravity-dependent area of constant blood flow (arterial pressure greater than alveolar pressure); zone 1 is the least gravity-dependent area of potentially no blood flow (alveolar pressure greater than arterial pressure). The interceding area is zone 2, an area of complex and varying intermittent blood flow. The presence or absence of blood flow in zone 2 depends primarily on the relationship of pulmonary artery pressure to alveolar pressure. Under normal circumstances, this is determined far more by the cardiac cycle (systole and diastole) than by the ventilatory cycle (inspiration and expiration).

Autoregulation.—The pulmonary vascular system is a low-pressure system and therefore would be more affected by gravitational forces than would the higher-pressure systemic vascular system. In addition, the systemic vascular system tends to react actively to changes in arterial pressure; that is, the vascular system attempts to actively control the distribution of blood flow in reaction to pressure changes. In contrast, the pulmonary vascular system tends to react passively to changes in pressure, thus accentuating the gravity effect on the distribution of pulmonary perfusion.

Cardiac Output

The amount of blood ejected by the right ventricle per unit time (cardiac output) is a major determinant of blood flow through the pulmonary vasculature. In general, *the greater the cardiac output, the greater the pulmonary artery pressure.* Thus, in the normal lung, as the cardiac output increases, zone 3 extends upward (see Fig 2–3); conversely, as the cardiac output decreases, zone 3 descends. Since the pulmonary vascular system tends to react *passively* to changes in arterial pressure, the gravity effect on the distribution of blood flow secondary to cardiac output changes is greater in the pulmonary system than in the systemic circulation.

Pulmonary Vascular Resistance

Although the pulmonary arterioles are less active in autoregulation than are their systemic counterparts, they are nonetheless capable of causing significant increases in resistance to blood flow.

Chronic Pulmonary Hypertension.—This is usually the result of periarteriolar fibrosis within the lung parenchyma. *Chronic pulmonary hypertension* results in increased right ventricular work. Over the long run, the right side of the heart meets these increased demands by musculature hypertrophy; that is, the right side of the heart becomes larger. Right ventricular hypertrophy due to chronic pulmonary hypertension is known as *cor pulmonale*—a common problem in patients with chronic lung diseases.

Acute Pulmonary Hypertension.—Acute increases in pulmonary vascular resistance usually result in acute pulmonary hypertension. Of course, acute pulmonary hypertension will result only if the right ventricle is capable of maintaining an adequate cardiac output; if not, the result is right ventricular failure.

Acute increase in pulmonary vascular resistance is a common phenomenon in critically ill patients. There are three factors that most commonly cause acute increases in pulmonary vascular resistance: (1) decreased alveolar oxygen tensions, (2) acidemia, and (3) arterial hypoxemia.

Decreased Alveolar Oxygen Tension.—Vasoconstriction occurs in vessels adjacent to alveoli with low oxygen tensions.[6] This local vaso-constriction is believed to play a significant role in diverting blood flow to lung areas where alveolar oxygen tensions are higher.

Acidemia.—Decreased blood pH tends to produce pulmonary vas-cular constriction. Acidemia is a common cause of acute pulmonary hypertension and may precipitate right ventricular failure.

Arterial Hypoxemia (decreased arterial oxygen tension).—Available evidence makes it reasonable to assume that severe hypoxemia may cause reflex-mediated increases in pulmonary vascular resistance.[7]

Certainly, combinations of the above three factors potentiate one another and result in marked pulmonary arteriolar vasoconstriction.

Ventilation to Perfusion Relationship

Gravity distribution of perfusion causes differences in perfusion pressures at various levels of the lung. In an erect human, at the lung bases the lateral wall pulmonary artery pressures are much higher than at the apices. Differences in intrapleural pressures result in the alveoli being smaller at the bases and larger at the apices.

At normal lung volumes, the greater portion of the tidal volume goes to the bases largely because of transpulmonary pressure differen-tials. In other words, small alveoli have larger volume changes per unit time than do larger alveoli. The net result is that under normal condi-tions, most of the air exchange takes place at the bases in coincidence with most of the blood flow. *Thus, in the normal lung most of the total ventilation and even more of the total blood flow go to the gravity-dependent areas.*

Of all the physiologic alterations resulting from pulmonary airway diseases, the problem of uneven distribution of ventilation is the most common and crucial. Any disease that causes pulmonary mucosal edema, inflammation, plugging of the bronchioles, or bronchospasm may result in uneven air distribution to alveoli.

Shunting and Deadspace

The basic pulmonary gas exchange unit is a single alveolus with its associated pulmonary capillary. This theoretical respiratory unit can exist in one of four relationships (Fig 2–4): (1) the *normal unit* is one in which ventilation and perfusion are relatively equal; (2) a *deadspace unit* is one in which the alveolus is normally ventilated but there is no blood flow

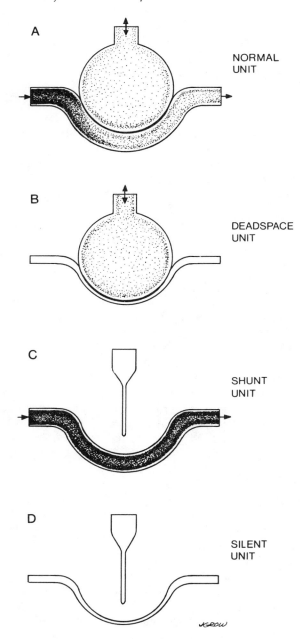

FIG 2–4.
The theoretical respiratory unit. **A,** normal ventilation, normal perfusion; **B,** normal ventilation, no perfusion; **C,** no ventilation, normal perfusion; **D,** no ventilation, no perfusion.

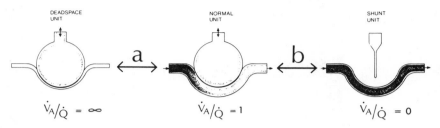

DEADSPACE UNIT

NORMAL UNIT

SHUNT UNIT

$\dot{V}_A/\dot{Q} = \infty$ $\dot{V}_A/\dot{Q} = 1$ $\dot{V}_A/\dot{Q} = 0$

FIG 2–5.
The spectrum of ventilation to perfusion relationships. As shown, *a* represents the spectrum of ventilation in excess of perfusion; *b* represents the spectrum of perfusion in excess of ventilation. The true deadspace unit is represented as infinite $\dot{V}_A/\dot{Q}$; the normal unit is represented as $\dot{V}_A/\dot{Q}$, equaling one; the shunt unit is represented as zero $\dot{V}_A/\dot{Q}$. (From Shapiro BA, Harrison RA, Kacmarek RM, Cane RD: *Clinical Application of Respiratory Care*, ed 2. Chicago, Year Book Medical Publishers Inc, 1985. Used by permission.)

through the capillary—the alveolar gas cannot participate in molecular blood gas exchange; (3) in a *shunt unit* the alveolus is completely un-ventilated while the adjacent capillary has blood flow—the blood goes from the right to the left side of the heart without undergoing gas ex-change; (4) a *silent unit* is one in which both the alveolus and the capillary are completely collapsed.

Any one of these absolute conditions may exist in the lungs at any time. An infinite number of ventilation-perfusion relationships may exist among the deadspace unit, the normal unit, and the shunt unit. This spectrum is illustrated in Figure 2–5. The complexities of the ventilation-perfusion relationships are primarily due to the spectrum between the two extremes of deadspace and shunt.

3

Metabolic Acid-Base Balance

Few subjects in clinical medicine have the aura of confusion and mystification as does acid-base balance. As discussed previously (see chap. 1), to evaluate acid-base balance one must measure at least two of the three Henderson-Hasselbalch parameters—i.e., pH, plasma bicarbonate concentration (HCO_3^-), or plasma carbonic acid concentration (H_2CO_3). The pH can be directly measured and the carbonic acid concentration can be indirectly obtained by measuring dissolved carbon dioxide (Pco_2) in the plasma. Thus, when measuring pH and Pco_2, plasma bicarbonate concentration can be calculated. Figure 3–1 reviews carbon dioxide transport and illustrates that the ratio of plasma bicarbonate concentration (primarily controlled by the kidneys) to plasma carbonic acid concentration (primarily controlled by the lungs) determines the pH.

Historically, the clinician could not readily measure any of these parameters. When serum electrolyte analysis became clinically available, the clinician attempted to reflect acid-base status based on electrolyte changes. This gave rise to a complex and bewildering "cult," which contributed to the confusion and difficulty of acid-base balance. Today, blood gas analysis is clinically available, and direct measurement of acid-base status is a reasonably simple procedure.

Some 50 years ago, pH and Pco_2 measurements were available to the research physiologist. At that time, clinical medicine had little to offer in terms of cardiopulmonary supportive care and, therefore, the importance of effective ventilation and cardiopulmonary homeostasis was not appreciated. The overwhelming interest was simply acid-base balance; thus, a simple nomenclature for *all* abnormalities (metabolic or respiratory) was developed. For this reason, blood gas measurements

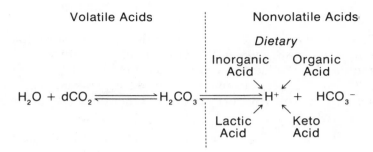

FIG 3–1.
Major sources of blood acids.

have been *traditionally* interpreted in relation to the acid-base state. In this chapter, the significant metabolic (nonrespiratory) factors that regulate acid-base balance are discussed.

THE CLINICAL SIGNIFICANCE OF ACID-BASE BALANCE

Intracellular metabolism requires a very narrow range of free hydrogen ion concentration (pH) within which enzymatic and biochemical processes function efficiently and appropriately. In addition, such critical functions as myocardial electrophysiology, central nervous system electrophysiology, and cellular responses to endogenous and exogenous chemical compounds (e.g., hormones and drugs) require a specific pH milieu. Significant deviations from these narrow ranges (especially when they occur over short intervals of time) are poorly tolerated and may be life-threatening. Therefore, an understanding of the homeostatic mechanisms working to maintain normal pH is essential.

REGULATION OF BLOOD ACIDS

A *volatile* substance is one that is capable of chemically varying between the liquid and gaseous states. The major blood acid, carbonic acid (H_2CO_3) is a volatile acid that is controlled by the ventilatory system. This subject will be discussed in detail in the following chapter.

All other potential sources of hydrogen ions are nonvolatile (or fixed) acids, and therefore, regulated by the kidneys and liver. The major sources of nonvolatile acids are (1) dietary acids, (2) lactic acids, and (3) keto acids (see Fig 3 – 1).

Dietary Acids

The normal food intake processed in the gastrointestinal tract tends to result in the absorption and metabolism of protein, which produces inorganic acids. The kidneys can normally be relied upon for excreting 50 to 100 mEq* of organic and inorganic acids generated each day. A normal diet in the presence of inadequate kidney function will eventually result in *renal acidosis*.

*The units mEq and mmol are essentially interchangeable units for acids and bases.

Lactic Acid

There is a normal production of lactic acid from red and white blood cells, skeletal muscle, and brain. Under normal circumstances, this lactic acid is circulated in the blood and metabolized primarily by the liver and excreted by the kidneys.

When adequate tissue oxygen is unavailable (hypoxia), intracellular metabolism continues by using biochemical pathways that do not require oxygen. Such *anaerobic* (non–oxygen-utilizing) pathways produce a lactate ion and a hydrogen ion as end products. When these ions enter the blood, they form lactic acid—a nonvolatile acid.

Lactic acidosis is the metabolic acidosis resulting from an accumulation of lactate ion and its accompanying hydrogen ion. The physiologic resolution to this lactic acid accumulation is the reestablishment of aerobic metabolism, which results in the lactate being metabolized primarily in the liver, with carbon dioxide and water as the ultimate metabolites.

Keto Acid

Normal aerobic metabolism uses the carbohydrate *glucose* ($C_6H_{12}O_6$ + $6O_2 \rightarrow 6CO_2 + 6H_2O$). *Insulin* is necessary for the utilization of glucose by the cell. When cellular glucose is inadequate, alternate aerobic pathways are used in which *keto acids* are the end products.

When adequate cellular glucose is unavailable due to lack of insulin, the resulting ketoacidosis is called *diabetic ketoacidosis*. Ketoacidosis can also result from starvation.

Ketoacidosis is resolved by providing adequate amounts of glucose to the cell. In starvation this would mean glucose administration; in the diabetic it would mean insulin and glucose administration. When normal metabolic pathways are resumed, the keto acids are recycled through metabolic pathways in the liver so that carbon dioxide and water are the metabolites.

REGULATION OF BLOOD BASE

The primary blood base is bicarbonate (HCO_3^-). Hydrogen ion is produced in the renal tubular cells by the following reaction:

$$CO_2 + H_2O \overset{CA}{\rightleftharpoons} H_2CO_3 \rightleftharpoons HCO_3^- + H^+$$

The presence of carbonic anhydrase in the renal tubular cells allows the reaction to take place rapidly and completely.

Renal Mechanism

It is the *total* amount of hydrogen ion secreted that is significant to metabolic acid-base balance. Since the kidneys have limited capability to acidify urine, the urine buffers play an important role in secreting large amounts of hydrogen ion.

The most important urine buffer is *phosphate*. In glomerular filtrate, 80% of the phosphate is in the dibasic form ($HPO_4^=$). In the urine, 99% of the phosphate is monobasic ($H_2PO_4^-$). The hydrogen ions attached to phosphate do not change urine pH. Ammonia and the ammonium ion is another important buffer system. *The time required for the kidneys to affect blood pH significantly is hours*, in contrast to the respiratory mechanism, which can make significant changes in seconds.

The renal mechanism is shown schematically in Figure 3 – 2. The steps are as follows:

Step 1.—Urine starts as glomerular filtrate with the same ionic concentrations and P_{CO_2} as plasma. Therefore, the bicarbonate ion concentration equals the plasma concentration since hydrogen ions attach to bicarbonate ions *first*; this means that bicarbonate ions are essentially moved from urine to blood, with hydrogen ions excreted in the urine.

Step 2.—When bicarbonate ions are no longer available in the urine, hydrogen ions attach to dibasic phosphates, once again adding bicarbonate ions to the blood.

Step 3.—Under certain circumstances, ammonium ions may be excreted in conjunction with a chloride ion.

Essentially, for each hydrogen ion secreted into the urine, the blood gains a bicarbonate ion. *It is this ability to add bicarbonate to the blood that is the kidney's main role in regulating acid-base balance.*

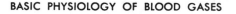

BASIC PHYSIOLOGY OF BLOOD GASES

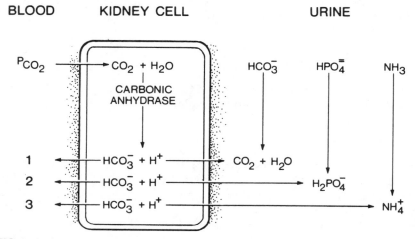

FIG 3–2.
Renal mechanism for blood base manipulation. Carbonic anhydrase exists in the kidney tubular cells and catalyzes the production of bicarbonate (HCO_3^-) and hydrogen ion (H^+) in quantities that are partly dependent on the blood P_{CO_2}. *(1)* Hydrogen ion combines with urine bicarbonate to produce carbon dioxide and water. The carbon dioxide is absorbed into the blood; the water is excreted in the urine. *(2)* Hydrogen ion attaches to dibasic phosphates and is excreted in the urine as $H_2PO_4^-$. *(3)* Under some circumstances, the kidney excretes ammonium ion (NH_4^+). In all these cases, a bicarbonate ion is added to the blood for each hydrogen ion secreted.

Electrolyte Mechanisms

The distribution of potassium ion (K^+) within intracellular and extracellular spaces influences acid-base balance. Most potassium is intracellular; if it leaves the cell, it must be replaced by a hydrogen ion from the extracellular fluid (plasma). Thus, *potassium leaving the cell provides a bicarbonate ion to the plasma.*

In addition, potassium can be exchanged for hydrogen ions in the distal tubules of the kidney. This may have a significant effect on acid-base balance in certain circumstances.

Chloride ion (Cl^-) is freely exchangeable in the kidney tubules; this is not true for most other anions (e.g., phosphates) that are primarily secreted into the urine. When chloride ions are not available in sufficient quantity, cation exchange at the renal tubular level can be adversely affected.

The primary electrolytes that are manipulated by the kidneys are:

Cations	Anions
Na$^+$	Cl$^-$
+	+
K$^+$	HCO$_3^-$

The necessity for electric neutrality may produce electrolyte changes when acid-base disturbances occur.* The meaning and importance of electrolyte changes are much easier to interpret when the acid-base status is known.

RENAL RESPONSE TO ACID-BASE IMBALANCE

Metabolic Alkalemia.—Increased plasma bicarbonate levels mean that some bicarbonate may actually be excreted in the urine. Thus, *the kidney may excrete base in response to excess blood base* if adequate chloride is available; it may excrete less H$^+$ if K$^+$ is available.

Metabolic Acidemia.—Decreased plasma bicarbonate means decreased urine bicarbonate ion. Thus, more bicarbonate is added to the blood as H$^+$ is excreted with phosphates.

Respiratory Acidemia.—Increased PCO_2 causes increased hydrogen ion excretion and bicarbonate reabsorption by the renal tubular cells. This adds base to the blood.

Respiratory Alkalemia.—Decreased PCO_2 causes decreased hydrogen ion excretion. Thus, less base is added to the blood.

STANDARD BICARBONATE

The clinical laboratory routinely includes some measurement of bicarbonate ion when reporting serum electrolytes. Historically this was a measurement of *standard bicarbonate*—the plasma bicarbonate concentration after the blood has been equilibrated to a PCO_2 of 40 mm Hg.[8] *Actual* plasma bicarbonate levels are calculated directly from pH and PCO_2.

---

*For instance, if Cl$^-$ is deficient, the kidneys may reabsorb excess HCO$_3^-$ into the blood. When total body K$^+$ is decreased, the kidneys may excrete excess H$^+$ into the urine.

TABLE 3–1.

The Henderson-Hasselbalch Parameters and Their Laboratory
Normal Ranges

	pH	$$pH \propto \frac{[HCO_3^-]p}{P_{CO_2}}$$ P_{CO_2} (mm Hg)	$[HCO_3^-]p$ (mEq/L)
Normal	7.35–7.45	35–45	22–28
Acidotic	<7.35	>45	<22
Alkalotic	>7.45	<35	>28

BASE EXCESS/DEFICIT

A far more satisfactory and clinically useful way to reflect the non-respiratory portion of acid-base balance is the calculation of base excess.[9] This calculation is an attempt to quantify the patient's *total base excess or deficit* from the normal buffer base at any given pH. The calculation is made from the measurement of pH, arterial carbon dioxide tension (Pa_{CO_2}), and hematocrit (inasmuch as the red blood cells contain the major blood buffers). It is reported as milliequivalents per liter (mEq/L) of base above or below the expected buffer base at that pH. Thus, a metabolic acidosis would have a negative base excess and is reported as such—e.g., a base excess of -10 mEq/L. A negative base excess is often referred to as a *base deficit*. Nonvolatile acid changes affect the base excess, while acute changes in carbonic acid concentration do not change base excess/deficit values. Thus, base excess is a true *nonrespiratory* reflection of acid-base status.[8]

When metabolic acid-base disturbances are treated, it may be desirable to partly correct the metabolic abnormality in a short time. In the case of metabolic acidosis, this is most commonly accomplished by the intravenous infusion of sodium bicarbonate ($NaHCO_3$) (see chap. 6). Metabolic alkalosis is most commonly treated by: (1) correcting the underlying electrolyte imbalance (e.g., potassium or chloride); (2) using ammonium chloride (NH_4Cl) in a manner similar to that described for sodium bicarbonate; and occasionally treated by (3) infusing dilute solutions of hydrochloric acid.

METABOLIC ACID-BASE INTERPRETATION

Blood gas studies provide us with all three Henderson-Hasselbalch parameters (Table 3–1). If normal ranges are known and the Henderson-

Hasselbalch equation is understood, metabolic acid-base interpretation becomes a straightforward exercise.

Blood pH measurement determines *acidemia* and *alkalemia*—an excess or deficit of free hydrogen ion activity in the arterial blood. The pathophysiologic states of *acidosis* and *alkalosis* are determined by the calculation of blood acid and blood base.

The following is a list of the standard nomenclature in regard to metabolic acid-base imbalance. The arrows indicate depressed or elevated values; N means normal; and BE is base excess.

Metabolic Acidosis

Nomenclature	pH	P_{CO_2}	$[HCO_3^-]_p$	BE
Uncompensated (acute)	↓	N	↓	↓ (−)
Partly compensated (subacute)	↓	↓	↓	↓ (−)
Completely compensated (chronic)	N	↓	↓	↓ (−)

Metabolic Alkalosis

	pH	P_{CO_2}	$[HCO_3^-]_p$	BE
Uncompensated (acute)	↑	N	↑	↑ (+)
Partly compensated (subacute)	↑	↑	↑	↑ (+)
Completely compensated (chronic)	N	↑	↑	↑ (+)

4

Respiratory Acid-Base Balance

CARBON DIOXIDE TRANSPORT

The arterial carbon dioxide tension (Pa_{CO_2}), directly reflects the adequacy of alveolar ventilation, i.e., it reflects how well air is exchanging with blood in the lungs. Only when the factors determining Pa_{CO_2} are thoroughly understood can the clinical usefulness of this measurement be appreciated.

Carbamino-CO_2 Mechanism

Carbamino compounds are formed when carbon dioxide chemically combines with amino acids. While only a fraction of the carbon dioxide entering the red blood cell combines directly with hemoglobin, it is the *difference* in the quantity of this substance in reduced and oxygenated hemoglobin that plays a significant role in CO_2 transport.[10] For a resting human at sea level, it has been estimated that 20% to 30% of the *change* in the carbon dioxide content of whole blood is due to carbamino-CO_2.[11] Thus, it is reasonable to conceive of this mechanism as being responsible for 20% to 30% of the blood's CO_2 transport capabilities.

Bicarbonate Ion Mechanism

Red blood cells and kidney tubular cells contain the enzyme *carbonic anhydrase*.[12] An enzyme is generally defined as a protein substance that speeds specific chemical reactions. The presence of carbonic anhydrase

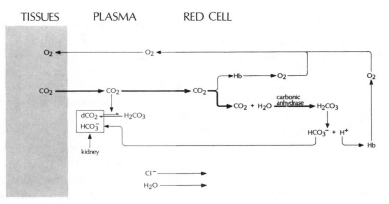

FIG 4–1.
A schematic representation of carbon dioxide transport in blood (see text). Note that only a small portion of plasma bicarbonate (HCO_3^-) is determined by this mechanism; the great majority of the plasma bicarbonate is determined by renal (kidney) mechanisms.

(CA) speeds the hydrating reaction of carbon dioxide to form carbonic acid:

$$CO_2 + H_2O \xrightarrow[CA]{} H_2CO_3 \rightarrow H^+ + HCO_3^-$$

The presence of carbonic anhydrase enables the red blood cells to carry carbon dioxide efficiently because carbonic acid is rapidly dissociated into hydrogen and bicarbonate ions. Since hemoglobin is an excellent buffer (see chap. 5), it allows great changes in hydrogen ion content to occur while minimizing the changes in free hydrogen ions (pH).

As carbon dioxide enters the blood (Fig 4–1), a small amount remains in physical solution in the plasma while the remainder enters the red blood cell. A portion of this carbon dioxide attaches directly to the hemoglobin to form carbamino-CO_2, while approximately 65% of the carbon dioxide is rapidly transformed to hydrogen and bicarbonate ions. The hydrogen ions are chemically bound to the hemoglobin.

Bicarbonate ions diffuse into the plasma because the *red blood cell to plasma gradient* becomes greater as the carbon dioxide content of the blood increases. Thus, as bicarbonate leaves the red blood cell, the laws of electrostatics result in the chloride ion migrating into the red blood cell to maintain electric neutrality. This decrease in plasma chloride concentration secondary to increased bicarbonate ion concentration is known as the *chloride shift*.

As the carbon dioxide content of blood increases, there is a corresponding increase in osmotically active particles within the red blood cells. Thus water tends to move from plasma into the erythrocytes, causing them to swell slightly as arterial blood becomes venous.

The most physiologically reflective blood gas measurement is the Pa_{CO_2}. It directly reflects the adequacy of alveolar ventilation; i.e., it tells how well air is exchanging with blood in the lungs. Only when the factors determining Pa_{CO_2} are thoroughly understood can the full clinical usefulness of this measurement be appreciated.

Most of the carbon dioxide in blood exists within the red blood cells in various reversible chemical combinations. A very small portion of blood carbon dioxide exists in physical solution and directly exerts a partial pressure (gas tension). Interrelationships between the dissolved and chemically combined carbon dioxide are very complex and usually referred to as "carbon dioxide transport."

As a review, three generalizations may be stated:

1. Almost all (approximately 95%) of the carbon dioxide in the blood is transported through buffering mechanisms in the red blood cell. A very small portion is actually dissolved in the plasma.

2. The *dissolved* carbon dioxide determines the blood partial pressure; thus, it is the only blood factor that participates in determining the carbon dioxide pressure gradient with alveolar air or tissue. This pressure gradient plays a major role in determining whether carbon dioxide enters or leaves the blood and at what rate it does so. In other words, *the dissolved carbon dioxide determines the blood portion of the pressure gradient.*

3. The quantity of carbon dioxide the blood is capable of accepting or giving up depends to a great extent on the buffering systems. In most circumstances, this natural blood-buffering capability is not exceeded, and therefore the carbon dioxide tension is the only significant determinant of the extent to which the blood accepts or gives up carbon dioxide. We will always assume this to be the case.

CARBON DIOXIDE HOMEOSTASIS

If one removes from the cardiopulmonary homeostatic schema (see Fig 2 – 1), all the factors that do not affect the moment-to-moment control of the arterial carbon dioxide tension, there remains an exquisitely simple relationship (Fig 4 – 2): *The metabolic rate of the body is balanced against the effectiveness of ventilation.* On the one hand, the metabolic rate determines the rate and amount of carbon dioxide that enters the venous blood; on the other, the effective ventilation determines the alveolar carbon dioxide

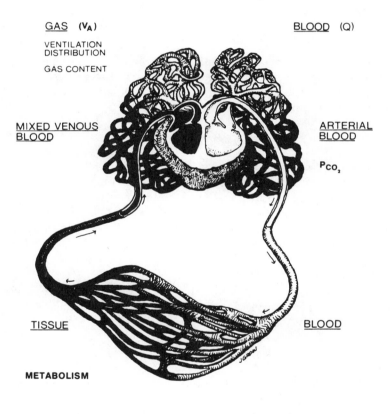

EXTERNAL RESPIRATION

PULMONARY CAPILLARY BED

GAS (V$_A$)

VENTILATION
DISTRIBUTION

GAS CONTENT

BLOOD (Q)

MIXED VENOUS
BLOOD

ARTERIAL
BLOOD

P$_{CO_2}$

TISSUE

BLOOD

METABOLISM

SYSTEMIC CAPILLARY BED

INTERNAL RESPIRATION

FIG 4–2.
The carbon dioxide homeostatic schema. This schema is the result of removing all factors in the cardiopulmonary homeostatic schema (see Fig 2–1) that do not affect carbon dioxide homeostasis. The arterial P$_{CO_2}$ is determined by the relationship between tissue metabolism and alveolar ventilation.

tension and, therefore, how much carbon dioxide will be excreted in the lung.

Total Ventilation

Ventilation is the mass movement of gases into and out of the pulmonary system. The most common clinical measurement of ventilation is either the tidal volume (VT) or minute volume (MV). The MV is the product of the VT and the respiratory rate.

Effective and Wasted Ventilation

A portion of the total ventilation respires — i.e., undergoes molecular gas exchange with pulmonary blood. Thus, the total ventilation per unit time is composed of gas that respires (alveolar ventilation) and gas that does not respire (deadspace ventilation):

$$\dot{V} = \dot{V}A + \dot{V}D$$

Alveolar Ventilation ($\dot{V}A$)

In general, only the portion of total ventilation that respires has positive physiologic significance; that is, it is the physiologically effective portion of the total ventilation. This *effective ventilation* is most commonly referred to as *alveolar ventilation — that portion of the total ventilation that undergoes molecular gas exchange with pulmonary blood.*

Deadspace Ventilation ($\dot{V}D$)

The portion of the total ventilation that does *not* respire is wasted ventilation—i.e., *not* physiologically effective. This wasted ventilation is most commonly called *deadspace ventilation—that portion of the total ventilation that does not undergo molecular gas exchange with pulmonary blood.*

Deadspace ventilation may result from one of three circumstances:

Anatomic Deadspace.—*The volume of air in the pulmonary conducting system* is the anatomic deadspace. In spontaneous breathing, the volume of the conducting system is fairly constant; this is to say that the volume of the conducting system is consistently related to normal body size. *The anatomic deadspace is usually equal to 1 ml/pound (2.2 ml/kg) of normal body weight.*

Alveolar Deadspace.—If an alveolus is being ventilated but the pulmonary capillary is not being perfused, the air in that alveolus is deadspace ventilation; i.e., the air is not exchanging with pulmonary blood.

Unlike anatomic deadspace, alveolar deadspace can be highly variable and unpredictable.

Deadspace Effect.—When ventilation in excess of perfusion exists, two results are theoretically possible. The greater air exchange in the alveolus may result in better alveolar ventilation; i.e., there is decreased PA_{CO_2} and Pa_{CO_2}. However, part or all of the increased alveolar air exchange may *not* respire. Such a ventilation-perfusion inequality may be due either to overventilation or to underperfusion. This is the component of deadspace ventilation that responds most markedly to changes in total ventilation or total pulmonary blood flow.

Ventilatory Pattern

Every tidal volume includes anatomic deadspace. The larger the tidal volume, the less significant the anatomic deadspace. The more rapid the respiratory rate, the greater the portion of the minute ventilation that will be anatomic deadspace. Figure 4–3 demonstrates how, in spite of a constant minute volume, changes in the ventilatory pattern alter the alveolar, or effective, ventilation. When we add the fact that total deadspace ventilation varies greatly with disease, *it becomes obvious that clinical observations of ventilation may be totally inadequate for assessing the physiologic adequacy of ventilation.*

ARTERIAL CARBON DIOXIDE TENSION (Pa_{CO_2})

The metabolic rate is a major determinant of tissue carbon dioxide tension and, therefore, is an important factor in determining the mixed venous (pulmonary artery) carbon dioxide tension ($P\bar{v}_{CO_2}$).

The movement of carbon dioxide from pulmonary blood to alveolar air is dependent on the carbon dioxide pressure gradient between pulmonary blood and the alveolus. Because carbon dioxide readily diffuses across the alveolar-capillary membrane, we may assume the carbon dioxide tensions are equal in alveolar air and arterial blood. This is shown schematically in Figure 4–4.

Arterial carbon dioxide tension (Pa_{CO_2}) is a direct reflection of how well the lungs are exchanging air with blood in relation to the metabolic rate. In other words, *the Pa_{CO_2} is the direct and immediate reflection of the adequacy of alveolar ventilation in relation to the metabolic rate.*

To emphasize the clinical importance of the arterial carbon dioxide tension measurement, remember that the physiologic criterion of ade-

VT 250 ml x RR 40/min = MV 10 L
VA = 4 L

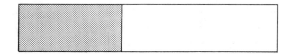

VT 500 ml x RR 20/min = MV 10 L
VA = 7 L

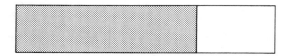

VT 1000 ml x RR 10/min = MV 10 L
VA = 8.5 L

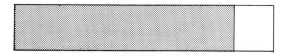

FIG 4–3.
The ventilatory pattern and alveolar ventilation. In all three examples, the minute volume (MV) is 10 L. Assuming an anatomic deadspace of 150 ml, the alveolar ventilation (VA) varies markedly with changes in ventilatory pattern (VT = tidal volume; RR = respiratory rate). Obviously, disease can add deadspaces other than the anatomic ones and can cause even greater variances in alveolar ventilation.

quate pulmonary function is how well the metabolic demands of the body are met. The assessment of adequate physiologic ventilation is accomplished through arterial carbon dioxide tension measurement. Differentiation and classification of pulmonary diseases are accomplished by pulmonary function studies and other methods, *but the physiologic assessment of the adequacy of ventilation is by* Pa_{CO_2} *measurement.*

In a normal human, metabolism produces approximately 12,000 mEq of hydrogen ion per day; less than 1% of this acid is excreted via the kidney because the normal metabolite is carbon dioxide, a substance transported as a volatile acid (H_2CO_3) and excreted via the lung. It was

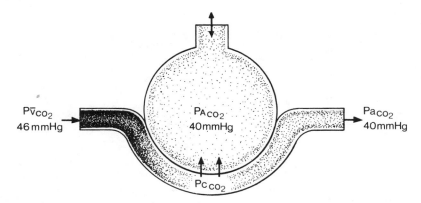

FIG 4–4.
Major factors determining alveolar carbon dioxide tension. Inspired air normally is void of a significant carbon dioxide tension; therefore alveolar carbon dioxide tension (PA_{CO_2}) must be the net result of fresh air exchange in the alveolus in relation to mixed venous carbon dioxide tension ($P\bar{v}_{CO_2}$). Carbon dioxide diffusion is normally so rapid that total equilibrium must occur between pulmonary capillary carbon dioxide tension (Pc_{CO_2}) and PA_{CO_2}. This means that arterial carbon dioxide tension (Pa_{CO_2}) should equal PA_{CO_2}. Normal values are illustrated.

noted many years ago that acid-base imbalance is not life-threatening for several hours to days following renal shutdown but becomes critical within minutes following the cessation of breathing. This essential role of *respiration* in the moment-to-moment maintenance of acid-base balance was fully appreciated more than 60 years ago. Since increases in blood carbon dioxide content (increased P_{CO_2}) cause increases in blood hydrogen ion concentration, the phenomenon was called *respiratory acidosis*; conversely, decreases in blood carbon dioxide cause decreases in blood hydrogen ion concentration, thus the term *respiratory alkalosis*. Table 4–1 denotes the criteria for the traditional nomenclature of *respiratory acidosis* and *respiratory alkalosis*.[13, 14]

There would be little purpose in introducing new nomenclature if a traditional nomenclature adequately served the modern clinician. In our opinion, this has not been the case for the past three decades, primarily due to advances in the technologic ability to monitor cardiopulmonary function (ECG monitor, arterial blood gases, central venous pressure, pulmonary artery catheterization, etc.) along with the improved capability of supporting and correcting cardiopulmonary malfunction (fluid and electrolyte therapy, cardiovascular pharmacology, ventilator care, positive end-expiratory pressure [PEEP] therapy, oxygen therapy, etc.).

Respiratory acid-base imbalance is primarily a ventilatory malfunction! Crit-

TABLE 4–1.

Traditional Respiratory Acid-Base Nomenclature

Nomenclature	pH	P_{CO_2}	$[HCO_3{}^-]p$	BE
Respiratory Acidosis				
Uncompensated (acute)	↓	↑	N	N
Partly compensated (subacute)	↓	↑	↑	↑
Compensated (chronic)	N	↑	↑	↑
Respiratory Alkalosis				
Uncompensated (acute)	↑	↓	N	N
Partly compensated (subacute)	↑	↓	↓	↓
Compensated (chronic)	N	↓	↓	↓

*Arrows indicate depressed or elevated levels; N is normal; and BE is base excess.

---

ical care medicine demands that a malfunction in respiration be specifically diagnosed, monitored, and supported, especially the differentiation of ventilation from oxygenation. Thus, we contend that a clinically oriented view of respiratory acid-base balance must be used that is based on cardiopulmonary physiology and clinical application.

RESPIRATORY FAILURE

A generally acceptable definition of organ failure is "the failure of an organ system to meet the metabolic demands of the body." In keeping with this definition, *heart failure* may be considered the failure of the heart to meet the metabolic demands of the body. This concept makes no reference to the cardiac output; that is, nothing is mentioned about whether the heart is putting out more blood, less blood, or the usual amount of blood. And in fact high-output cardiac failure is not only possible but quite common.

In terms of cardiopulmonary homeostasis, heart failure refers only to the relationship between metabolic demand and the ability of the heart to meet that demand. The measurement of cardiac output does not provide an objective measurement of physiologic adequacy, and therefore the clinical diagnosis of heart failure must be a matter of clinical judgment and deduction. This is true only because a single clinical objective measurement is not available.

The failure of the kidneys to meet the body's metabolic demands is called *renal failure*. As with heart failure and cardiac output, the measurement of urine output is not always diagnostic; high-output renal failure does exist. Fortunately, certain laboratory measurements (blood urea nitrogen, creatinine) may be used to diagnose and follow the course of renal failure. For this reason, the clinical judgment of renal failure is far less subjective than is the assessment of heart failure.

Respiration has been defined for almost 100 years as the movement of gas molecules across permeable membranes. Although respiration may fail to meet metabolic demands at the internal as well as the external level (see chap. 2), clinical tradition and practicality dictate that the term *respiratory failure* denote failure of adequate gas exchange at the pulmonary level. Accepting this statement, we may define respiratory failure as *failure of the pulmonary system to meet the metabolic demands of the body.* This logically leads to the clinical assumption that *respiratory failure* means the lungs are inadequately providing oxygen and/or carbon dioxide exchange.

As such, respiratory failure is a broad and poorly delineated *clinical diagnosis* that makes no pretense of specifying or quantifying the pathophysiology. The limitations of such a clinical diagnosis are that it does not *document, specify,* or *quantitate* the disease process. The clinician attempts to accomplish these things through laboratory testing and other means. The following are several examples to illustrate this vitally important concept.

Acute Myocardial Infarction and the Electrocardiogram

A 40-year-old man enters the emergency room complaining of severe chest pain radiating to the left arm, shortness of breath, tachycardia, and "thready" pulse. He is clinically diagnosed as having an acute myocardial infarction. Of course, other diagnoses may be entertained, but acute myocardial infarction is certainly a reasonable clinical diagnosis. One important laboratory test would be the 12-lead electrocardiogram because: (1) it may *document* the clinical diagnosis of acute myocardial ischemia; (2) it may further *specify* the insult (e.g., localize the area of injury); and (3) it may *quantitate* the insult so that serial measurements may be used to follow the course of the pathology.

The term *acute myocardial infarction* is a useful and legitimate clinical diagnosis; however, *acute inferior wall injury* is an electrocardiographic diagnosis that documents, specifies, and quantitates the clinical diagnosis.

Acute Respiratory Failure and Blood Gas Measurement

1. A 60-year-old man enters the emergency room complaining of shortness of breath. He is tachypneic, tachycardiac, sweaty, and cy-

anotic. A diagnosis of acute respiratory failure is made and several laboratory tests are ordered (arterial blood gases, chest x-ray, and so on). Arterial blood gas results show the P_{CO_2} is well below normal, the pH is alkalemic, and the arterial P_{O_2} is very low.

The blood gases have *documented* the gas exchange inadequacy (respiratory failure), *specified* this inadequacy to be a primary oxygenation problem, and *quantified* the severity of the gas exchange abnormality. The clinical diagnosis of acute respiratory failure is appropriate but limited in its usefulness. The arterial blood gases have documented, specified, and quantitated the physiologic insult and will lead to appropriate supportive measures if properly interpreted.

2. A 60-year-old man enters the emergency room with complaints similar to the man in the example above. Again, a diagnosis of acute respiratory failure is appropriately made. Arterial blood gases reveal a very high P_{CO_2}, a low pH, and a moderately low P_{O_2}.

The blood gases have *documented* acute respiratory failure, *specified* the pathophysiology as primarily ventilatory, and *quantitated* the severity of the insult. Surely this information will lead to different supportive care than in the previous example of respiratory failure.

The concept of respiratory failure is limited in its clinical usefulness and application; it must be accepted only as a general and nonspecific diagnosis. Arterial blood gas measurements are mandatory to document, specify, and quantitate the physiologic insult. Most important, one must differentiate primary oxygenation deficiencies from primary ventilatory deficiencies.

Oxygenation Versus Ventilation

Tissue oxygenation may be considered the prime factor in the cellular life process. Logically, tissue oxygenation has traditionally been considered the prime function of the pulmonary system. For this reason, *respiratory failure* has traditionally been thought of primarily in terms of oxygenation.

In Chapter 5 it is discussed how complex and difficult the clinical assessment of tissue oxygenation can be, even when blood gas measurements are available. This means that the assessment of respiratory failure in terms of tissue oxygenation must be a completely subjective clinical judgment. In addition, subtle clinical signs are easily missed, making respiratory failure a clinically unreliable diagnosis short of extremis. Experience teaches that clinical evaluation of respiratory failure is far more difficult, unreliable, and unpredictable than the clinical evaluation of heart failure. In addition, tissue oxygenation may be totally unrelated to lung function; hypoxia can exist in many circumstances where the pulmonary system is functioning adequately.

Ventilation and oxygenation must be considered two separate entities! However, a complicated interrelationship exists between them. A significant change in one may affect the other — the extent of the effect is variable and complex, depending on the capabilities of the reflex mechanisms and the work capacities of the cardiopulmonary system. It is very important to distinguish clinically between ventilation and oxygenation, because the proper application of supportive modalities depends on this distinction.

THE CONCEPT OF VENTILATORY FAILURE

The adequacy of alveolar ventilation is directly reflected in the arterial P_{CO_2}. Even though the disease state causing abnormal alveolar ventilation may have its etiology outside of the pulmonary system, we are still dealing with the inability of the pulmonary system to meet the metabolic demands as far as carbon dioxide is concerned.

If the physiologic assessment of the pulmonary system is considered in terms of carbon dioxide homeostasis, the concept of *ventilatory failure* results.[15] Respiratory failure includes the assessment of oxygenation and ventilation. *Ventilatory failure involves ventilation only;* oxygenation is assessed separately.

Defining Ventilatory Failure

The metabolic rate is reflected in the respiratory quotient (RQ), which represents the relationship of gas exchange in the systemic capillaries; for the amount of oxygen consumed, an amount of carbon dioxide is produced. The carbon dioxide is carried by the venous blood to the lungs, where the moment-to-moment control of arterial carbon dioxide tension is determined. If arterial carbon dioxide tensions are to remain normal, the air exchange in the alveoli being perfused must increase as carbon dioxide production increases. *The arterial carbon dioxide tension directly reflects the adequacy of alveolar ventilation; therefore, it provides an objective measurement of physiologic lung function.* Blood gases give us the objective measurement with which to diagnose ventilatory failure.

Ventilatory failure is defined as the condition in which the lungs are unable to meet the metabolic demands of the body as far as carbon dioxide homeostasis is concerned. Because alveolar ventilation is a reflection of how well the ventilatory demand is being met, ventilatory failure is the condition of inadequate alveolar ventilation in relation to the metabolic rate. The diagnosis *cannot* be made without arterial blood gas measurement; it is made without regard to the arterial or tissue oxygenation state.

Respiratory Acidosis

Table 4–2 demonstrates that both *ventilatory failure* and *respiratory acidosis* are terms describing an increased arterial PCO_2. In other words, *ventilatory failure and respiratory acidosis are the same thing!* In the modern care of the critically ill patient, the term *ventilatory failure* is preferred because it refers to the *primary* cardiopulmonary abnormality; that is, it refers directly to the physiologic function in need of support.

Acute Ventilatory Failure

If the arterial carbon dioxide tension rises, plasma carbonic acid must correspondingly increase in concentration. The increase in carbonic acid results in a drop in blood pH. The kidneys respond by excreting more hydrogen ion and thereby add more bicarbonate ion to the venous blood (see chap. 3). Given enough time, this renal mechanism will gradually correct the pH to near normal.

If the arterial carbon dioxide tension is suddenly increased from 40 mm Hg to 80 mm Hg, the pH changes from 7.40 to 7.20; the pH change is an *immediate* reflection of arterial carbon dioxide change. This arterial carbon dioxide tension to pH relationship may be changed by renal mechanisms over time.

Obviously, then, an arterial carbon dioxide tension change that is accompanied by an appropriate pH change must be a recent event; i.e., ventilatory failure (respiratory acidosis) accompanied by an acidemia must be an *acute* event.

Acute ventilatory failure (*acute* respiratory acidosis) is the presence of a high arterial carbon dioxide tension with acidemia. It is usually accompanied by hypoxemia and must be considered a dire clinical emergency!

TABLE 4–2.

Nomenclature for Ventilatory Abnormalities

Respiratory Acidosis	=	*Ventilatory Failure*
Acute (uncompensated)		Acute
Chronic (compensated)		Chronic
Respiratory Alkalosis	=	*Alveolar Hyperventilation*
Acute (uncompensated)		Acute
Chronic (compensated)		Chronic

Chronic Ventilatory Failure

If ventilatory failure has existed for a long time or has developed very gradually over a long time, it will not be accompanied by an acidemia. *Ventilatory failure is chronic when metabolic compensation of the acidemia has occurred.* In other words, *chronic* ventilatory failure (*chronic* respiratory acidosis) is a high arterial carbon dioxide tension with a near-normal blood pH.

The differentiation of acute and chronic ventilatory failure is of more than academic interest. Basic biochemical cellular processes are affected by *sudden* environmental changes far more than by gradual changes. For example, cellular function is disrupted to a far greater degree by a sudden pH change than by the gradual development of that same pH change. Acute ventilatory failure is far more life-threatening than chronic ventilatory failure, not only because an acidemia exists but also because the change has been sudden. *The severity of ventilatory failure must be judged by the degree of the accompanying acidemia.*

ALVEOLAR HYPERVENTILATION (RESPIRATORY ALKALOSIS)

Disease states may affect the cardiopulmonary homeostatic schema in such a way that normal alveolar air exchange is insufficient to meet metabolic demands. The patient is stimulated to breathe more, and he will do so if he possesses the muscular power. This results in an *alveolar hyperventilation* — i.e., an arterial carbon dioxide tension below normal. *Alveolar hyperventilation* and *respiratory alkalosis* both describe a decrease in arterial carbon dioxide tension (see Table 4–2). The term *alveolar hyperventilation* is preferred to remain consistent with the concept of referring to the *primary* cardiopulmonary malfunction.

Acute and Chronic

The alkalemia accompanying a sudden decrease in arterial carbon dioxide tension reflects the acuteness of ventilatory change. Thus, *acute* alveolar hyperventilation (*acute* respiratory alkalosis) is the occurrence of a decreased P_{CO_2} with alkalemia, and *chronic* alveolar hyperventilation (*chronic* respiratory alkalosis) is the occurrence of a decreased P_{CO_2} with a near-normal pH.

Causes of Alveolar Hyperventilation

Numerous disease processes may result in alveolar hyperventilation (respiratory alkalosis). A meaningful approach is to consider that the decreased arterial carbon dioxide tension occurs in response to three general pathophysiologic states: (1) arterial oxygenation deficits severe enough to stimulate peripheral chemoreceptors (see chap. 5); (2) metabolic acidosis severe enough to stimulate the peripheral and/or central chemoreceptors; and (3) abnormal stimulation of the ventilatory centers of the central nervous system.

Ventilatory failure (respiratory acidosis) is always a form of respiratory failure because carbon dioxide exchange is inadequate. However, alveolar hyperventilation (respiratory alkalosis) can be considered a form of respiratory failure only when it is the result of an oxygen exchange deficiency (arterial oxygenation deficit).

CAUSES OF VENTILATORY FAILURE

Almost any disease that is severe enough, or present in a person with limited abilities to compensate, may result in ventilatory failure.[15, 16] Figure 4–5 outlines the essential factors that allow for adequate alveolar ventilation.

Respiratory Center
↓
Ventilatory Motor Nerves
↓
Neuromuscular Junction
↓
Ventilatory Muscles
↓
Thoracic Cage
↓
Lungs
↓
Airways and Blood Vessels
↓
Ventilation Perfusion Relationship

FIG 4–5.
Ventilatory pathway.

PATHOGENESIS OF VENTILATORY FAILURE

Diseases that affect the efficiency or capability of the various factors as previously illustrated (see Fig 4–5) may lead to ventilatory failure. In general, such disease may be classified as cardiopulmonary, central nervous system, neurologic, musculoskeletal, hepatorenal, and fatigue. Ventilatory failure may be considered to follow a general pathophysiologic pattern regardless of its cause.

Acute Ventilatory Failure

A sudden increase in the work of breathing or a sudden decrease in ventilatory reserves may result in the pulmonary system being incapable of meeting the normal carbon dioxide homeostatic demands. Although this usually occurs in conjunction with clinical changes, it may occur with little change in the clinical status. Such a patient may imperceptibly go into acute ventilatory failure (acute respiratory acidosis) without significant clinical change until cardiopulmonary collapse ensues. With acute ventilatory failure (acute respiratory acidosis), the supportive and therapeutic care will be immediate and obvious. However, in chronic lung disease, a chronic ventilatory failure (chronic respiratory acidosis) often exists in which the understanding of its pathogenesis is crucial to its support and therapy.

Chronic Ventilatory Failure

There are at least three physiologic factors that lead to increased work of breathing in persons with chronic obstructive pulmonary disease (COPD).

1. An *increased functional residual capacity* means a constant state of hyperinflation, which decreases the efficiency of air exchange at the alveolar level. Thus, more ventilatory work is required to achieve adequate physiologic ventilation.

2. Degenerative alveolar changes (emphysema) result in less area for exchange between alveolar air and pulmonary blood. Thus, a greater portion of the alveolar gas does not exchange with blood. Increased deadspace ventilation requires increased work of breathing.

3. Bronchitic, asthmatic, and emphysematous diseases lead to *uneven distribution of ventilation*, creating hypoventilated areas in relation to blood flow. This results in less than optimal oxygenation of the blood perfusing that area of lung—arterial hypoxemia; this causes the car-

diopulmonary system to increase work to meet the organism's metabolic demands.

Increased work of breathing, decreased efficiency in the distribution of ventilation, decreased efficiency in the distribution of pulmonary perfusion, and hypoxemia may lead to chronic carbon dioxide retention.

Figure 4–6 depicts the generalized pathogenesis of this ventilatory failure in chronic obstructive pulmonary disease. This teleologic discussion assumes the heart will not fail to meet the increased demands placed upon it and the CNS is appropriate for allowing CO_2 retention. The early disease process results in a progressive arterial hypoxemia secondary to the ventilation-perfusion deterioration at point *A*. When the arterial oxygen tension reaches some minimal level *B*, usually around 60 mm Hg, the peripheral chemoreceptors experience decreased tissue oxygen supply and respond by stimulating both the ventilatory muscles and the myocardium. This stimulation produces the amount of myocardial and ventilatory work necessary to maintain the arterial oxygen tension at a level minimizing chemoreceptor tissue hypoxia.

Maintaining the arterial oxygen tension at a level where the peripheral chemoreceptors are minimally stimulated in the face of progressive

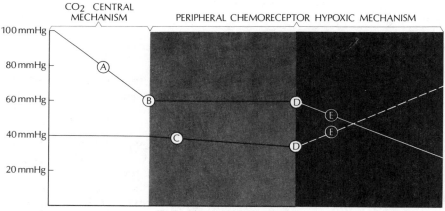

FIG 4–6.
A theory on the pathogenesis of ventilatory failure in chronic obstructive pulmonary disease. *A*, decreasing arterial Po_2 due to early disease process; *B*, peripheral chemoreceptor stimulation begins and becomes the primary drive to breathe; *C*, arterial Po_2 level remains fairly constant while arterial Pco_2 level may decrease to some degree; *D*, theoretic points at which work of breathing is so costly that a decreased arterial Po_2 is unavoidable (see text); *E*, arterial Po_2 begins to decrease and arterial Pco_2 begins to increase.

disease necessitates increasing ventilatory and myocardial work. The increasing ventilatory work is reflected by a somewhat decreasing arterial carbon dioxide tension at point *C* (see Fig 4 – 6). The increased ventilatory and myocardial work continues to maintain the minimal arterial oxygen tension that "satisfies" the chemoreceptors.

Point *D* is reached when the work of breathing uses so much oxygen that increasing total ventilation actually consumes more oxygen than is gained. In other words, physiologic deadspace is so great and shunting is so significant that a further increase in alveolar ventilation (seldom below 35 mm Hg) produces a net loss in arterial oxygen tension. It is essential to understand that at point *D* the organism faces a decrease in arterial oxygen tension, whether ventilation is unchanged, increased, or decreased, for the following reasons:

1. *Unchanged* alveolar ventilation leads to decreased arterial Po_2 because of increasing shunting and shunt effect.

2. *Increased* alveolar ventilation requires a great increase in ventilatory muscle work because there is much "wasted" ventilation (physiologic deadspace). In addition, the vital capacity is decreased and airway resistance is increased. These factors lead to an oxygen consumption for increased ventilatory work that is greater than the oxygen gained from the increased alveolar ventilation.

3. *Decreased* alveolar ventilation decreases the oxygen consumed for the work of breathing, but this oxygen gain is not great enough to offset the oxygen loss from the decreased alveolar ventilation.

The organism obviously chooses the alternative that results in the smallest arterial oxygen loss for the least energy expended. As shown at points *E* (see Fig 4 – 6), alveolar ventilation slowly decreases as arterial Po_2 slowly decreases. The cardiopulmonary homeostatic mechanisms dictate that the organism decreases effective ventilation and adjusts to the hypoxemia.

SUMMARY

Respiratory failure is a useful clinical term referring to the failure of the pulmonary system to provide adequate gas exchange. Arterial blood gas measurements are necessary to document, specify, and quantitate the malfunction. The concept of ventilatory failure recognizes the physiologic malfunction as one of ventilation rather than the secondary effect of acid-base imbalance. By changing the focus from the general concepts of acid-base balance to a specific ventilatory function of the pulmonary system, a far more applicable and meaningful physiologic understanding is achieved in the clinical setting.

Clinical assessment of the ventilatory status is difficult and unreliable except *in extremis*. The difference between a person with a given disease state manifesting alveolar hyperventilation or ventilatory failure may be the presence or absence of the muscular ability to increase total ventilation.

Pulmonary function studies alone are of minimal assistance because total ventilation does not necessarily reflect alveolar ventilation. For example, a high minute volume gives no information concerning alveolar ventilation unless the physiologic deadspace is known. A high minute volume and high physiologic deadspace may be thought of as "high-output ventilatory failure."

The diagnosis of ventilatory failure can be made only by arterial blood gas analysis! For example, a patient in status asthmaticus may have an unchanging disease state for several days. Due to lack of sleep and the great work of breathing, the patient may enter a serious fatigue state without showing any clinical signs of change. In other words, the patient may go imperceptibly from alveolar hyperventilation to ventilatory failure. This acute ventilatory failure (acute respiratory acidosis) increases in severity but becomes clinically obvious only in the extreme state when the patient is on the verge of cardiopulmonary collapse. The best way to reliably detect such subclinical, gradual, and critical ventilatory change is by serial blood gas measurement.

5

Arterial Oxygenation

Tissue hypoxia exists when cellular oxygen tensions are inadequate to meet cellular oxygen demands. This requires some cellular metabolism to be accomplished by other than oxidative mechanisms. These *anaerobic* mechanisms are undesirable because they are far less efficient and produce metabolites other than carbon dioxide. Since technology to measure intracellular PO_2 clinically is not available, the diagnosis of tissue hypoxia is a clinical judgment that greatly depends on the appropriate interpretation of the *arterial* oxygenation status.

DEFINING HYPOXEMIA

Hypoxemia is traditionally defined as "a relative deficiency of oxygen in the blood"; in other words, a state of oxygenation in the arterial blood that is less than normal. Over the past 30 years, the Pa_{O_2} measurement has become the primary tool for the clinical evaluation of the arterial oxygenation status.

Keeping in mind that arterial oxygen content involves more than the oxygen tension, in this text hypoxemia is defined as *a relative deficiency of oxygen tension in the arterial blood*. Such a definition is completely compatible with the current medical literature and lends itself most readily to the clinical care of acutely ill patients. It is essential that the hemoglobin content be evaluated and considered in a clinical judgment. For the remainder of this discussion, we shall assume that the hemoglobin content is normal.

Thus, hypoxemia denotes that the arterial oxygen tension is below an acceptable range. Hypoxemia does not necessarily mean that tissues are hypoxic. It is possible to have normal tissue oxygenation in conjunction with hypoxemia, just as it is possible to have normal arterial oxygen tensions and still have tissue hypoxia. The clinical application of the Pa_{O_2} measurement is based primarily on the concept of arterial blood oxygenation, which demands a thorough understanding of hemoglobin.

HEMOGLOBIN

Hemoglobin is the main component of the red blood cells and is responsible for the red color of blood. A single red blood cell contains approximately 280 million molecules of hemoglobin. Each hemoglobin molecule is approximately 64,500 times the weight of one hydrogen atom and is composed of more than 10,000 atoms of hydrogen, carbon, nitrogen, oxygen, and sulfur. In addition, each hemoglobin molecule contains four atoms of iron—the most significant factor in its ability to carry oxygen. Without hemoglobin, large organisms could neither supply adequate oxygen to their tissues nor transport the carbon dioxide from the tissues to the lungs.

The Chemistry of Hemoglobin

The exact chemical structure of hemoglobin is not entirely known; however, chemical and x-ray analyses have revealed much of the structure and have made even more fascinating the study of this crucial molecule.[17] For those interested in the physiologic process of respiration, an appreciation of this "oxygen carrier" molecule is fundamental.

When four pyrrole rings are cyclically linked through methylene bridges, a *porphyrin* results (Fig 5–1). These porphyrin substances are important in biologic systems primarily because they are capable of forming complexes with metals. A basic theory of chemistry states that chemical compounds may be formed through *covalent bonds*. Covalent bonds are formed between the electrons of two or more atoms. The *ferrous ion* generally has six valence bonds available (Fig 5–2,A). When a ferrous ion (Fe^{++}) binds to a porphyrin ring, each iron atom is attached by covalent bonds to the four nitrogens on the pyrrole groups. The result is a substance known as *heme* (see Fig 5–1).

Amino acids may chemically link to one another to form long chains. Chains of amino acids (polypeptide chains) are known as *protein molecules*. When four specific amino acid chains are combined (two alpha chains and two beta chains), the protein *globin* is the result. This protein molecule contains imidazole nitrogen groups that are capable of forming covalent bonds with metal ions.

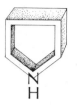

pyrrole

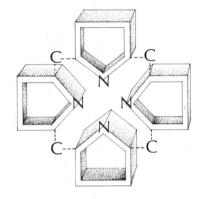

porphyrin

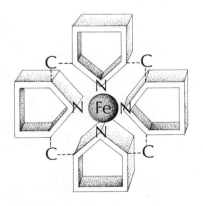

heme

C--- methylene
     bridge

FIG 5–1.
The chemical structure of heme.

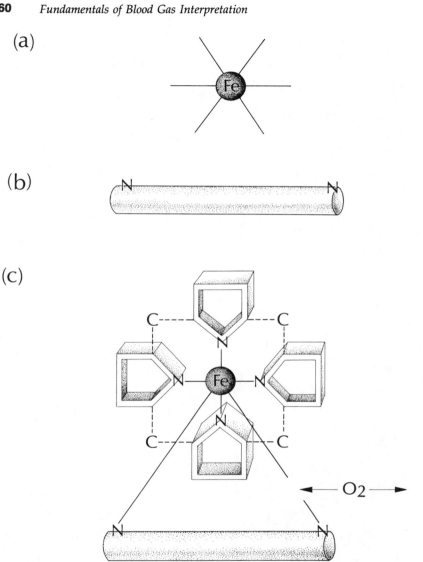

FIG 5–2.
a, the ferrous ion (Fe^{++}) with six potential valence bonds. **b,** schematic representation of a polypeptide chain with two imidazole nitrogens that are capable of forming covalent bonds with metal ions. A protein molecule containing two alpha and two beta polypeptide chains is known as a globin molecule. **c,** heme molecule attached to polypeptide chain. Four heme molecules attached to the four polypeptide chains of a globin molecule constitute the molecule hemoglobin.

Each of the four heme groups in the hemoglobin molecule is believed to be attached to the large protein (globin) (Fig 5–2,B) by a fifth valence bond. In other words, four of the six available ferrous valence bonds are attached to the pyrrole nitrogens; the fifth is attached to globin (see Fig 5–2,C). *The sixth covalent bond of the iron is available for reversible combination with oxygen.* The linkage of the iron atom in heme to the globin protein confers on the iron the unique power of reacting reversibly with oxygen by means of a neighboring valence bond.

Each of the four atoms of iron in the hemoglobin molecule can reversibly bind to one molecule of oxygen. When this occurs, the hemoglobin changes color; that is, *oxyhemoglobin* (HbO_2) makes arterial blood appear scarlet. Oxygen-free hemoglobin imparts a purplish hue to the blood and is commonly referred to as *reduced hemoglobin* (Hb). The term *reduced* is a misnomer since to the chemist that term means that electrons have been added to an atom or a group of atoms. In fact, the iron atoms in both reduced and oxygenated hemoglobin are in the same electronic condition—the ferrous (Fe^{++}) state. Although chemically incorrect, the term *reduced hemoglobin* is so well established that its use will be retained to denote the *oxygen-free form of the hemoglobin molecule.*

The Stereochemistry of Hemoglobin

Chemical theory has long recognized the possibility that spatial relationships between molecules and atoms within molecules may affect chemical activity. Few molecules attest to this theory more than hemoglobin. It is essential to conceive of this large molecule not only in terms of its chemistry but also in terms of its three-dimensional spatial relationships (*stereo*chemistry). Although the stereochemistry of hemoglobin is not completely understood, x-ray analyses have elucidated the basics upon which a firm concept may be developed.[18]

Each of the four iron atoms in the hemoglobin molecule lies in the center of the porphyrin ring and is known as heme (see Fig 5–1). In turn, each of the four heme groups is enfolded in one of the four chains of amino acids that collectively constitute the protein portion of the molecule (globin). The four chains contain approximately 574 amino acid units, making it possible for these very large chains to surround and appear to engulf the heme molecules.

Two of the four chains shift back and forth so that the gap between them narrows as oxygen molecules are bound. Conversely, the space between the heme groups widens as oxygen is released from the molecule. This has been described as a "molecular lung" by one of the pioneers in x-ray analysis of the hemoglobin molecule.[18]

The ability of hemoglobin to reversibly combine with oxygen atoms greatly increases the blood's capability of carrying oxygen from the lungs to the tissues. Thus, delivery of oxygen to the cell depends in good measure on the *affinity* with which hemoglobin binds and releases oxygen from the red blood cell.

The physicochemical equilibria of hemoglobin with oxygen are only partially delineated at present; however, some generalizations may be safely made if one remembers that they are based on mathematical theory (primarily Hill's equation and Adair's intermediate compound equation) that has been "adjusted" to explain more readily the observed phenomenon of hemoglobin-oxygen relationships in human red blood cells. Three major factors are known to have significant effect on the hemoglobin-oxygen affinity relationships in man: (1) the heme-heme interaction, (2) allosteric interactions, and (3) intra-red blood cell enzyme systems.

Heme-Heme Interaction

Each of the four iron-binding sites in the hemoglobin molecule is affected by the oxygenation status of the other three sites. As each successive heme iron moiety is occupied by oxygen, the distance between them is decreased. These spatial relationships are believed to affect significantly the ability of the unoxygenated heme moieties to combine with oxygen. In essence, the more heme groups that are oxygenated, the smaller is the molecule—resulting in a diminished affinity for oxygen. This physicochemical relationship is probably the major basis for the sigmoid shape of the hemoglobin dissociation curve.

Allosteric Interactions

The status of the globin portion of the molecule may affect the spatial relationships of the heme groups. For example, the content of carbon dioxide and hydrogen ion within the red blood cell affects the globin and thereby predictably affects the hemoglobin-oxygen equilibrium.[19] Temperature is believed to affect the mobility and activity of the amino acid chains, thus affecting the heme spatial relationships. The predictable effects of hydrogen ion concentration, carbon dioxide concentration, and temperature on the hemoglobin-oxygen relationship have been known for many years.

Red Blood Cell Enzyme Systems

Certain intracellular organic phosphate compounds (e.g., 2,3-diphosphoglycerate) exert profound effects on the release and binding of oxygen from hemoglobin.[20] These reactions have been described only recently and the full impact of their activity has yet to be determined.

Hemoglobin Variants

The above three factors are certainly the major physicochemical relationships that affect the *normal* hemoglobin-oxygen equilibria. Numerous conditions are encountered in clinical medicine that alter these equilibria. Of course, any abnormality in the amino acid sequence of the globin chains (hemoglobinopathies) may alter the oxygen affinity. In addition to the hemoglobinopathies, three cases are so significant that they demand specific consideration: (1) carbon monoxide, (2) methemoglobin, and (3) fetal hemoglobin.

Carbon Monoxide (CO)

Carbon monoxide is capable of forming covalent bonds with the ferrous ion. When this occurs to one or more of the heme groups, *carboxyhemoglobin* (HbCO) is formed. Heme groups combined with carbon monoxide are incapable of combining with oxygen since the carbon monoxide occupies the sixth covalence position.[21]

The affinity of the hemoglobin for carbon monoxide is approximately 200 to 250 times as great as the affinity for oxygen. The greater the number of heme sites bound to carbon monoxide, the greater is the affinity of the remaining heme sites for oxygen.[22]

In addition, both oxygen and carbon monoxide affinities are affected by the partial pressures of the gases to which the hemoglobin is exposed. Stated simplistically, the greater the partial pressure of oxygen, the less hemoglobin affinity for carbon monoxide; and conversely, the greater the partial pressure of carbon monoxide, the less hemoglobin affinity for oxygen.[23]

Methemoglobin (Met Hb)

Methemoglobin exists when a ferrous ion (Fe^{++}) is oxidized to the ferric (Fe^{+++}) state. This oxidation process causes the hemoglobin to turn brown. Methemoglobin is incapable of combining reversibly with oxygen and thus cannot act as an oxygen carrier. Like carboxyhemoglobin, methemoglobin increases the affinity for oxygen of the remaining iron sites.

Fetal Hemoglobin (HbF)

Fetal hemoglobin comprises approximately 85% of the hemoglobin in the full-term fetus and differs chemically from adult hemoglobin (HbA) in that the two *beta* polypeptide chains are absent and two *gamma* polypeptide chains are present.[24] The gamma chains are believed to affect the physicochemical relationships in such a way that the affinity for oxygen is *increased*.[25, 26] Hemoglobin F is more easily oxidized to met-

↑ affinity - shift to (L)

hemoglobin than hemoglobin A, and there is evidence that the phosphorylase enzyme systems are less active in red blood cells containing hemoglobin F.[27]

Bohr and Haldane Effects

Bohr first described the underlying chemical factor governing the hemoglobin molecule's reaction to oxygen and CO_2. *Oxygenated hemoglobin is a stronger acid than deoxygenated hemoglobin.* In simplistic terms, this chemical observation means that as arterial (oxygenated) blood begins to give up oxygen to the tissues, the loss of oxygen from the hemoglobin makes the molecule a weaker acid (i.e., more capable of binding with hydrogen ions). This phenomenon obviously increases the blood's ability to transport the carbon dioxide that is entering the blood at this time. Conversely, as the blood passes through the lungs, the oxygenation of the hemoglobin makes it a stronger acid (i.e., less capable of binding with hydrogen ion). This phenomenon aids the reversal of the bicarbonate ion and carbamino mechanisms, allowing carbon dioxide to be reformed and excreted through the lungs as the blood is oxygenated.

The effects of Bohr's observation have been used over the years to describe the intricacies of the interrelationships of oxygen and CO_2 transport mechanisms as they relate to hemoglobin. The so-called *Bohr effect* most commonly refers to the phenomenon that the addition of carbon dioxide to the blood enhances oxygen release from hemoglobin. The *Haldane effect* most commonly refers to the phenomenon that the addition of oxygen to the blood enhances the release of carbon dioxide from the hemoglobin.[28]

Obviously, these are simply alternative ways to describe the chemical interrelationships of oxygen, CO_2, and the hemoglobin molecule. From a chemical viewpoint, it is reasonable to state that the effect of oxygenation on carbon dioxide transport is several times more important than the effect of carbon dioxide on oxygen transport.

HEMOGLOBIN DISSOCIATION CURVE

The normal range of hemoglobin in the adult is 12 to 16 gm/100 ml blood—expressed as grams percent (gm%). Under normal conditions, hemoglobin exists primarily in two forms: oxyhemoglobin (HbO_2) and reduced hemoglobin (Hb).

Exposing a solution such as blood to a given partial pressure of oxygen results in oxygen molecules moving into the blood (see Henry's

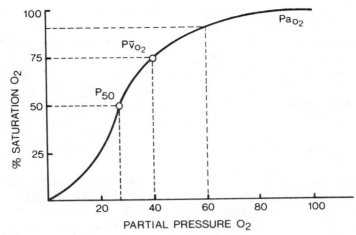

FIG 5–3.
The hemoglobin dissociation curve. This curve shows the relationship of plasma oxygen partial pressure to the degree to which potential oxygen-carrying hemoglobin sites have oxygen attached (% saturation oxygen). This nonlinear relationship accounts for most of the oxygen reserves in blood. Normally, hemoglobin is 50% saturated at a plasma PO_2 of approximately 27 mm Hg; this is designated P_{50}. Normal mixed venous blood has an oxygen partial pressure ($P\bar{v}_{O_2}$) of 40 mm Hg and an oxyhemoglobin saturation of 75%. A PO_2 of 60 mm Hg normally results in approximately 90% saturation. Normal arterial blood has an oxygen partial pressure (Pa_{O_2}) of 97 mm Hg and an oxyhemoglobin saturation of 97%.

law in chap. 1). Most of the entering oxygen attaches immediately to the hemoglobin molecule. Oxygen continues to move from the alveoli into the blood until a pressure gradient between the alveoli and the pulmonary capillary blood no longer exists. At this equilibrium point, the hemoglobin is maximally saturated for that blood oxygen tension.

Exposing the hemoglobin to increasing oxygen tensions results in increasing oxyhemoglobin saturation until eventually nearly all the hemoglobin is saturated with oxygen. A sigmoid curve results at oxygen tensions between 0 and 100 mm Hg; this curve is characterized as the *hemoglobin dissociation curve* (Fig 5–3). For oxygen tensions between 20 and 60 mm Hg, large amounts of oxygen may be carried and released by the blood with relatively small changes in blood oxygen tensions.

To summarize, the partial pressure of oxygen is critical since it determines the pressure gradient between systemic capillary blood and tissue (as well as between pulmonary capillary blood and alveoli). The quantity of oxygen that may move into (or out of) the blood is dependent on three factors: the amount of dissolved oxygen, the amount of oxygen that is carried by the hemoglobin, and the degree to which the hemoglobin attracts the oxygen molecule. Under normal conditions, the quantity of dissolved oxygen is relatively small compared with the total oxygen carried by the blood (Fig 5–4).

Conditions may exist where partial pressures of oxygen are increased up to 1 atm or more (e.g., high concentrations of inspired oxygen or hyperbaric conditions). In such cases, a metabolically significant amount of oxygen may be carried in the dissolved state. It is essential to make the distinction between oxygen *tension* and oxygen *content*.

OXYGEN CONTENT

Early laboratory studies determined that 1 gm of hemoglobin fully saturated with oxygen could carry 1.34 ml oxygen. These measurements involve techniques in which the red blood cells remained intact. Later work with hemolyzed blood suggests that a value of approximately 1.39 ml of oxygen may be more representative. Throughout this text, the traditional value of 1.34 ml of oxygen will be used.

The quantity of *dissolved* oxygen that may be carried by the blood

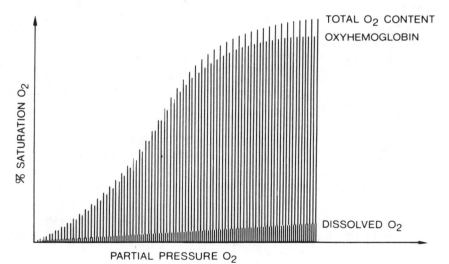

FIG 5–4.
Oxygen content and hemoglobin saturation. Total oxygen content is shown, along with the portion attached to hemoglobin and the portion dissolved in plasma. As long as the hemoglobin is not fully saturated, great increases in oxygen content are seen with small increases in P_{O_2}. In this range, almost all the increase in oxygen content is due to oxygen attached to hemoglobin. When hemoglobin is maximally saturated, large increases in P_{O_2} are accompanied by small increases in oxygen content, because only increases in dissolved oxygen are possible.

TABLE 5-1.

Calculating Oxygen Content

Grams percent (gm%) = grams of hemoglobin per 100 ml blood

Volumes percent (vol%) = milliliters of oxygen per 100 ml blood

Steps
1. Hemoglobin content (gm%) × 1.34* × So_2 = oxygen attached to hemoglobin (vol%)
2. Po_2 × 0.003* = oxygen dissolved in plasma (vol%)
3. Steps 1 + 2 = *oxygen content* (vol%)

Example 1: Hb 15 gm%, Po_2 100 mm Hg, So_2 100%
    1. 15 × 1.34 × 1.00 = 20.10 vol%
    2. 100 × 0.003   = <u>0.30 vol%</u>
    3.   20.40 vol%

Example 2: Hb 15 gm%, Po_2 50 mm Hg, So_2 85%
    1. 15 × 1.34 × 0.85 = 17.09 vol%
    2. 50 × 0.003   = <u>0.15 vol%</u>
    3.   17.24 vol%

*For the derivation of these constants, see text.

can be obtained from the Bunsen solubility coefficient for oxygen in blood. For each 100 ml of blood at BTPS* 0.003 ml of oxygen can be dissolved for each 1 mm Hg of oxygen tension. Thus, 100 ml of blood with an oxygen tension of 100 mm Hg contains 0.3 ml of dissolved oxygen. Milliliters of oxygen dissolved per 100 ml blood is expressed as volumes percent (vol%) or milliliters per deciliter (ml/dl).

The oxygen content represents the sum of the oxygen attached to hemoglobin and that dissolved in plasma. Thus, blood at BTPS with 15 gm of hemoglobin and 100% saturation has an oxygen content of 20.4 vol%. Steps in the calculation of oxygen content are illustrated in Table 5-1.

OXYGEN AFFINITY

Hemoglobin has a strong affinity for oxygen. It is this property of hemoglobin that allows poorly oxygenated blood to oxygenate readily in the pulmonary capillary bed. On the other hand, this affinity for oxygen may make the hemoglobin less able to release oxygen at the tissue level. Certain factors in the blood alter the affinity and, in so doing, change the normal relationship between hemoglobin saturation and oxygen tension (Fig 5-5). In other words, a change in the hemo-

*Body temperature, atmospheric pressure, fully saturated with water vapor (see chap. 1).

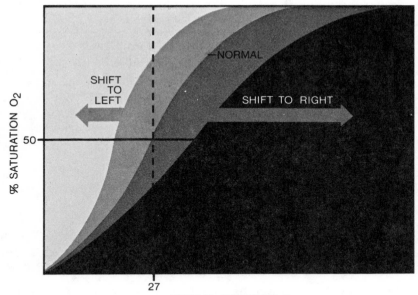

FIG 5–5.
Hemoglobin affinity for oxygen. Increased oxygen affinity *(shift to the left)* means there will be a higher oxygen content at any given Po_2. Conversely, decreased oxygen affinity *(shift to the right)* means there will be a lower oxygen content at any given Po_2. A shift to the left is the result of alkalemia (decreased H^+), hypothermia (cold), hypocarbia (decreased Pco_2), and decreased 2,3-diphosphoglycerate. A shift to the right is the result of acidemia (increased H^+), hyperthermia (fever), hypercarbia (increased Pco_2), and increased 2,3-DPG.

globin affinity for oxygen changes the position of the hemoglobin dissociation curve.

Decreased Oxygen Affinity

This is most often referred to as a *shift of the oxygen dissociation curve to the right*. In other words, for any given oxygen tension, there is decreased oxyhemoglobin relative to the normal state. Therefore, for any given oxygen tension, the oxygen transport capability of the blood is decreased because the oxygen content is decreased. A shift to the right aids oxygen movement from blood to tissue in the peripheral capillaries. However, an *extreme* shift to the right almost always results in a decreased arterial oxygen content, which limits the amount of oxygen that may be given to the tissue regardless of how easily it can dissociate from the hemoglobin.

Increased Oxygen Affinity

This is most commonly referred to as a *shift of the dissociation curve to the left*. In other words, for any given oxygen tension, there is increased oxyhemoglobin saturation. At any given oxygen tension, the oxygen transport capability of the blood is increased since there is increased oxyhemoglobin present. The tissue oxygenation significance of an increased hemoglobin affinity is *potentially* profound. Hemoglobin may be thought of as an oxygen magnet in the blood—the stronger the magnet, the less effective is any given blood to tissue tension gradient for transferring oxygen to the tissues. In other words, the greater the hemoglobin affinity for oxygen, the less potential effectiveness any arterial oxygen tension has in delivering oxygen to the tissues.

Clinical Significance

Physiologic factors such as changes in hydrogen ion concentration, carbon dioxide tension, and temperature affect the hemoglobin affinity for oxygen.[29] An increase in any of these factors produces a shift of the oxygen dissociation curve to the right (see Fig 5–5). Conversely, a decrease in any of these factors produces a shift to the left. Under normal circumstances, these factors work to the physiologic benefit of the organism. For example, tissue metabolism produces hydrogen ions and carbon dioxide, which result in a slight shift of the oxygen dissociation curve to the right and a slight decrease in the affinity of hemoglobin for oxygen. This process results in increased amounts of oxygen available for transfer to the tissues. However, in disease states, these relationships may not benefit the organism. For example, when there is a sudden *severe* shift to the right, there is a resultant decrease in arterial oxygen available for the tissues. Thus, sudden and severe acidemia and/or hypercarbia cause decreased arterial oxygen *content* and, therefore, potentially decreased oxygen availability to the tissues.

P_{50}

Studies of red blood cells have revealed that certain enzyme systems are responsible for aiding the dissociation of oxygen from hemoglobin. Many phosphorylase enzyme systems seem to be involved, but the most completely studied is the enzyme producing the substrate 2,3-diphosphoglycerate (2,3-DPG). This enzyme system enhances the dissociation of oxygen from hemoglobin by competing with oxygen for the iron-binding site.[30] Thus, lowered levels of the enzyme will produce an increased hemoglobin affinity for oxygen, which has the same effect as shifting the curve to the left. The laboratory ability to measure such changes led to the development of the P_{50} measurement.

The P_{50} is defined as the oxygen tension at which 50% of the hemoglobin is saturated under very specific conditions of laboratory measurement: 37°C, PCO_2 40 mm Hg, and pH 7.40.[31, 32] Figure 5–6 illustrates the concept of the P_{50} measurement. Whatever the laboratory method for determining P_{50}, the conditions of a pH of 7.40, a PCO_2 of 40 mm Hg, and a body temperature of 37°C must be included. In most laboratories, PCO_2 and pH are calculated in the final determination.[33] It must be emphasized that pH, PCO_2, and temperature changes in the patient will affect the hemoglobin affinity for oxygen (see Fig 5–5) but will not affect the P_{50} measurement.

The normal adult P_{50} is approximately 27 mm Hg; in other words, normal adult hemoglobin is 50% saturated at a PO_2 of 27 mm Hg when the temperature is 37°C, the PCO_2 is 40 mm Hg, and the pH is 7.40.[34] A reduced P_{50} means an increased hemoglobin affinity for oxygen. This phenomenon has been studied in stored blood in which 2,3-DPG activity is reduced.[35] The clinical phenomenon has also been observed in septic patients and other critically ill patients. An increased P_{50} means a decreased hemoglobin affinity for oxygen. This phenomenon has been observed in patients with chronic anemia.[36] The clinical application of

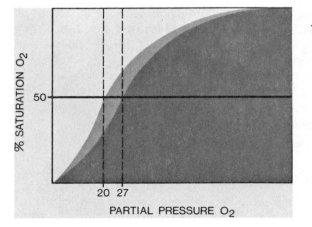

handwritten: ↓ 2,3 DPG   shift to ⊝

FIG 5–6.
P_{50}, a measurement of oxygen affinity. At normal pH and temperature, the hemoglobin curve will be such that 50% of the hemoglobin will be saturated at a PO_2 of 27–28 mm Hg. If hemoglobin affinity for oxygen is increased for some reason other than alkalemia, cold, or hypocapnia, hemoglobin will be 50% saturated at a lower PO_2. Thus, a P_{50} of 20 mm Hg means the oxygen affinity is increased.

P_{50} is not clear at present; in fact, some doubt there is any clinical usefulness for the measurement.[37]

CYANOSIS

The term *cyanosis* indicates bluish coloration of the skin, mucous membranes, and nail beds, usually associated with an above-normal amount of reduced hemoglobin. Many studies have correlated cyanosis with the presence of 5 gm reduced hemoglobin per 100 ml blood. Other studies have revealed that the clinical detection of cyanosis varies widely with different observers and varying light conditions.[38] The presence of cyanosis must suggest a high probability of tissue hypoxia; however, the absence of cyanosis does not mean there is no tissue hypoxia. *Severe states of tissue hypoxia are possible without cyanosis.*

An increased number of red blood cells is called *polycythemia*. Polycythemic states are also correlated to a high degree with chronic hypoxemic conditions. Thus, it is not uncommon for a polycythemic patient who is hypoxemic to be cyanotic because of the presence of more than 5 gm reduced hemoglobin. However, because of the increased quantity of oxygenated hemoglobin per 100 ml of blood, there is usually adequate tissue oxygenation.

The clinical importance of cyanosis may be summarized by stating that its presence demands a careful and thorough clinical evaluation for the possibility of tissue hypoxia, whereas its absence should not be taken as an indication that there is adequate tissue oxygenation.

CAUSES OF HYPOXEMIA

Blood that does not exchange effectively with alveolar air always enters the left ventricle with a lower oxygen content than the blood that has effectively exchanged. In the case where a zero ventilation/perfusion (V/Q) ratio exists, the blood enters the left ventricle unchanged from pulmonary artery blood. This relatively desaturated hemoglobin mixes with the oxygenated blood, and the new oxygen content equilibrium results in arterial hypoxemia.

Intrapulmonary shunting is the most common manifestation of pulmonary disease and is usually responsible for the arterial hypoxemia accompanying pulmonary disease. However, *it is incorrect to assume that all hypoxemia is caused by increased intrapulmonary shunting alone*; limited cardiovascular capability (i.e., limited ability to increase cardiac output) is often associated with significant hypoxemia.* Therefore, in persons with excellent cardiovascular reserve, it is possible to have a significant increase in shunting and a minimal arterial hypoxemia. The pathophysiologic causes of hypoxemia may be simplified and categorized into the following three major areas (Table 5–2).

Decreased Alveolar Oxygen Tensions

This results in decreased pulmonary capillary oxygen tensions secondary to reduced oxygen gradients, automatically leading to decreased arterial oxygen tensions. These regional areas of inadequate ventilation are among the most common causes of hypoxemia. This phenomenon has been referred to as *shunt effect*, or *ventilation/perfusion inequality*.

Increased Zero V/Q

This pathophysiologic cause of hypoxemia is the result of totally unchanged venous (pulmonary artery) blood mixing with saturated blood. This type of arterial hypoxemia is often severe and "notably refractory" to oxygen therapy (refractory hypoxemia).

Decreased Mixed Venous Oxygen Content

Any mechanism that causes more oxygen extraction in the systemic capillaries may result in more desaturated hemoglobin in the venous blood. Therefore, the simultaneous presence of any degree of intrapulmonary shunting will result in an eventual decrease in the arterial oxygen

---

TABLE 5–2.

Pathophysiologic Causes of Hypoxemia

1. Decreased $P_{A_{O_2}}$
   a. Hypoventilation
   b. Breathing less than 21% oxygen
   c. Underventilated alveoli (venous admixture)
2. Zero V/Q
3. Decreased mixed venous oxygen content
   a. Increased metabolic rate
   b. Decreased cardiac output
   c. Decreased arterial oxygen content

---

*This concept is explained further in the development of the shunt equation (see chap. 9).

content if no compensatory mechanisms interfere. In other words, *the effect of any intrapulmonary shunt on the arterial oxygen tension is directly related to the degree of desaturation of the venous blood that is being shunted.* There are three major causes for mixed venous blood having decreased oxygen content.

Increased Metabolic Rate.—Higher oxygen consumption leads to a lowered mixed venous oxygen content unless the organism is able to compensate by increasing the cardiac output.

Decreased Cardiac Output.—This phenomenon is the most common cause of a decrease in mixed venous oxygen content..Less blood flow per unit time through the capillary bed requires a greater degree of oxygen extraction per unit volume of blood if the tissue oxygen consumption is to remain unchanged.

Decreased Arterial Oxygen Content.—This is most often secondary to an existent hypoxemia or to a significant anemia. Again, the organism's primary compensatory mechanism is dependent on increased cardiac output.

CARDIOPULMONARY COMPENSATION FOR HYPOXEMIA

Chemoreceptors

The peripheral chemoreceptors are small clusters of nervelike tissue located in the arch of the aorta and the bifurcation of the internal and external carotid arteries. They are referred to as the *carotid and aortic bodies*.[39] This small tissue mass has an exceptionally high metabolic rate and a very large blood supply; it is these properties that make them exceptionally sensitive to any decrease in oxygen supply. Thus, when the chemoreceptors' oxygen tension drops for any reason (such as decreased arterial oxygen content, decreased arterial oxygen tension, or decreased blood flow), the response is to initiate afferent (sensory) signals to the brain. Efferent (motor) signals are then sent to the pulmonary system, which responds by increasing the total ventilation. The goal is that the increased ventilation resulting in an increased alveolar oxygen tension will in turn lead to a greater blood oxygen tension and content, thereby relieving the chemoreceptor stimulus. The peripheral chemoreceptors also play an important role in stimulating the heart in response to decreased oxygen supply.

Pulmonary Response to Hypoxemia

Normally the 159 mm Hg oxygen tension in inspired air results in an ideal alveolar gas oxygen tension of 101 mm Hg (this assumes an alveolar P_{CO_2} of 40 mm Hg). In general, the alveolar oxygen tension rises as the degree of effective alveolar ventilation increases. The efficiency of this compensatory mechanism is limited in two major ways:

1. The mechanism has minimal effect on hypoxemia secondary to absolute shunting inasmuch as the blood that is effectively exchanging with alveolar air is already adequately oxygenated. In other words, the slight increase in alveolar oxygen tensions adds little content to the capillary blood that is exchanging and obviously has no effect on the shunted blood.

2. A point is reached, especially with large increases in total ventilation, at which the increased oxygen consumption due to the increased work of breathing negates any gain in available oxygen for general tissue use.

As a general rule, increasing inspired oxygen concentrations (up to 50% to 60%) by oxygen therapy is a far more efficient method of increasing alveolar oxygen tension (see chap. 7). While this method does not require any increased ventilatory work, its effectiveness is limited by the presence of any absolute shunt.

Cardiac Response to Hypoxemia

The most important compensatory mechanism available to the body to correct hypoxemia is increasing cardiac output. This concept may be more easily understood if it is assumed that the body's metabolic demand for oxygen is held constant. If the cardiac output increases while the metabolic rate is stable, the amount of oxygen extracted from any given quantity of blood decreases. The effect of this mechanism is to increase the venous oxygen tension and the amount of hemoglobin still saturated with oxygen.

When hypoxemia is due to intrapulmonary shunting, the effect of the shunt on arterial blood is dependent on the degree of desaturation of the shunted blood. As shown in Table 5–3, the heart may compensate for a shunt by increasing cardiac output. The venous hemoglobin saturation level is increased, and thereby the hypoxemic effect of the shunted blood is decreased. The information presented (see Table 5–3) must be completely understood to comprehend the clinical importance of cardiac and pulmonary compensatory mechanisms for hypoxemia. The following conditions are shown:

TABLE 5–3.

Cardiopulmonary Compensation for Hypoxemia

Table of values at 10 gm% hemoglobin and pH 7.40

P_{O_2} (mm Hg)	250	150	100	60	45	37	31	27	23
S_{O_2}%	100	100	98	90	80	70	60	50	40
Content (vol%)	14.1	13.8	13.4	12.4	11.0	9.7	8.3	7.0	5.6

1. Normal shunt, ventilation, cardiac ouput, metabolic rate

$\dot{Q}_{SP}/\dot{Q}_T$ = 5% $P_{A_{O_2}}$ 100 mm Hg $S\bar{v}_{O_2}$ 70%

95% $\dot{Q}c$ at 13.4 vol%
5% $\dot{Q}s$ at 9.7 vol%

Ca_{O_2} = 13.2 vol%

Sa_{O_2} = 97%

Pa_{O_2} 95 mm Hg

2. Increased shunt, normal ventilation, cardiac output, metabolic rate

$\dot{Q}_{SP}/\dot{Q}_T$ = 10% $P_{A_{O_2}}$ 100 mm Hg $S\bar{v}_{O_2}$ 70%

90% $\dot{Q}c$ at 13.4 vol%
10% $\dot{Q}s$ at 9.7 vol%

Ca_{O_2} = 13.0 vol%

Sa_{O_2} = 95%

Pa_{O_2} 72 mm Hg

3. Decreased cardiac output, normal shunt, ventilation, metabolic rate

$\dot{Q}_{SP}/\dot{Q}_T$ = 5% $P_{A_{O_2}}$ 100 mm Hg $S\bar{v}_{O_2}$ 50%

95% $\dot{Q}c$ at 13.4 vol%
5% $\dot{Q}s$ at 7.0 vol%

Ca_{O_2} = 13.0 vol%

Sa_{O_2} = 95%

Pa_{O_2} 72 mm Hg

4. Increased shunt, cardiac output; normal ventilation and metabolic rate

$\dot{Q}_{SP}/\dot{Q}_T$ = 10% $P_{A_{O_2}}$ 100 mm Hg $S\bar{v}_{O_2}$ 80%

90% $\dot{Q}c$ at 13.4 vol%
10% $\dot{Q}s$ at 11.0 vol%

Ca_{O_2} = 13.2 vol%

Sa_{O_2} = 97%

Pa_{O_2} 95 mm Hg

5. Increased shunt, oxygen therapy; normal cardiac output and metabolic rate

$\dot{Q}_{SP}/\dot{Q}_T$ = 10% $P_{A_{O_2}}$ 250 mm Hg $S\bar{v}_{O_2}$ 70%

90% $\dot{Q}c$ at 14.1 vol%
10% $\dot{Q}s$ at 9.7 vol%

Ca_{O_2} = 13.7 vol%

Sa_{O_2} = 100%

Pa_{O_2} 140 mm Hg

1. Normal cardiopulmonary homeostasis.
2. Hypoxemia due to increased physiologic shunt.
3. Hypoxemia due to decreased cardiac output.
4. Increased physiologic shunt compensated for by increased cardiac output. Note that increased cardiac output results in increased mixed venous oxyhemoglobin saturation.
5. Increased physiologic shunt compensated for by oxygen therapy.

In conclusion, it is necessary to understand the clinical manifestations of cardiac and pulmonary compensatory mechanisms for hypoxemia. It must be stressed again that intrapulmonary shunting and its effect on arterial hypoxemia cannot always be equated as cause and effect.

6

Clinical Approach to Interpretation of Arterial Blood Gases

INTERPRETIVE GUIDELINES

Laboratory Normal Ranges

Measurements of a specific biologic function tend to be similar but not identical in a given population. For example, a laboratory test performed on a large normal population will show a *range* of results—the variability within this range tending to be distributed in a symmetric manner. Figure 6–1 graphically illustrates a symmetric distribution; such a distribution is known as bell shaped. The *bell-shaped curve* represents the normal biologic system's distribution of variability in a particular measurement; the arithmetic average (the mean), the median (the middle number), and the mode (the number that appears most often) are all the same number. In a symmetric distribution, the *mean* represents the exact center of the population, with equal numbers above and below this center point.

A computation can be made that includes approximately two thirds of the total population with the mean as the center. On a graph this includes two thirds of the area under the curve and is called *one standard deviation from the mean* (see Fig 6–1). *Two standard deviations from the mean* would include 95% of the total population, or 95% of the area under the curve with the mean as the center. In other words, two standard deviations from the mean would include all but 5% of the population—$2^1/_2\%$ on each extreme.

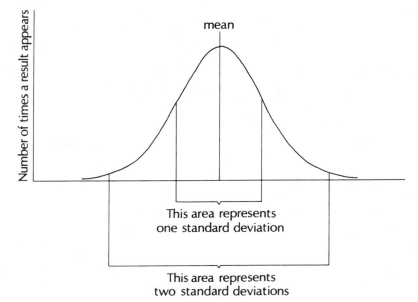

FIG 6–1.
A bell-shaped curve representing symmetric distribution (see text). The mean represents the exact center of the population. One and two standard deviations from the mean are depicted.

These statistical relationships are used in medical laboratories to establish "normal ranges." A *laboratory normal* is determined by performing these statistical calculations on a large series of measurements for a representative population. The computed mean is considered the laboratory normal value, with one or two standard deviations from the mean considered the normal ranges.[40]

pH and Pa_{CO_2} Laboratory Normals

The laboratory normal ranges for arterial carbon dioxide tension and pH are well documented and listed in Table 6–1.[41, 42] These are universally accepted and must be memorized. Most clinical laboratories consider two standard deviations from the mean as the normal range since it includes 95% of the normal population.

Clinically Acceptable Ranges

For the clinician attempting to decide when to institute cardiopulmonary supportive measures or attempting to estimate cardiopulmonary homeostatic adequacy, small variations from the normal ranges of ar-

TABLE 6–1.

Laboratory Normal Ranges

	Mean	1 SD	2 SD
Pa_{CO_2} (mm Hg)	40	38–42	35–45
pH	7.40	7.38–7.42	7.35–7.45

TABLE 6–2.

Acceptable Therapeutic Ranges

Pa_{CO_2} (mm Hg)	30–50
pH	7.30–7.50

terial carbon dioxide tension and pH are most often not clinically significant.[43, 44] This is no more than recognition of the fact that hospitalized patients requiring blood gas measurements are by and large seriously ill and are suspected of having various degrees of acid-base, ventilatory, or oxygenation abnormalities. Much discussion has taken place among physicians in respiratory care and critical care medicine over such questions as: At what pH abnormality should one intervene with supportive measures?; or, how high must arterial carbon dioxide tension rise before mechanical support of ventilation should be seriously considered? The past 30 years have taught these physicians that clinical therapeutic judgments are rarely influenced by minor variations from the normal ranges of arterial carbon dioxide tension and/or pH measurements.

It is from this clinical reality that the concept of "acceptable ranges" for arterial carbon dioxide tension and pH emerged (Table 6–2). These broader acceptable ranges are not attempts to replace the normal ranges; rather, they recognize that minor variations from normal in the seriously ill patient are seldom therapeutically significant. In the clinical application of blood gas measurement, these acceptable therapeutic ranges for arterial carbon dioxide tension and pH have proved dependable and practical. We shall use these ranges throughout the remainder of this text, hoping the reader will remember that we are not proposing that the normal ranges (see Table 6–1) be replaced or forgotten.

Our criteria for using the terms *acidemia, alkalemia, ventilatory failure,* and *alveolar hyperventilation* are listed in Table 6–3. These are clinical terms for blood gas interpretation and therefore are determined by clinically unacceptable ranges of arterial carbon dioxide tension and pH.

Arterial Carbon Dioxide–pH Relationship

The pH is essentially the result of the plasma bicarbonate-plasma carbonic acid relationship (see chap. 3). When acute changes in ventilation occur, a predictable relationship between pH and plasma carbonic acid results. This chemically represents the pH change due to variations in alveolar ventilation (Pa_{CO_2})—i.e., respiratory acid-base change. Although the relationship is not linear, within clinical ranges it is linear enough to assume an easy-to-remember guideline—when starting at an arterial PCO_2 of 40 mm Hg: for every 20 mm Hg increase in Pa_{CO_2}, the pH will decrease by 0.10 unit; for every 10 mm Hg decrease in Pa_{CO_2}, the pH will increase by 0.10 unit (Table 6–4). This guideline will prove helpful in quickly estimating the degree of abnormality that is due to *acute* ventilatory change.

Total Ventilation to Alveolar Ventilation Relationship

In Chapter 4 the observation was presented that total ventilation ($\dot{V}$) must be composed of a portion that respires—alveolar ventilation ($\dot{V}A$)—and a portion that does not respire—deadspace ventilation ($\dot{V}D$). If minute ventilation (MV) is accepted as a measurement of total ventilation, the relationship may be written: $MV = \dot{V}A + \dot{V}D$.

It is well documented that in normal exercising man, the physiologic

TABLE 6–3.

Nomenclature for Pa_{CO_2} and pH Outside of Acceptable Range

pH > 7.50	Alkalemia
pH < 7.30	Acidemia
Pa_{CO_2} > 50 mm Hg	Ventilatory failure (respiratory acidosis)
Pa_{CO_2} < 30 mm Hg	Alveolar hyperventilation (respiratory alkalosis)

TABLE 6–4.

Approximate Pa_{CO_2} – pH Relationship

Pa_{CO_2} (mm Hg)	pH	$[HCO_3{}^-]p$ (mEq/L)
80	7.20	28
60	7.30	26
40	7.40	24
30	7.50	22
20	7.60	20

TABLE 6–5.

Expected Minute Volume to Arterial Carbon Dioxide
Tension Relationships in the Normal Nonexercising Man

MV	Pa_{CO_2} (mm Hg)	Range (mm Hg)
Normal	40	35–45
Twice normal	30	25–35
Quadruple normal	20	15–25

deadspace either decreases or remains unchanged.[45] This results in the arterial carbon dioxide tension remaining the same or decreasing to a small degree. In other words, in normal exercising man, alveolar ventilation does not change in relation to the metabolic rate because the metabolic rate and cardiac output have increased in a proportionate manner to the increase in ventilation.[46, 47]

The normal nonexercising man who is spontaneously hyperventilating is not well studied. One would expect the deadspace ventilation to increase as total ventilation increases because the cardiac output and metabolic rate would not be expected to increase in proportion to the total ventilation. An increase in deadspace ventilation is well documented in the hyperventilated person on positive-pressure ventilation.[48, 49]

In persons with adequate cardiopulmonary reserves, clinical experience has shown that diseases producing increases in minute ventilation without producing increases in physiologic deadspace result in a decreased arterial PCO_2—e.g., pneumonia. The expected relationship between total ventilation and alveolar ventilation in these persons is shown in Table 6–5.

Many patients with adequate cardiopulmonary reserves manifest increases in total ventilation with an alveolar ventilation response less than that predicted (see Table 6–5). It seems reasonable to assume that these patients may have increases in deadspace ventilation. Conversely, the patient who manifests a decreased alveolar ventilation (increased Pa_{CO_2}) without a decrease in total ventilation may be assumed to have an increased deadspace ventilation.

The previous guideline (see Table 6–5) is useful for the spontaneously hyperventilating patient with adequate cardiopulmonary reserves. The existence of a significant *minute volume to* PCO_2 *disparity* should alert the clinician to the possibility that a deadspace-producing pathology may be present (see chap. 10).

Arterial Oxygen Tensions

In the healthy adult at sea level (760 mm Hg atmospheric pressure), the laboratory normal for arterial oxygen tension is usually stated as 97 mm Hg. Variations in arterial P_{O_2} above 80 mm Hg seldom affect therapeutic clinical judgment since the oxygen saturation of hemoglobin is seldom significantly affected at a P_{O_2} above 80 mm Hg. Thus, we consider the acceptable therapeutic range for Pa_{O_2} at sea level as greater than 80 mm Hg (Table 6–6), and *hypoxemia is defined as an arterial P_{O_2} less than 80 mm Hg* at sea level in an adult breathing room air.

There are two major exceptions to this rule that has been shown (see Table 6–6): (1) the normal newborn infant breathing room air usually has an arterial oxygen tension range of 40–70 mm Hg,[50] and (2) the normal arterial oxygen tension levels decrease with age.[51] Lung degeneration is a normal part of the aging process and the alveolar degenerative processes are believed to cause hypoxemia. A general guideline is to subtract 1 mm Hg from the minimal 80 mm Hg level for every year over 60 years of age. This means that an arterial oxygen tension of 70 mm Hg in a 70-year-old person and 60 mm Hg in an 80-year-old person are acceptable. The guideline is not applicable in persons over 90 years of age.

Inspired Oxygen Concentration–Arterial Oxygen Tension Relationship (FI_{O_2}-Pa_{O_2})

Hypoxemia is defined as an arterial P_{O_2} below an acceptable range *when breathing room air.* Oxygen therapy is a common feature in the

TABLE 6–6.

Acceptable Arterial Oxygen Tensions at Sea Level Breathing Room Air (21% Oxygen)

Adult and Child	
Normal	97 mm Hg
Acceptable range	>80 mm Hg
Hypoxemia	<80 mm Hg
Newborn	
Acceptable range	40–70 mm Hg
Aged	
Acceptable range	
60 years old	>80 mm Hg
70 years old	>70 mm Hg
80 years old	>60 mm Hg
90 years old	>50 mm Hg

TABLE 6–7.

Generalized Inspired Oxygen-Arterial Tension
Relationship*

$F_{I_{O_2}}$ (%)	Predicted Minimal Pa_{O_2} (mm Hg)
30	150
40	200
50	250
80	400
100	500

*If Pa_{O_2} is less than $F_{I_{O_2}} \times 5$, the patient can be assumed
to be hypoxemic at room air.

treatment of patients who need blood gas analysis. A common question
is: Should oxygen be withheld so that the patient can breathe room air
during blood gas sampling? There is a widely held notion that a "room
air blood gas" is essential as a baseline; this is not true! To withhold
oxygen therapy from a hypoxemic patient until a blood gas sample is
drawn is as wrong as withholding an anti-arrhythmic drug from a patient
who has serious ventricular arrhythmia until a complete 12-lead ECG is
obtained. Although a room air baseline blood gas measurement is extremely helpful, it is by no means essential for the proper supportive
care of the critically ill patient.

Increasing the inspired oxygen concentration by 10% means increasing the inspired oxygen tension by approximately 75 mm Hg (10% of
760 mm Hg). In the normal lung, this means increasing the *ideal alveolar
oxygen* tension by approximately 50 mm Hg. Table 6–7 outlines an approximate relationship between inspired oxygen concentration and minimally acceptable arterial oxygen tensions in normal man. The minimally
acceptable arterial P_{O_2} at each 10% rise in $F_{I_{O_2}}$ increases by approximately
50 mm Hg. A simple way to remember this is to multiply the $F_{I_{O_2}}$ by 5;
the result will be a minimally acceptable P_{O_2} for that oxygen therapy. If
that tension is not present, it may be assumed that the patient will be
hypoxemic at room air.

Determining Base Excess/Deficit

The Pa_{CO_2}-pH relationship shown previously (see Table 6–4) demonstrates that if a baseline P_{CO_2} of 40 mm Hg and a pH of 7.40 are
assumed, an acute 10 mm Hg increase in the Pa_{CO_2} results in a pH
decrease of 0.05 unit, and an acute decrease in the Pa_{CO_2} of 10 mm Hg
results in a pH increase of 0.10 unit. This relationship allows us to

determine a "predicted" respiratory pH—i.e., the expected pH if the only abnormality is the respiratory component (Pco_2 change).

Determining the Predicted Respiratory pH

1. Determine the difference between the measured Pa_{CO_2} and 40 mm Hg; then move the decimal point two places to the left.

2. If the Pco_2 is greater than 40, subtract half the difference from 7.40.

3. If the Pco_2 is less than 40, add the difference to 7.40.

These simple steps result in the predicted respiratory pH. For example,

$$a.\ pH\ 7.04,\ Pa_{CO_2}\ 76$$
$$76 - 40 = 36 \times \tfrac{1}{2} = 0.18$$
$$7.40 - 0.18 = 7.22$$

$$b.\ pH\ 7.21,\ Pa_{CO_2}\ 90$$
$$90 - 40 = 50 \times \tfrac{1}{2} = 0.25$$
$$7.40 - 0.25 = 7.15$$

$$c.\ pH\ 7.47,\ Pa_{CO_2}\ 18$$
$$40 - 18 = 22$$
$$7.40 + 0.22 = 7.62$$

Determining the Metabolic Component

Under normal circumstances, a 10 mEq/L variance from the normal buffer baseline represents a pH change of approximately 0.15 unit. If we move the pH decimal point two places to the right, we have a 10 (10 mEq/L) to 15 (0.15 unit) relationship, which can be expressed as a *$\tfrac{2}{3}$ relationship*.

The difference between the measured pH and the predicted respiratory pH is the metabolic pH change. If we determine that difference and move the decimal point two places to the right, two thirds of that number will estimate the mEq/L variation from the buffer baseline. In other words, we will have calculated the base excess/deficit.

Table 6–8 reviews the three steps of the process. Following are some examples. When you understand the system, you will find it easy, useful, and reliable.

$$a.\ pH\ 7.04,\ Pa_{CO_2}\ 76,\ predicted\ pH\ 7.22$$
$$7.22 - 7.04 = 0.18 \times \tfrac{2}{3} = 12\ mEq/L\ base\ deficit$$

$$b.\ pH\ 7.21,\ Pa_{CO_2}\ 90,\ predicted\ respiratory\ pH\ 7.15$$
$$7.21 - 7.15 = 0.06 \times \tfrac{2}{3} = 4\ mEq/L\ base\ excess$$

TABLE 6–8.

Three Steps for Determining Base Excess/Deficit

1. *Determine* P_{CO_2} *variance:* Difference between measured P_{CO_2} and 40; move decimal point two places to the left.
2. *Determine predicted pH:* If P_{CO_2} over 40, subtract half P_{CO_2} variance from 7.40. If P_{CO_2} under 40, add P_{CO_2} variance to 7.40.
3. *Estimate base excess/deficit:* Determine difference between measured and predicted pH. Move decimal point two places to the right. Multiply by two thirds.

Base excess: Measured pH greater than predicted pH.
Base deficit*: Measured pH less than predicted pH.

*Often referred to as a "minus base excess"—i.e., base excess–15 mEq/L.

TABLE 6–9.

Quantifying Extracellular Bicarbonate Deficit

1. Base deficit is the mEq of bicarbonate that is deficient per liter of extracellular water.
2. Approximately 25% of the adult's total body weight in kilograms is equivalent to the number of liters of extracellular water.

$$\frac{\text{Base deficit} \times \text{weight (kg)}}{4} = \text{deficient mEq of bicarbonate}$$

---

   c. pH 7.47, Pa_{CO_2} 18, predicted respiratory pH 7.62
      $7.62 - 7.47 = 0.15 \times {}^2\!/_3 = 10$ mEq/L base deficit

Guidelines for Bicarbonate Administration in the Adult

1. Do *not* routinely treat a base deficit of less than 10 mEq/L.
2. Do *not* routinely treat an arterial pH greater than 7.20 unless there is cardiovascular instability.
3. When sodium bicarbonate is deemed necessary, calculate the deficiency as outlined in Table 6–9. Give half the calculated dose and repeat blood gas measurements in 5 minutes.

INTERPRETIVE APPROACH

The value of laboratory measurements is dependent on the ability of the clinician to apply them for the benefit of patient care. No matter how useful these measurements may be potentially, their actual benefit depends on their clinical interpretation and application. One cannot expect to interpret the complex or unusual case without experience and special training. However, the situation need not be as confusing as it seems to most students and clinicians.

Based on the material presented in the previous chapters, we will outline and discuss a method of blood gas interpretation that is orderly, sensible, and reasonably simple. *The method is clinically very useful because the interpretation will delineate the primary life-threatening physiologic abnormality.* Furthermore, the interpretation will aid greatly in indicating the proper cardiopulmonary supportive measures needed. The interpretation also will allow subsequent blood gas measurements to guide the patient's continued supportive therapy.

Structured approaches to interpretation are necessary for the novice and useful to the initiated. Such categorized approaches are accepted in the teaching of radiologic and electrocardiographic interpretation, and they are no less applicable and necessary in the teaching of arterial blood gas interpretation.

Three basic steps should be followed when considering any set of blood gases:

Step 1: Assessment of the ventilatory status. This will automatically lead to assessment of the metabolic acid-base balance when indicated.

Step 2: Assessment of the hypoxemic state.

Step 3: Assessment of the tissue oxygenation state.

Table 6–10 defines the clinical nomenclature used in this system.

Step 1: Evaluation of the Ventilatory Status

The primary step in arterial blood gas interpretation should be to classify the carbon dioxide tension. This measurement is the direct reflection of the adequacy of alveolar ventilation. As shown in Table 6–11, the arterial carbon dioxide tension must be in one of three categories:

1. Less than 30 mm Hg: alveolar hyperventilation (respiratory alkalosis).
2. Between 30 and 50 mm Hg: acceptable alveolar ventilation.
3. Greater than 50 mm Hg: ventilatory failure (respiratory acidosis).

Assessment of the arterial pH in relation to the arterial carbon dioxide tension classification allows the determination of whether we are dealing with a primary ventilatory problem (respiratory acid-base imbalance) or a primary metabolic acid-base problem.

TABLE 6–10.

Nomenclature for Clinical Interpretation of Arterial Blood Gas Measurements

Clinical Terminology	Criteria
Ventilatory failure (respiratory acidosis)	Pa_{CO_2} above acceptable limit (50 mm Hg)
Alveolar hyperventilation (respiratory alkalosis)	Pa_{CO_2} below acceptable limit (30 mm Hg)
Acute ventilatory failure	Pa_{CO_2} above acceptable limit (50 mm Hg), pH below acceptable limit (7.30)
Chronic ventilatory failure	Pa_{CO_2} above acceptable limit (50 mm Hg), pH within acceptable limits (7.30–7.50)
Acute alveolar hyperventilation	Pa_{CO_2} below acceptable limit (30 mm Hg), pH above acceptable limit (7.50)
Chronic alveolar hyperventilation	Pa_{CO_2} below acceptable limit (30 mm Hg), pH within acceptable limits (7.40–7.50)
Acidemia	pH below acceptable limit (7.30)
Alkalemia	pH above acceptable limit (7.50)
Acidosis	Pathophysiologic state where a significant base deficit is present (plasma bicarbonate below normal limit)
Alkalosis	Pathophysiologic state where a significant base excess is present (plasma bicarbonate above normal limit)

TABLE 6–11.

Evaluation of Ventilatory Status and Metabolic Acid-Base Status

Classification of Pa_{CO_2}

Pa_{CO_2} < 30 mm Hg	Alveolar hyperventilation (respiratory alkalosis)
Pa_{CO_2} 30–50 mm Hg	Acceptable alveolar ventilation
Pa_{CO_2} > 50 mm Hg	Ventilatory failure (respiratory acidosis)

Classification of Ventilatory State in Conjunction With pH

1. Alveolar hyperventilation (Pa_{CO_2} < 30 mm Hg)

    a. pH > 7.50   *Acute* alveolar hyperventilation
    b. pH 7.40–7.50   *Chronic* alveolar hyperventilation
    c. pH 7.30–7.40   *Compensated* metabolic acidosis
    d. pH < 7.30   *Partly compensated* metabolic acidosis

2. Acceptable alveolar ventilation (Pa_{CO_2} 30–50 mm Hg)

    a. pH > 7.50   Metabolic alkalosis
    b. pH 7.30–7.50   Acceptable ventilatory and metabolic acid-base status
    c. pH < 7.30   Metabolic acidosis

3. Ventilatory failure (Pa_{CO_2} > 50 mm Hg)

    a. pH > 7.50   *Partly compensated* metabolic alkalosis
    b. pH 7.30–7.50   *Chronic* ventilatory failure
    c. pH < 7.30   *Acute* ventilatory failure

1. Alveolar Hyperventilation and pH.—

a. Acute Alveolar Hyperventilation.—With an arterial carbon dioxide tension below 30 mm Hg and the arterial pH above 7.50, adequate renal compensation has not been elicited and, therefore, the alveolar hyperventilation is assumed to be recent. The pH change is secondary to the ventilatory change.

b. Chronic Alveolar Hyperventilation.—In the presence of alveolar hyperventilation, an arterial pH between 7.40 and 7.50 most probably represents a long-standing hyperventilation with renal compensation for the respiratory alkalemia; that is, the kidney has decreased plasma HCO_3^- to compensate for decreased H_2CO_3. The primary physiologic problem is the ventilatory status change that is assumed to have existed for at least 24 hours.

c. Completely Compensated Metabolic Acidosis.—Alveolar hyperventilation in the presence of an arterial pH between 7.30 and 7.40 probably reflects a primary metabolic acidosis in which the ventilatory system has normalized the pH by creating a respiratory alkalosis. It would be extremely unusual for this to represent a *primary* alveolar hyperventilation, inasmuch as this would mean the kidneys had overcompensated. *It is very unusual for either the renal system or the respiratory system to overcompensate.* It is a fairly safe clinical assumption that an alveolar hyperventilation accompanied by a pH of 7.30 to 7.40 is a completely compensated metabolic acidosis.

d. Partly Compensated Metabolic Acidosis.—An alveolar hyperventilation in the presence of an arterial pH less than 7.30 usually does not represent a *primary* ventilatory change. This represents a primary metabolic acidemia to which the ventilatory system has responded by alveolar hyperventilating. Either the metabolic acidosis is very severe or the ventilatory system is incapable of doing the work necessary to completely compensate for the situation.*

2. Acceptable Alveolar Ventilation and pH.—

a. Metabolic Alkalosis.—An arterial carbon dioxide tension within an acceptable range accompanied by a pH greater than 7.50 most likely

---

*Steps 2 and 3 may lead us to change this interpretation to alveolar hyperventilation if severe hypoxemia and hypoxia are present. This would be a lactic acidosis—i.e., a metabolic acidosis due to accumulation of nonvolatile blood acids.

represents a primary metabolic alkalosis for which the ventilatory system has not compensated.*

b. Acceptable Ventilatory and Metabolic Acid-Base Status.—An acceptable arterial carbon dioxide tension accompanied by an acceptable arterial pH must represent an acceptable ventilatory and acid-base state.

c. Metabolic Acidosis.—An acceptable arterial carbon dioxide tension accompanied by an arterial pH less than 7.30 represents a metabolic acidosis for which the ventilatory system has not compensated.

3. Ventilatory Failure and pH.—

a. Partly Compensated Metabolic Alkalosis.†—An inadequate alveolar ventilation accompanied by an arterial pH greater than 7.50 probably represents a primary metabolic alkalosis for which the ventilatory system has partly compensated by producing an alveolar hypoventilation. In an alert person whose central nervous system is intact, it is rare for the P_{CO_2} to rise above 60 mm Hg in response to metabolic alkalosis. However, in obtunded or comatose patients, the P_{CO_2} may rise much higher.[52]

b. Chronic Ventilatory Failure.—An inadequate alveolar ventilation accompanied by a pH in the acceptable range probably represents a primary ventilatory change that has existed long enough for the renal mechanisms to have compensated.

c. Acute Ventilatory Failure.—An inadequate alveolar ventilation accompanied by an arterial pH below 7.30 probably represents an acute change in the ventilatory state.

Review of Step 1

At the completion of step 1, all blood gases must fall within one of the seven primary classifications outlined in Table 6–12. There are four primary ventilatory classifications and three primary acid-base classifi-

---

*We shall see later that this interpretation may change when accompanied by hypoxemia. (See acute alveolar hyperventilation superimposed on chronic ventilatory failure, chap. 7).

†This may represent acute alveolar hyperventilation superimposed on chronic ventilatory failure. Steps 2 and 3 will delineate this circumstance. (See chap. 7).

TABLE 6–12.

Seven Primary Blood Gas Classifications*

Classification	Pa$_{CO_2}$	pH	[HCO$_3^-$]p	BE
Primary ventilatory				
1. Acute ventilatory failure	↑	↓	N	N
2. Chronic ventilatory failure	↑	N	↑	↑
3. Acute alveolar hyperventilation	↓	↑	N	N
4. Chronic alveolar hyperventilation	↓	N	↓	↓
Primary acid-base				
1. Uncompensated acidosis	N	↓	↓	↓
Uncompensated alkalosis	N	↑	↑	↑
2. Partly compensated acidosis	↓	↓	↓	↓
Partly compensated alkalosis	↑	↑	↑	↑
3. Compensated alkalosis or acidosis	↑ or ↓	N	↑ or ↓	↑ or ↓

*Arrows indicate depressed or elevated values; N is normal; and BE is base excess.

cations. In other words, after step 1 the basic differentiation has been made as to whether the clinical pathology is primarily cardiopulmonary or primarily acid-base and whether the process is acute or chronic.

It is essential that the methodology presented thus far be completely mastered. The following exercises give sample blood gas results. The reader should test himself or herself on placing these results in one of the seven primary classifications and should not proceed further in this chapter until this is completely mastered and understood.

Exercises

Do *not* attempt any correlation with clinical situations; simply interpret each set of values in accordance with step 1. For clarity, the units are omitted. They are understood to be:

P$_{CO_2}$	mm Hg
Plasma bicarbonate (PBic)	mEq/L
Base excess (BE)	mEq/L

All values are arterial.

	1	2	3	4	5	6	7
pH	7.26	7.52	7.60	7.44	7.38	7.20	7.56
P$_{CO_2}$	56	28	55	24	76	25	44
PBic	24	22	51	16	42	9	38
BE	−4	+1	+26	−6	+14	−17	+14

1. Acute ventilatory failure (acute respiratory acidosis).
2. Acute arterial hyperventilation (chronic respiratory alkalosis).
3. Partly compensated metabolic alkalosis.
4. Chronic alveolar hyperventilation (chronic respiratory alkalosis).
5. Chronic ventilatory failure (chronic respiratory acidosis).
6. Partly compensated metabolic acidosis.
7. Uncompensated metabolic alkalosis.

	8	9	10	11	12	13	14
pH	7.36	7.60	7.35	7.56	7.55	7.20	7.46
P_{CO_2}	25	25	95	40	58	78	26
PBic	15	24	49	34	49	30	18
BE	-10	$+4$	$+15$	$+11$	$+20$	0	-4

8. Completely compensated metabolic acidosis.
9. Acute alveolar hyperventilation.
10. Chronic ventilatory failure.
11. Uncompensated metabolic alkalosis.
12. Partly compensated metabolic alkalosis.
13. Acute ventilatory failure.
14. Chronic alveolar hyperventilation.

	15	16	17	18	19	20	21
pH	7.36	7.54	7.24	7.20	7.42	7.24	7.10
P_{CO_2}	83	29	60	38	28	28	95
PBic	48	24	26	15	18	12	29
BE	$+15$	$+3$	-2	-13	-5	-15	-5

15. Chronic ventilatory failure.
16. Acute alveolar hyperventilation.
17. Acute ventilatory failure.
18. Uncompensated metabolic acidosis.
19. Chronic alveolar hyperventilation.
20. Partly compensated metabolic acidosis.
21. Acute ventilatory failure.

	22	23	24	25	26	27	28
pH	7.39	7.48	7.40	7.24	7.54	7.55	7.24
P_{CO_2}	25	24	56	44	25	52	32
PBic	15	18	34	18	21	44	14
BE	-7	-4	$+7$	-7	0	$+17$	-13

22. Completely compensated metabolic acidosis.
23. Chronic alveolar hyperventilation.
24. Chronic ventilatory failure.
25. Uncompensated metabolic acidosis.
26. Acute alveolar hyperventilation.
27. Partly compensated metabolic alkalosis.
28. Uncompensated metabolic acidosis.

	29	30	31	32	33	34	35
pH	7.35	7.52	7.48	7.16	7.28	7.46	7.55
Pco_2	25	44	20	83	20	58	20
PBic	14	39	16	29	9	40	18
BE	−11	+14	−7	−3	−17	+11	−3

29. Completely compensated metabolic acidosis.
30. Uncompensated metabolic alkalosis.
31. Chronic alveolar hyperventilation.
32. Acute ventilatory failure.
33. Partly compensated metabolic acidosis.
34. Chronic ventilatory failure.
35. Acute alveolar hyperventilation.

Step 2: Assessment of the Hypoxemic State

Evaluation of the hypoxemic state must *follow* evaluation of the ventilatory and acid-base status. Only by knowing the specific pathophysiologic state of the patient's ventilatory system and his acid-base status can one obtain meaningful clinical information concerning arterial oxygen tensions.

The only direct information obtained from the arterial oxygen tension measurement is the indication of the existence or absence of *arterial hypoxemia*. Hypoxemia makes the existence of tissue hypoxia a distinct possibility but does not assure its presence. Of equal importance is the fact that hypoxemia may *cause* ventilatory and acid-base disturbances.

Arterial hypoxemia is an arterial oxygen tension less than the minimally acceptable limit (see Table 6–6). These are values derived from normal subjects breathing room air, which means that the *actual diagnosis of hypoxemia can be made only when the patient is breathing room air;* however, hypoxemia may be assumed and evaluated while breathing enriched oxygen atmospheres. Table 6–13 lists the suggested ranges and nomenclature on room air and with oxygen therapy. Since many patients are already on oxygen therapy when blood gas samples are obtained, it is essential that the *probable hypoxemic state* be assessed so that the adequacy of the oxygen therapy can be evaluated. Even more important is to assess the effect the oxygen therapy is having on the ventilatory status (see chap. 7). Do *not* interrupt the oxygen therapy to assess hypoxemia; that is not necessary and may be dangerous.

1. Uncorrected Hypoxemia.—Despite increased inspired oxygen concentrations, the arterial PO_2 remains less than the room air minimal limits; i.e., it remains in the hypoxemic range. Any patient who is "room air hypoxemic" may have uncorrected hypoxemia with proper oxygen therapy. In other words, *uncorrected hypoxemia does not necessarily mean the oxygen therapy is inadequate* (see chap. 7). The tissue oxygenation state must be assessed before changing the oxygen therapy.

2. Corrected Hypoxemia.—This is the condition in which oxygen therapy has corrected the arterial hypoxemia; i.e., the oxygen therapy has restored the arterial PO_2 to an acceptable range. In this situation, hypoxemia must exist at room air, because the Pa_{O_2} is below the predicted normal level for that oxygen therapy.

3. Excessively Corrected Hypoxemia.—This is the condition in which the Pa_{O_2} is greater than 100 mm Hg with oxygen therapy. Hypoxemia must exist at room air, because the Pa_{O_2} is not as high as one would expect with the administered FI_{O_2}. Too much oxygen is being adminis-

TABLE 6–13.

Evaluation of Hypoxemia (Step 2)

Room Air: Patient Under 60 Years Old	
Mild hypoxemia	$Pa_{O_2} < 80$ mm Hg
Moderate hypoxemia	$Pa_{O_2} < 60$ mm Hg
Severe hypoxemia	$Pa_{O_2} < 40$ mm Hg

For each year over 60 years, subtract 1 mm Hg for limits of mild and moderate hypoxemia. At any age, a Pa_{O_2} less than 40 mm Hg indicates severe hypoxemia.

Oxygen Therapy	
Uncorrected hypoxemia	$Pa_{O_2} <$ room air acceptable limit
Corrected hypoxemia	$Pa_{O_2} >$ room air minimal acceptable limit; < 100 mm Hg
Excessively corrected hypoxemia	$Pa_{O_2} > 100$ mm Hg; $<$ minimal predicted (see Table 6–7)

tered; in most circumstances a Pa_{O_2} greater than 100 mm Hg is excessive. This usually indicates the need to reduce the oxygen delivered.

When the arterial PO_2 is greater than the theoretically minimal Pa_{O_2} for that FI_{O_2}, it means one of two things: (1) oxygen therapy may not be needed because hypoxemia may not exist, or (2) oxygen consumption is greatly reduced.

As stated previously (see Chapter 5), arterial hypoxemia results from one of three physiologic causes: decreased alveolar oxygen tensions, increased absolute shunting, or decreased mixed venous oxygen content.

Exercises

The following exercises are specifically for learning and practicing step 2—assessment of the hypoxemic state. (Step 1 is necessarily a part of these exercises.) Do *not* attempt any correlation with clinical situations; simply interpret each set of values. For clarity, the units are omitted. They are understood to be:

PCO_2	mm Hg
Plasma bicarbonate (PBic)	mEq/L
Base excess (BE)	mEq/L
PO_2	mm Hg
FI_{O_2}	percent
Age	years

All values are arterial.

	1	2	3	4	5
pH	7.60	7.20	7.44	7.38	7.28
PCO_2	25	78	24	76	20
PBic	24	30	16	42	9
BE	+4	0	−6	+14	−17
PO_2	65	50	58	50	110
FI_{O_2}	21	21	21	21	21
Age	30	45	40	70	35

1. Acute alveolar hyperventilation (acute respiratory alkalosis) with mild hypoxemia.
2. Acute ventilatory failure (acute respiratory acidosis) with moderate hypoxemia.
3. Chronic alveolar hyperventilation with moderate hypoxemia.

4. Chronic ventilatory failure with hypoxemia.
5. Partly compensated metabolic acidosis without hypoxemia.

	6	7	8	9	10
pH	7.48	7.54	7.48	7.24	7.46
Pco_2	28	25	33	60	58
PBic	20	21	24	26	40
BE	−1	0	+1	−2	+11
Po_2	65	90	85	50	45
Fi_{O_2}	21	21	50	21	21
Age	40	40	40	45	70

6. Chronic alveolar hyperventilation with mild hypoxemia.
7. Acute alveolar hyperventilation without hypoxemia.
8. Acceptable ventilatory status with corrected hypoxemia.
9. Acute ventilatory failure with hypoxemia.
10. Chronic ventilatory failure with hypoxemia.

	11	12	13	14	15
pH	7.24	7.42	7.54	7.16	7.36
Pco_2	32	28	29	83	83
PBic	14	18	24	29	48
BE	−13	−5	+3	−3	+15
Po_2	100	50	65	30	45
Fi_{O_2}	21	40	21	40	21
Age	40	50	45	40	80

11. Uncompensated metabolic acidosis without hypoxemia.
12. Chronic alveolar hyperventilation with uncorrected hypoxemia.
13. Acute alveolar hyperventilation with mild hypoxemia.
14. Acute ventilatory failure with severe uncorrected hypoxemia.
15. Chronic ventilatory failure with hypoxemia.

	16	17	18	19	20
pH	7.48	7.24	7.46	7.40	7.48
Pco_2	33	28	26	56	33
PBic	24	12	18	34	24
BE	+1	−15	−4	+7	+1
Po_2	75	90	70	55	50
Fi_{O_2}	50	21	21	21	50
Age	70	40	75	60	30

16. Acceptable ventilatory status with corrected hypoxemia.
17. Partly compensated metabolic acidosis without hypoxemia.
18. Chronic alveolar hyperventilation without hypoxemia (75-year-old person; minimal normal Po_2 is 65 mm Hg).
19. Chronic ventilatory failure with hypoxemia.
20. Acceptable ventilatory status with uncorrected hypoxemia.

	21	22	23	24	25
pH	7.48	7.55	7.26	7.56	7.10
Pco_2	33	20	56	32	95
PBic	24	18	24	28	29
BE	+1	−3	−4	+6	−5
Po_2	160	45	50	100	35
Fi_{O_2}	50	21	21	21	21
Age	30	40	40	40	50

21. Acceptable ventilatory status with excessively corrected hypoxemia.
22. Acute alveolar hyperventilation with moderate hypoxemia.
23. Acute ventilatory failure with hypoxemia.
24. Uncompensated metabolic alkalosis without hypoxemia.
25. Acute ventilatory failure with severe hypoxemia.

	26	27	28	29	30
pH	7.48	7.20	7.32	7.48	7.52
Pco_2	20	25	95	20	28
PBic	16	9	49	16	22
BE	−7	−17	+15	−7	+1
Po_2	90	100	40	90	55
Fi_{O_2}	50	21	21	21	21
Age	30	40	75	50	40

26. Chronic alveolar hyperventilation with corrected hypoxemia.
27. Partly compensated metabolic acidosis without hypoxemia.
28. Chronic ventilatory failure with hypoxemia.
29. Chronic alveolar hyperventilation without hypoxemia.
30. Acute alveolar hyperventilation with moderate hypoxemia.

Step 3: Assessment of the Tissue Oxygenation State

The evaluation of the hypoxemic state is of critical importance in patient care and is essential to the application of proper supportive respiratory care. The need to evaluate the tissue oxygenation state is likewise essential, and it cannot be separated from the hypoxemic evaluation. To accomplish the assessment of the tissue oxygenation state, one must clinically assess (1) the cardiac status, (2) the peripheral perfusion status, and (3) the blood oxygen transport mechanism.

The assessment of cardiac output and microcirculatory perfusion is usually clinical; i.e., it depends on vital signs and physical examination. Some key factors are blood pressure, pulse pressure, heart rate, ECG, skin color and condition, capillary fill, sensorium, electrolyte balance, and urine output. More sophisticated methods for evaluating cardiac output and perfusion are discussed elsewhere (see chap. 8). *If cardiac output and microcirculatory perfusion are adequate, only the blood oxygen transport mechanism can be interfering with proper tissue oxygenation.* This mechanism is composed of three factors: (1) arterial oxygen tension, (2) blood oxygen content, and (3) hemoglobin-oxygen affinity.

1. Arterial Oxygen Tension.—The arterial oxygen tension determines the initial oxygen blood-tissue gradient in the peripheral capillary. This gradient is an important factor in determining how fast, and for how long, oxygen will pass from blood to tissue. Hypoxemia means the blood side of the pressure gradient is less than normal. Tissue hypoxia is quite probable. If hypoxia is to be avoided in the presence of hypoxemia, the cardiovascular system must provide an increased rate of tissue perfusion or an increased hemoglobin content (polycythemia) must be present.

2. Blood Oxygen Content.—The blood oxygen content determines how much oxygen may leave the blood for a given decrease in oxygen tension. This means it will be an important factor in determining how much oxygen may leave the blood before the pressure gradient is no longer adequate for blood-tissue exchange. As the arterial oxygen content decreases, there is a decrease in the amount of oxygen that may leave the capillary blood for any given decline in oxygen tension. If no increase in cardiac output occurs, the decreased oxygen content may result in insufficient oxygen delivery to the tissues. Factors affecting blood oxygen content are:

a. Hypoxemia, which results in decreased hemoglobin saturation (and thus a decreased oxygen content).

b. Hypercarbia, acidemia, and hyperthermia, which cause a hemoglobin curve shift to the right. This means the hemoglobin is less saturated at any given arterial oxygen tension.

c. Hypoxemia and acidemia, in combination, may drop oxygen contents to critically low levels. *Whenever hypoxemia and acidemia coexist, tissue hypoxia should be assumed.*

d. Anemia obviously decreases oxygen content because there is less hemoglobin per 100 ml blood. Factors other than decreased hemoglobin content can cause this; among such factors are methemoglobinemia and carbon monoxide poisoning.

3. Hemoglobin-Oxygen Affinity.—Various factors affect the strength with which hemoglobin attaches to (and holds on to) oxygen molecules. This is important because *the greater the hemoglobin-oxygen affinity, the less effective is a given oxygen blood-tissue gradient in transferring oxygen to tissue.*

a. Alkalemia and hypothermia increase hemoglobin-oxygen affinity. This shift to the left may be very significant clinically when alkalemia coexists with hypoxemia or a decreased oxygen content (see Chapter 5).

b. Lowered P_{50} means that at pH 7.40, the hemoglobin is 50% saturated at a P_{O_2} of less than 27 mm Hg; i.e., oxygen affinity is increased (see chap. 9).

Evaluation of the tissue oxygenation state is not a simple task! It is a clinical evaluation process that is significantly enhanced with the proper interpretation of blood gas measurements.

PART II.

Blood Gas Analysis Applied to Patient Care

7

Hypoxemia and Oxygen Therapy

Hypoxemia is defined as an arterial Po_2 less than 80 mm Hg when breathing room air (see chap. 5). The administration of increased oxygen atmospheres is the oldest and still most common therapy for attempting to treat hypoxemia. Although blood gas measurements give us the means of properly monitoring arterial oxygenation, too few physicians, nurses, and allied health personnel understand oxygen therapy. Thus, before considering the proper monitoring of oxygen as a drug, it is necessary to state clearly the objectives of oxygen therapy and explain oxygen administration.

GOALS OF OXYGEN THERAPY

Before hospitals were air conditioned it was common practice to place a patient in an oxygen tent on a warm day, primarily to cool him. Unfortunately, many physicians believed this was the *only* purpose of oxygen administration. Another common practice was to place an oxygen apparatus on the critically ill patient to alleviate emotional stress. Undoubtedly there is some psychologic value in this, but it is by no means the basic advantage of proper oxygen therapy, which is its physiologic value.

The only direct effects of breathing fractions of inspired oxygen (FI_{O_2}) above 21% are:

1. The alveolar oxygen tensions may be increased.
2. The work of breathing required to maintain a given alveolar oxygen tension may be decreased.

3. The myocardial work necessary to maintain a given arterial oxygen tension may be decreased.

Thus there are three clinical goals that can be accomplished with proper oxygen therapy.

Treat Hypoxemia.—When arterial hypoxemia is a result of decreased alveolar oxygen tensions, that hypoxemia may be dramatically improved by increasing the inspired oxygen fractions.

Decrease the Work of Breathing.—Increased ventilatory work is a common response to hypoxemia or hypoxia. Enriched inspired oxygen atmospheres may allow a more normal alveolar gas exchange to maintain adequate alveolar oxygen levels. The result is a decreased need for total ventilation, which means a decreased work of breathing at no expense to the oxygenation status.

Decrease Myocardial Work.—The cardiovascular system is a primary mechanism for compensation of hypoxemia or hypoxia. Oxygen therapy can effectively support many disease states by decreasing or preventing the demand for increased myocardial work.

ADMINISTRATION OF OXYGEN

Fraction of Inspired Oxygen

The assessment of the adequacy and effectiveness of oxygen therapy is a matter of clinical evaluation and blood gas measurement—as long as the administration of oxygen is consistent and predictable. This necessitates a knowledge of oxygen devices and techniques.

Normal variances in the distribution of ventilation and pulmonary blood flow make the measurement of alveolar oxygen concentrations impractical and complex. Significant variation in oxygen concentration may occur throughout the inspiratory and expiratory cycle; it is not universally agreed on where and when to make the measurement. Sampling tracheal gas is now technically accurate, but the clinical application of an "invasive" technique remains difficult to justify for routine use. The necessity exists for having a measurement that can easily, practically, and consistently be used in the clinical setting to reflect inspired oxygen concentrations. The *fractional inspired oxygen concentration* (FI_{O_2}) is the clinical standard.

Clinical Definition of $F_{I_{O_2}}$.—Because the final judgment of the adequacy of oxygen therapy is made by blood gas analysis and clinical examination, the major requisites of oxygen administration are *consistency* and *control*. Logic dictates that the most reasonable approach is to define the $F_{I_{O_2}}$ as the *measurable* or *calculable* concentration of oxygen delivered to the patient; that is, if a tidal volume (VT) of 500 ml is composed of 250 ml oxygen, the $F_{I_{O_2}}$ will be considered 0.5 (50%). In other words, we will not be concerned with how the gases are distributed throughout the tracheobronchial tree and the lung parenchyma; the concern will be solely with the fact that 50% of the entire inspired atmosphere is oxygen. This provides us with a consistent, practical, and understandable terminology that is easily applied to any method of oxygen therapy. With this accepted arbitrary definition, reliable oxygen therapy becomes a matter of methodology and thorough understanding of oxygen delivery systems.

Gas Delivery Systems

The advent of anesthetic gases and their clinical administration necessitated the development of gas delivery systems to meet various needs. The past century has seen a myriad of techniques developed for delivering controlled gas concentrations. All these techniques fall into one of two categories: nonrebreathing and rebreathing systems.

Nonrebreathing Systems (Fig 7–1).—A *nonrebreathing system* is designed so that exhaled gases have minimal contact with inspiratory gases. In most cases, this is simply a matter of venting the exhaled gases to the atmosphere via one-way valves. A primary advantage to nonrebreathing systems is that exhaled carbon dioxide is not involved in the inspiratory gas system. However, a gas flow sufficient to meet the requirements of the minute volume and peak flow rate must be supplied. This usually is accomplished by an inspiratory reservoir that allows an additional amount of gas to be available during the transient times when inspiratory demands are beyond the capabilities of the uniform flow rates delivered by the apparatus.

To meet this problem of sufficient gas delivery better, nonrebreathing systems have been developed, in which a one-way valve allows room air to enter if the system itself is not adequate to meet the ventilatory demands. In this way, adequate minute volume and peak inspiratory flow volume are assured. This is accomplished at the expense of diluting the initially delivered gas concentrations with room air.

A nonrebreathing system in which the minute volume, flow rates,

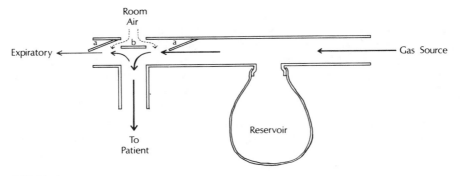

FIG 7–1.
A model nonrebreathing system. The gas source must supply a volume at least equal to the patient's minute ventilation. A reservoir bag serves to make gas available to meet peak flow requirements. A one-way valve system (at point *a*) ensures the patient will inhale only fresh gas and exhale only to the room atmosphere. A one-way valve *(b)* will allow room air to supply a portion of the inspiratory volume if the gas source and reservoir prove inadequate.

and reservoir system are adequate to meet the total ventilatory needs of the patient is called a *fixed performance high-flow system.*[53, 54] Whenever room air must enter the system to meet total gas requirements, the system is considered a *variable performance low-flow system.*[53, 54] In other words, *low-flow nonrebreathing systems do not allow inspired gas mixtures to be determined precisely.*

Rebreathing Systems.—A *rebreathing system* is one in which a reservoir exists on the expiratory line and a carbon dioxide absorber is present so that the exhaled air minus the CO_2 can reenter the inspiratory system. Rebreathing systems gained popularity in anesthesiology because of their potential for conserving expensive anesthetic gases and because many anesthetic gases were explosive.

During induction of anesthesia, the rebreathing system is often used as a high-flow, nonrebreathing system. By preventing exhaled gases from diluting fresh inspired gas, the concentration of anesthetic gases delivered to the patient is kept constant. In other words, anesthesiology has long recognized that high-flow, nonrebreathing systems are most desirable for precise control of inspired gas mixtures.[55]

Oxygen Delivery Systems

Modern oxygen therapy is properly administered by *nonrebreathing systems* because (1) oxygen is a nonexplosive agent, (2) the expense is not prohibitive, and (3) rebreathing CO_2 is easily avoided. Since we are dealing with oxygen delivery and nonrebreathing systems, we may think in terms of high-flow and low-flow systems.

The *high-flow system* is defined as one in which the gas flow of the apparatus is sufficient to meet all inspiratory requirements. A *low-flow system* is one in which the gas flow of the apparatus is *in*sufficient to meet all inspiratory requirements. Thus, room air must be used to provide part of the inspired atmosphere.

Most of the confusion surrounding oxygen therapy results from referring to the *technique* rather than to the *device*. Low-*concentration* oxygen techniques were unfortunately described in terms of oxygen *flow rate* through a nasal cannula. This "low-flow oxygen administration" has led much of the medical world to believe that low flow is synonymous with low concentration. *Because it is the fraction of inspired oxygen that is important, oxygen flow should be considered only in relation to the total gas flow.* The concentration of oxygen delivered by any oxygen flow rate is determined solely by the apparatus and patient.

High-Flow Oxygen Systems.—A high-flow oxygen system is one in which the flow rate and reservoir capacity are adequate to provide the total inspired atmosphere. In other words, the patient is breathing only the gas that is supplied by the apparatus. The characteristics of a high-flow oxygen delivery system are distinct from the *concentration* of oxygen provided; both high and low oxygen concentrations may be administered by high-flow systems.

Most high-flow oxygen delivery systems use a method of gas entrainment to provide a specific $F_{I_{O_2}}$ and adequate flows. Traditionally, these were referred to as "Venturi" devices because they were believed to be governed by the Bernoulli principle of gas flow, which states that a rapid velocity of gas exiting from a restricted orifice will create subatmospheric lateral pressures resulting in atmospheric air being entrained into the mainstream. This physical behavior can also be explained by the principle of *constant-pressure jet mixing*, which states that a rapid velocity of gas through a restricted orifice creates "viscous shearing forces" that entrain air into the mainstream. This theory better explains the behavior of high-flow oxygen delivery systems[56] because the rapid flow of oxygen from the orifice creates viscous shearing forces that entrain room air at a specific ratio so that variation in orifice or entrainment port size will result in variation of the $F_{I_{O_2}}$, whereas variation of the oxygen flow rate will determine the total volume of gas provided by the device.

Figure 7–2 illustrates an air entrainment device in which pressurized oxygen is forced through a constricted orifice. For any $F_{I_{O_2}}$, room air to oxygen ratios are fixed as illustrated in Table 7–1. The $F_{I_{O_2}}$ is determined in the air entrainment device by altering the size of the entrainment port, whereas the total gas flow is determined by the oxygen flow to the device. The $F_{I_{O_2}}$ values from 0.24 to 0.40 are most frequently provided by air entrainment masks; $F_{I_{O_2}}$ values greater than 0.40 are best provided by large volume nebulizers and wide bore tubing.

A high-flow system must be capable of meeting the patient's peak inspiratory flow to ensure consistent $F_{I_{O_2}}$. Although the reservoir of the device is important, the flow rate is undoubtedly the most important

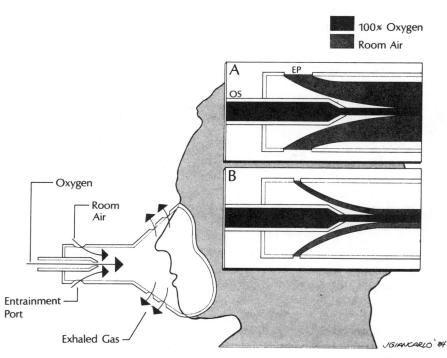

FIG 7–2.
Principle of an air entrainment device. Pressurized oxygen is forced through a constricted orifice; the increased gas velocity distal to the orifice creates a shearing effect that causes room air to be entrained through the entrainment ports (see text). The high flow of gas fills the mask that has holes allowing both exhaled and delivered gas to escape. Insets **A** and **B** illustrate that the size of the entrainment ports (EP) determine the amount of room air to be entrained; OS is the oxygen source. **A** illustrates large ports resulting in relatively low $F_{I_{O_2}}$. **B** illustrates small ports resulting in relatively higher $F_{I_{O_2}}$. For any size entrainment port, the $F_{I_{O_2}}$ is stable; however, the total gas flow will vary with the pressurized oxygen flow (see text).

TABLE 7–1.

Approximate Air Entrainment Ratio

Oxygen Concentration (%)	Air*/100% O_2
24	25/1
28	10/1
34	5/1
40	3/1
60	1/1
70	0.6/1

Examples:
  a. 40% air entrainment—10 L/min O_2 flow will produce a total gas flow of approximately 40 L/min.
  b. 28% air entrainment—4 L/min O_2 flow will produce a total gas flow of approximately 44 L/min.

*Room air is assumed to be 20.9% oxygen.

factor.[57–59] This is best accomplished clinically by ensuring that the device delivers at least four times the patient's measured minute volume.[60–62]

High-flow systems have two major advantages: (1) consistent and predictable $F_{I_{O_2}}$ values are provided as long as the system is applied properly, and thus changes in the patient's ventilatory pattern do not affect the $F_{I_{O_2}}$, and (2) because the entire inspired atmosphere is provided, the temperature and humidity of the gas may be controlled.

The $F_{I_{O_2}}$ can be measured directly in a high-flow system with an oxygen analyzer and the patient's minute volume with a portable spirometer. Numerous analyzers and spirometers are commercially available and most are reliable and accurate when used and maintained properly. The fact that oxygen concentration can be *measured* in a high-flow system is a significant advantage for critically ill patients. If not for the disadvantages of economics and patient comfort, high-flow systems would certainly be the method of choice for all oxygen therapy.

Low-Flow Oxygen Systems.—The low-flow system does not provide sufficient gas to supply the entire inspired atmosphere; therefore, part of the V_T must be supplied by breathing room air. Any concentration of oxygen from 21% to 80+% can be provided by such a system. The variables controlling $F_{I_{O_2}}$ are (1) the size of the available oxygen reservoir; (2) the oxygen flow (L/min); and (3) the patient's ventilatory pattern. These systems are used because of tradition, familiarity, patient comfort, economics, and availability—*not* because of accuracy or dependability.

In principle, low-flow systems depend primarily on the existence of a *reservoir* of oxygen and its dilution with room air. To demonstrate how one may estimate theoretically the Fi_{O_2} provided by a low-flow system, consider a "normal" person with a "normal" ventilatory pattern:

Vт	500 ml
Ventilatory rate (RR)	20/min
Inspiratory time	1 sec
Expiratory time	2 sec
Anatomic reservoir	50 ml

The anatomic reservoir is composed of the nose, the nasopharynx, and the oropharynx (Fig 7–3). It is assumed for the purpose of this calculation that the volume of the anatomic reservoir is one third of the anatomic deadspace; therefore, $1/3 \times 150$ ml = 50 ml.

A nasal cannula with an oxygen flow of 6 L/min (100 ml/sec) is placed on this patient. We can assume that most of the expired flow occurs during the first 1.5 seconds (75%) of the expiratory time; that is, the last 0.5 second of expiration has negligible expired gas flow. This allows the anatomic reservoir to fill completely with 100% oxygen because the flow rate is 50 ml/0.5 sec (100 ml/sec).

Assuming all oxygen supplied by the cannula and contained in the anatomic reservoir is inspired by the patient, the next 500 ml Vт that takes 1 second is composed of:

• 50 ml of 100% oxygen from the anatomic reservoir.
• 100 ml of 100% oxygen supplied by the cannula flow rate.
• 350 ml of 20% oxygen (room air); thus, 0.20×350 ml = 70 ml oxygen.

The 500 ml of inspired gas contains 220 ml of 100% oxygen: 50 ml + 100 ml + 70 ml = 220 ml. Thus:

$$\frac{220 \text{ ml oxygen}}{500 \text{ ml}} = 0.44 \text{ ml oxygen}$$

This means that a patient with an "ideal ventilatory pattern" who received 6 L/min of oxygen flow by nasal cannula is receiving an Fi_{O_2} of 0.44 ml.

If we compute for this person all flows from 1 L to 6 L by nasal cannula or catheter, we see that for every liter-per-minute change in flow rate there is approximately an 0.04 (4%) change in the inspired oxygen fraction (Table 7–2).

For practical application, guidelines for "estimating" the $F_{I_{O_2}}$ that a given low-flow apparatus with a given oxygen flow will deliver to a patient are established. However, it is essential to understand that *the*

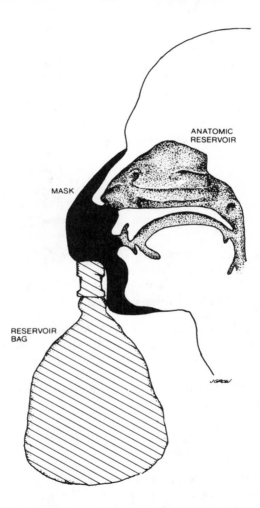

FIG 7–3.
Reservoirs in low-flow oxygen therapy. The *anatomic reservoir* consists of the nose, the nasopharynx, and the oropharynx. This reservoir is estimated to be approximately one third of the anatomic deadspace. The *appliance reservoir* consists of (1) the mask: 100 ml–200 ml volume, depending on the appliance; and (2) the reservoir bag: 600 ml–1,000 ml of added volume.

TABLE 7–2.

Guidelines for Estimating FI_{O_2} With Low-Flow Oxygen Devices*

100% O_2 Flow Rate (L)	FI_{O_2}
Nasal cannula or catheter	
1	0.24
2	0.28
3	0.32
4	0.36
5	0.40
6	0.44
Oxygen mask	
5–6	0.40
6–7	0.50
7–8	0.60
Mask with reservoir bag	
6	0.60
7	0.70
8	0.80
9	0.80 +
10	0.80 +

*Note: Normal ventilatory pattern is assumed.

FI_{O_2} in a low-flow system varies tremendously with changes in V_T, respiratory rate, minute volume, and ventilatory pattern.

Let us consider the same patient with a reduced V_T by half: 250 ml instead of 500 ml. The quantities now are

- 50 ml of 100% oxygen from the anatomic reservoir.
- 100 ml of 100% oxygen determined by the cannula flow rate.
- 100 ml of 20% oxygen (room air): 0.20 × 100 = 20 ml oxygen.

Thus, the 250 ml of inspired gas contains 170 ml of 100% oxygen: 50 ml + 100 ml + 20 ml = 170 ml.

$$\frac{170 \text{ ml oxygen}}{250 \text{ ml}} = 0.68 \text{ ml oxygen}$$

In a low-flow system, the larger the V_T, or the faster the respiratory rate, the lower the FI_{O_2}, the smaller the V_T, or the slower the respiratory rate, the higher the FI_{O_2},

$$\uparrow MV \rightarrow \downarrow FI_{O_2}$$

$$\downarrow MV \rightarrow \uparrow FI_{O_2}$$

A low-flow system delivers consistent oxygen concentrations as long as the ventilatory pattern is unchanged. However, it is erroneous to assume that a nasal cannula guarantees low-concentration oxygen. Obviously, a 1-L or 2-L oxygen flow in a patient breathing shallowly can deliver much higher oxygen concentrations than one would be led to believe.

A nasal cannula can be used as long as the nasal passages are patent because mouth breathing does not affect FI_{O_2}. The airflow in the oropharynx creates a jet mixing effect in the nasopharynx, and air is inspired through the nose. Remember, the *nasal passages must be patent.*

A nasal cannula or catheter with more than a 6-L flow does little to increase inspired oxygen concentrations, primarily because the anatomic reservoir is filled. Thus, to provide a higher FI_{O_2} with a low-flow system, one has to increase the size of the oxygen reservoir. This is accomplished by placing a mask over the nose and mouth, thus increasing the volume of the potential oxygen reservoir (see Fig 7–3). This type of apparatus gives the inspired oxygen concentration previously shown as long as the ventilatory pattern is normal (see Table 7–2).

An oxygen mask should never be run at less than a 5-L flow; otherwise, exhaled air accumulating in the mask reservoir might be rebreathed. Above 5 L/min, most of the exhaled air will be flushed from the mask. Above an 8-L flow there is little increase in the inspired oxygen concentration because the reservoir is filled. Of course, changes in ventilatory pattern are as important in affecting the inspired oxygen concentrations as they are with the cannula and the catheter.

To deliver more than 60% oxygen by a low-flow system, one must again increase the oxygen reservoir (see Fig 7–3). This is accomplished by attaching a reservoir bag to the mask (see Table 7–2). Without a one-way valve between the bag and mask, this apparatus is called a *partial rebreathing mask.* This bag is neither a carbon dioxide reservoir nor a rebreathing bag. It is meant to be an *oxygen reservoir;* therefore, the bag must never be totally collapsed during inspiration. The very early exhaled air (the first one third of exhalation) will go back into the bag. This is deadspace air from the mouth and the trachea and contains little carbon dioxide. Again, it must be remembered that this is a low-flow system, in which the inspired oxygen concentrations vary according to the ventilatory pattern. At flow rates from 6 to 10 L/min, a close-fitting mask with reservoir bag gives approximately 60% to 80 + % oxygen.

With these basic guidelines for oxygen administration in mind, one can readily provide a patient with a consistent and predictable oxygen concentration. Increasing or decreasing the inspired oxygen concentrations within reasonably predictable limits is possible, and, most important, we can deliver a *consistent* oxygen concentration. A patient with a shallow, deep, or irregular ventilatory pattern should receive oxygen therapy from a high-flow system rather than from a low-flow system. It must be clearly understood that even though the term *low-flow oxygen* generally is considered to mean low-concentration oxygen, this may not be the case. The ventilatory pattern must be assessed. *As long as oxygen administration is consistent and predictable, clinical observation plus blood gas measurement will ensure proper oxygen therapy.*

HYPOXEMIA AND OXYGEN THERAPY

In the most simplistic terms possible, hypoxemia is secondary to either *true shunt* mechanisms (mixed venous blood entering the left side of the heart) or *shunt effect* mechanisms (alveolar P_{O_2} values are less than ideal) (see chaps. 5 and 9). Shunt effect has little clinical significance if the alveolar P_{O_2} values are great enough to saturate the exposed hemoglobin fully (> 80 mm Hg).

Figure 7–4 demonstrates theoretically how shunt effect mechanisms of hypoxemia are affected by the patient's breathing 100% oxygen. Alveolus **A** represents a shunt effect unit, whereas alveolus **B** is normal. The *denitrogenation* process results in nearly identical alveolar P_{O_2} values (**A'** and **B'**); therefore, any impact on arterial oxygenation secondary to the shunt effect mechanism essentially is removed.

Increasing the $F_{I_{O_2}}$ by 10% at sea level increases the ideal alveolar P_{O_2} by approximately 45 mm Hg. As illustrated in Figure 7–5, increasing the $F_{I_{O_2}}$ from room air to 30% oxygen theoretically increases all alveolar P_{O_2} values by 45 mm Hg. If we understand that in actuality the under-ventilated alveolus would have a lesser increase in alveolar P_{O_2} than depicted, we can see that whatever that increase may be it will have considerable impact on the saturation of exposed hemoglobin.

Oxygen therapy should greatly affect arterial hypoxemia secondary to shunt effect mechanisms. Indeed, this "responsiveness" to oxygen therapy is a clinical reality, as exemplified by the chronic obstructive pulmonary disease (COPD) patient whose arterial hypoxemia is exquisitely responsive to small increments in $F_{I_{O_2}}$.

On the other hand, hypoxemia due to true shunting is not nearly so responsive to increased inspired oxygen concentrations.[63] Alveolar oxygen tensions in the undiseased lung are usually greater than 80 mm Hg; thus, little additional oxygen can be added to the exposed blood by increasing these alveolar oxygen tensions. The true shunt blood is not exposed to alveolar air and therefore is unaffected by alveolar oxygen tensions. *The primary compensatory mechanism for hypoxemia secondary to true shunt mechanisms is an increase in cardiac output.*

Refractory Hypoxemia

All hypoxemia cannot be treated adequately simply by increasing the concentrations of inspired oxygen. Because excessive concentrations of inspired oxygen are potentially harmful, it is desirable to clinically

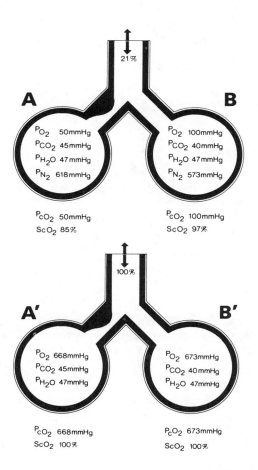

FIG 7–4.
Alveoli **A** and **A'** represent diminished ventilation with normal perfusion; Alveoli **B** and **B'** represent normal ventilation and perfusion. After 15 minutes of breathing 100% oxygen, the lung is denitrogenated (**A'** and **B'**). Note that any meaningful Pa_{O_2} difference is ablated after denitrogenation.

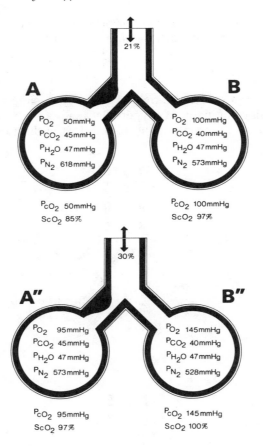

FIG 7–5.
Shunt effect and 30% FI_{O_2}. Alveoli **A** and **B** represent room air breathing. Alveoli **A″** and **B″** represent alveolar gases following 30% oxygen administration for 15 minutes. The **A″** alveolar oxygen tension has been increased to the point where end pulmonary capillary Po_2 is 95 mm Hg and ScO_2 is 97%. The hypoxemia of the shunt effect mechanism is gone. This is the principle behind low-concentration oxygen therapy and shunt effect mechanisms.

identify hypoxemic states that are relatively refractory to oxygen therapy. In the following discussion, a clinical schema is presented that we have found reliable in differentiating those patients with refractory hypoxemia (*true shunt* mechanisms) from those that are adequately responsive to oxygen therapy (*shunt* effect mechanisms).

Figure 7–6 illustrates the Pa_{O_2}–FI_{O_2} relationships for three theoretical true shunt lines (0%, 15%, and 30%). These calculations are made assuming that only true shunt is present, the hemoglobin concentration

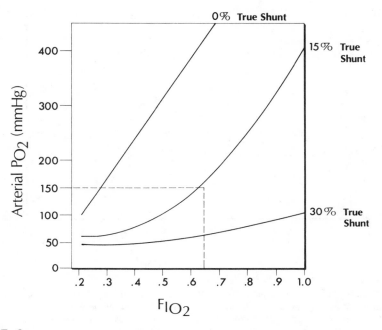

FIG 7–6.

Comparison of the theoretical F_{IO_2}–Pa_{O_2} relationships in 0%, 15%, and 30% true shunts. These relationships were calculated assuming normal lung ventilation, a hemoglobin of 15 gm%, AV O_2 content difference of 5 vol%, as well as normal cardiac output, metabolic rate, pH, and Pco_2. This schema assumes that only true shunting exists, i.e., no shunt effect is present. The 0% true shunt line reveals a Pa_{O_2} of 100 mm Hg at room air. There is a predictable increase in Pa_{O_2} for incremental increases in F_{IO_2}, because the arterial hemoglobin is nearly fully saturated at room air. Because all the blood exchanges with alveolar gas, incremental increases in alveolar oxygen tensions produce similar increases in arterial oxygen tensions. Note that, with 15% true shunt, the arterial Po_2 is approximately 60 mm Hg (90% saturation) because 15% of the cardiac output enters the left side of the heart with approximately a 75% hemoglobin saturation. Incremental increases in alveolar Po_2 result in small increases in oxygen content (dissolved oxygen) in 85% of the cardiac output, while 15% of the cardiac output continues to enter the left side of the heart with a hemoglobin saturation of approximately 75%. Note that the arterial blood does not approach 100 mm Hg (near complete hemoglobin saturation) until the F_{IO_2} approaches 0.5. With incremental F_{IO_2} increases above 0.5, near linear increases in Pa_{O_2} occur, but at a slightly lesser slope than with 0% true shunt. Thirty percent true shunt produces an arterial Po_2 of approximately 45 mm Hg at room air. This degree of true shunt does not allow an arterial Po_2 of 100 mm Hg, even at 100% inspired oxygen concentration.

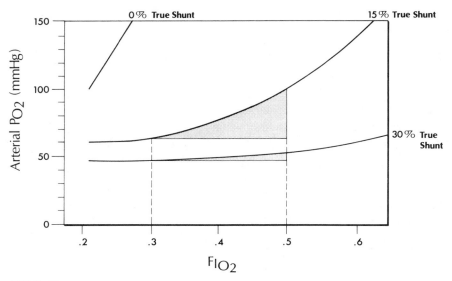

FIG 7–7.
The oxygen challenge principle. The lower left portion of Figure 7–6 is shown in greater detail. *Shaded areas* depict the change in arterial Po$_2$ with an increase in F$_{IO_2}$ from 0.3 to 0.5. An increase in F$_{IO_2}$ of 0.2 theoretically results in an alveolar Po$_2$ increase of approximately 100 mm Hg. Note that the arterial Po$_2$ increase with 15% true shunt is considerably greater than 10 mm Hg, while the increase is considerably less than 10 mm Hg with 30% true shunt. The same would be true if the oxygen challenge were administered from room air (0.21) to 0.4 F$_{IO_2}$. An arterial Po$_2$ response of less than 10 mm Hg to a 0.2 oxygen challenge is arbitrarily designated as refractory hypoxemia (see text).

is 15 gm%, the arterial–venous oxygen content difference is 5 vol%, the metabolic rate is normal, and the pH and Pco$_2$ values are normal. Fifteen percent true shunt represents a degree of intrapulmonary pathology that is seldom life-threatening, whereas 30% true shunt may be life-threatening.

At sea level, an increase in F$_{IO_2}$ of 0.2 is associated with an increase in the ideal alveolar oxygen tension of approximately 90 mm Hg to 100 mm Hg. Such an "oxygen challenge" should significantly increase the alveolar Po$_2$ of all ventilated alveoli. This would hold true whether the oxygen challenge was administered from a baseline at room air (21%) or at some oxygen therapy baseline such as 30% (F$_{IO_2}$ 0.3). Figure 7–7 demonstrates that in response to an oxygen challenge (F$_{IO_2}$ increase from 0.3 to 0.5), the Pa$_{O_2}$ increases more than 10 mm Hg when 15% true shunt exists and significantly less than 10 mm Hg when 30% true shunt exists. *We shall arbitrarily define a Pa$_{O_2}$ increase of less than 10 mm Hg to an oxygen challenge of 0.2 as a refractory hypoxemia.* Therefore, the hypoxemia secondary to a 30% true shunt that is shown was *refractory* to oxygen challenge (see Fig 7–7).

Figure 7–8 illustrates a circumstance more representative of that found in clinical practice, in which both true shunt and shunt effect coexist. Let us assume that we are confronted with two patients manifesting a room air arterial P_{O_2} of 40 mm Hg. In one case, the severe hypoxemia is secondary to a 30% true shunt accompanied by some shunt effect, whereas the other case manifests a severe hypoxemia secondary to a great deal of shunt effect plus a 15% true shunt. Although the oxygen challenge could be administered at a room air baseline, this example assumes the patient already is receiving 30% oxygen (see Fig 7–8). The patient with 15% true shunt responds to the oxygen challenge

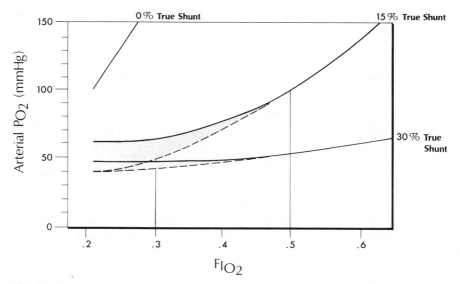

FIG 7–8.
Theoretical representation of two patients with a room air arterial P_{O_2} of 40 mm Hg. One patient has 15% true shunting and, in addition, significant shunt effect resulting in severe hypoxemia; the severe hypoxemia of the second patient is attributed primarily to a 30% true shunt with a minimal degree of shunt effect. A shunt calculation in both patients inspiring room air would be approximately 40%. *Broken lines* represent each patient's arterial P_{O_2}–$F_{I_{O_2}}$ relationship; *solid lines* represent the P_{O_2} values attributable to true shunt alone. *Shaded areas* accentuate the difference in hypoxemia secondary to shunt effect in these two patients. As the $F_{I_{O_2}}$ approaches 0.5, the hypoxemic effect of shunt effect diminishes. An oxygen challenge of 0.2 beginning at 30% oxygen or less will result in an arterial P_{O_2} increase of greater than 10 mm Hg in the patient with 15% true shunt. Of greater significance is the fact that the patient with 30% true shunt will have an arterial P_{O_2} response of significantly less than 10 mm Hg. The latter patient is designated as having refractory hypoxemia (see text).

TABLE 7–3.

Common Pathologies Causing
Refractory Hypoxemia

Cardiovascular
  Right to left intracardiac shunts
  Pulmonary arteriovenous fistula
Pulmonary
  Consolidated pneumonitis
  Lobar atelectasis
  Large neoplasm
  Adult respiratory distress syndrome

with a Pa_{O_2} increase greater than 10 mm Hg. The patient with the 30% true shunt has less than a 10 mm Hg rise in arterial Po_2. The latter patient is considered to have a *refractory hypoxemia*.

Clinical Relevance

The previous theoretical concept is readily applicable to any patient who is breathing less than 35% oxygen at sea level with a Pa_{O_2} less than 55 mm Hg.* When the baseline FI_{O_2} is increased by 0.2 and assuming no other therapy is instituted that may alter gas exchange, the arterial blood gas measurement is repeated in 10 to 15 minutes. If the Pa_{O_2} increases less than 10 mm Hg, the primary pathophysiology responsible for the hypoxemia is most likely a true shunt mechanism. This clinical assumption is valid because the hypoxemia is refractory to oxygen challenge.

Table 7–3 lists the most common true shunt mechanisms. These pathologies usually can be differentiated by careful clinical history, physical examination, and chest x-ray after oxygen challenge indicates that a refractory hypoxemia exists.

To summarize, refractory hypoxemia most likely is present when either: (1) the Pa_{O_2} is less than 55 mm Hg at FI_{O_2} values greater than 0.35, or (2) the Pa_{O_2} is less than 55 mm Hg at FI_{O_2} values less than 0.35 and the response to oxygen challenge is less than 10 mm Hg. In a refractory hypoxemia, the primary pathology responsible for the arterial oxygenation deficit is creating true shunting. Arterial Pa_{O_2} values less than 60 mm Hg at FI_{O_2} values of 0.5 or greater are reflective of true shunting mechanisms.

---

*Patients that must be excepted are the chronic CO_2 retainers! These patients may severely hypoventilate in response to increased oxygen administration.

Limitations of Oxygen Therapy

The therapeutic range of oxygen administration is realistically limited to less than 50%. The primary reason for this limitation is the existence of refractory hypoxemia; however, there are several other situations in which oxygen concentrations between 50% and 100% are not of benefit to the patient. Two of these circumstances are worthy of detailed discussion because of their present clinical relevance, namely, denitrogenation absorption atelectasis and oxygen toxicity.

HYPOXIC PULMONARY VASOCONSTRICTION

A mechanism for producing arteriolar constriction is known to exist concomitant with lung pathology. This diminished pulmonary blood flow to diseased areas of lung is known to occur in response to low alveolar oxygen tensions and is termed *hypoxic pulmonary vasoconstriction* (HPV). Although vasoconstricting and dilating agents are known to alter this response, the existence of chemical mediators that are responsible for HPV have yet to be demonstrated. Present knowledge must assume the existence of unidentified oxygen-sensitive receptors (probably located on or near the epithelium) that modulate pulmonary arteriolar and capillary smooth muscle contraction.

Classic HPV physiology is based on data from animal models, in which one lung is ventilated with 100% oxygen, whereas the other is ventilated with varying concentrations of oxygen. Blood flow and vascular resistance are measured for each lung. As alveolar P_{O_2} values fall below 80 mm Hg (15% FI_{O_2}), increasing pulmonary vascular resistance can be measured; as the FI_{O_2} decreases, the resistance increases and blood flow decreases.[64, 65] This phenomenon is maximal when the lung is ventilated with pure nitrogen. Making the lung atelectatic results in less resistance and more blood flow than when the lung is ventilated with pure nitrogen.[66] Recently, more sophisticated models have shown that HPV in the atelectatic lung is modulated by the pulmonary arterial (mixed venous) P_{O_2}.[67, 68]

It is reasonable to conclude from the known data that while the patient is breathing room air, shunt effect mechanisms would result in HPV. The diminished blood flow would minimize the decrease in V/Q and therefore minimize the arterial oxygenation deficit resulting from the shunt effect pathology. On the other hand, true shunt mechanisms would vary with mixed venous P_{O_2}, that is, the greater the $P\bar{v}_{O_2}$, the less the HPV. Since $P\bar{v}_{O_2}$ tends to increase as cardiac output increases (see chap. 8), one would expect increased true shunting with increased cardiac output.

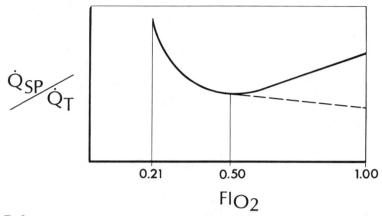

FIG 7–9.
The general relationship between intrapulmonary shunt fractions (Qsp/Q_T) and increasing inspired oxygen concentration (F$_{IO_2}$). The shunt fraction diminishes as the F$_{IO_2}$ is increased from 0.21 (room air) toward 0.50. This is readily attributed to the decreasing hypoxemic effect of low V/Q as the alveolar PO_2 values increase. As the F$_{IO_2}$ is increased from 0.50 toward 1.0, the shunt fraction increases. The *broken line* depicts what would be anticipated if all low V/Q alveoli remained open as the F$_{IO_2}$ increased. The observed increase in shunt fraction must be attributed to increased true shunt.

DENITROGENATION ABSORPTION ATELECTASIS

Figure 7–9 depicts the documented relationship between the physiologic shunt calculation (Qsp/Q_T) and F$_{IO_2}$ values. Although pulmonary disease, positive pressure ventilation, and positive end-expiratory pressure (PEEP) may shift the position or alter the shape of this curve, almost all circumstances show (1) a higher Qsp/Q_T at 100% oxygen than at 50% oxygen, and (2) the lowest Qsp/Q_T between 40% and 60% oxygen.[69–74]

The physiologic shunt calculation reflects the hypoxemic effects of both true shunting (zero V/Q) and shunt effect (low V/Q) mechanisms. Therefore, the significant decrease in Qsp/Q_T from room air to 50% oxygen is attributable to the oxygen therapy diminishing the hypoxemic effect of shunt effect mechanisms. Clearly the greatest benefit of oxygen therapy is expected to occur in concentrations from 22% to 50%!

As F$_{IO_2}$ increases from 0.5 to 1.0, alveolar PO_2 values in shunt effect areas will nearly equalize with PO_2 values in normal alveoli (see Fig 7–4). Therefore, one would assume that the shunt calculation would continue to decline and remain minimal when the person is breathing 100% oxygen (see Fig 7–9, shown by the broken line). The documented increase in physiologic shunting at higher F$_{IO_2}$ values can be attributed only to an increase in true shunt. These observations are best explained by the process referred to as *denitrogenation absorption atelectasis (DAA)*.

Nitrogen, an inert gas, does not enter into chemical reactions in the body. Because nitrogen freely distributes throughout the total body water, nitrogen tensions (PN_2) are nearly equal in the alveoli, blood, and cellular water under steady-state conditions. When 100% oxygen is administered, most of the nitrogen will be eliminated from the body within 15 minutes.[74] This "denitrogenation" process can result in some underventilated alveoli collapsing because of absence of gas volume.[75]

Figure 7–10 illustrates a theoretical steady-state condition at an FI_{O_2} of 0.21, comparing a normally ventilated lung unit with a poorly ventilated lung unit. Pulmonary physiology dictates that the underventilated lung unit will have a low alveolar PO_2, an increased alveolar PCO_2, diminished gas volume, and a PN_2 greater than that in the normal lung unit.[75] The alveolar hypoxia has caused local vasoconstriction with greatly diminished blood flow to the underventilated lung unit.

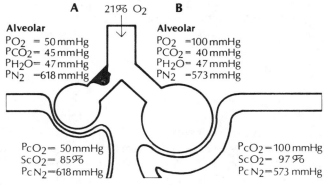

A   21% O_2 **B**

Alveolar
PO_2 = 50 mmHg
PCO_2 = 45 mmHg
PH_2O = 47 mmHg
PN_2 = 618 mmHg

Alveolar
PO_2 = 100 mmHg
PCO_2 = 40 mmHg
PH_2O = 47 mmHg
PN_2 = 573 mmHg

PcO_2 = 50 mmHg
ScO_2 = 85%
PcN_2 = 618 mmHg

PcO_2 = 100 mmHg
ScO_2 = 97%
PcN_2 = 573 mmHg

FIG 7–10.
Schematic representation of steady-state gas exchange in a normal alveolar capillary unit **(B)** and a severely underventilated alveolar capillary unit **(A)**. Compared to unit **B**, unit **A** has a severely decreased alveolar PO_2 and mildly increased alveolar PCO_2 and PN_2. Although both alveoli maintain the same total gas pressure (760 mm Hg), unit **A** has a significantly diminished gas volume. Thus, although less nitrogen is present in alveolus **A** than in alveolus **B**, the nitrogen constitutes a greater proportion of the total gas volume in alveolus **A**. The volume of oxygen is greatly reduced in alveolus **A** because it constitutes a significantly smaller proportion of a greatly diminished gas volume. Continuing depletion of alveolar oxygen in unit **A** is limited by the profound constriction of this juxta-alveolar capillary resulting from the alveolar hypoxia. Thus, although the end capillary blood of unit **A** is significantly desaturated, its adverse effect on the systemic arterial oxygenation status is minimized because the blood flow to this unit is greatly reduced. The steady-state result is that the V/Q relationship of unit **A** is only slightly lower than that of unit **B**, that is, unit **B** is well ventilated and well perfused, whereas unit **A** is poorly ventilated and poorly perfused. Thus, the hypoxemic effect of unit **A** is minimized, and the residual nitrogen provides enough gas volume to prevent the alveolus from collapsing.

An increased FI_{O_2} would result in an increasing PO_2 and a decreasing PN_2 in the alveoli and blood. These factors could result in two simultaneous phenomena as illustrated in Figure 7–11: (1) significantly improved alveolar PO_2 reduces HPV and results in increased blood flow to the still poorly ventilated lung unit, and (2) a rapid decrease in the alveolar PN_2 in the well-ventilated lung unit results in decreased blood PN_2 that, when presented to the poorly ventilated unit, results in rapid removal of nitrogen via the blood. Barometric pressure is maintained in these underventilated units by diminishing alveolar volumes. They may lose enough gas volume to collapse. Thus, poorly ventilated and poorly profused lung units at room air may become poorly perfused collapsed lung units at 100% oxygen.

The laws of physics and pulmonary physiology dictate that the process of denitrogenation must occur whenever the FI_{O_2} is increased. It is most probable that the resultant phenomenon of DAA is a major factor responsible for the clinical observation previously illustrated (see Fig 7–9). Thus, the laws of physics and pulmonary physiology may be the primary reasons that oxygen therapy usually is clinically beneficial in concentrations up to 50%, yet seldom beneficial for prolonged periods of time at over 50% concentration.

Clinical Relevance

As previously demonstrated (see Fig 7–6), the arterial oxygen tension almost always increases to some degree with the application of 60% to 100% inspired oxygen concentrations. However, many patients do not maintain these improved arterial tensions for more than several hours. This clinical phenomenon is illustrated in the following case study.

A 63-year-old woman was admitted to the hospital at 5:00 P.M. with a diagnosis of acute bacterial pneumonia. Except for a significant smoking history and chronic bronchitis, her medical history was unremarkable. Her acute illness began 48 hours prior to admission with symptoms of dyspnea, fever, cough, and right-sided chest pain on inspiration. On admission she complained of severe shortness of breath and was using accessory muscles of respiration. She had no cyanosis; her skin was warm and dry, and her temperature was 103°F. Fine and coarse rales were heard over the right lower hemithorax. A chest x-ray revealed an alveolar infiltrative pattern in the right middle and lower lobes. Her white blood cell (WBC) count was 17,500/mm³. Her sputum was yellow, and a Gram stain revealed numerous leukocytes and intracellular gram-positive bacteria. Other factors are given below (BP = blood pressure, P = pulse, and RR = respiratory rate):

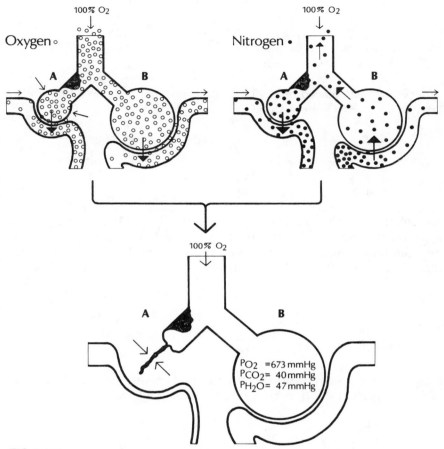

FIG 7–11.
Schematic representation of primary mechanisms causing DAA. The two top drawings represent the alveolocapillary units depicted in Figure 7–10 shortly after administration of 100% inspired oxygen. *White circles* represent oxygen molecules that have increased in concentration in both units **A** and **B**. The ablation of alveolar hypoxia in unit **A** results in loss of HPV with considerably increased blood flow. The increased blood flow to this still poorly ventilated alveolus results in significantly increased oxygen extraction, which results in diminished gas volume. *Black circles* represent nitrogen, which is rapidly depleted from all units secondary to the fact that inspired nitrogen concentration is now zero. Initially, more nitrogen leaves the blood and the body via unit **B** because it is better ventilated. As the blood P_{N_2} level progressively decreases, however, nitrogen will start to leave alveolus **A** via the blood. This results in further loss of gas volume from alveolus **A** because it remains poorly ventilated but well perfused. Thus, nitrogen is depleted from all units within 5 to 15 minutes. The bottom drawing represents the final steady state in which increased oxygen and nitrogen extraction has caused the alveolus to collapse. Thus, a poorly ventilated, poorly perfused unit **A** (see Fig 7–10) becomes a nonventilated, poorly perfused unit after administration of 100% inspired oxygen.

FI_{O_2}	0.21	BP	140/100
pH	7.51	P	126/min
PCO_2	28 mm Hg	RR	36/min
PO_2	46 mm Hg		

The patient was placed on a 40% hi-flow system mask, and 15 minutes later the readings were as follows:

FI_{O_2}	0.4	BP	126/98
pH	7.46	P	104/min
PCO_2	35 mm Hg	RR	24/min
PO_2	65 mm Hg		

She related that she felt better. By 8:00 P.M. she had been started on an appropriate antibiotic, Tylenol, and intravenous fluid. She began to cough up even larger amounts of purulent sputum, and her temperature decreased to 100°F. At 12:00 midnight, these were the measurements:

FI_{O_2}	0.4	BP	126/90
pH	7.45	P	96/min
PCO_2	34 mm Hg	RR	24/min
PO_2	52 mm Hg		

Despite her subjective and objective improvement, she was increased to 50% oxygen. Twenty minutes later, the readings were

FI_{O_2}	0.5	BP	124/90
pH	7.46	P	98/min
PCO_2	35 mm Hg	RR	24/min
PO_2	62 mm Hg		

At 7:00 A.M. the following morning, the following readings were obtained:

FI_{O_2}	0.5	BP	126/94
pH	7.46	P	96/min
PCO_2	34 mm Hg	RR	26/min
PO_2	49 mm Hg	Temp	99°F

The oxygen therapy was increased to 60%. The physician's note stated that although the patient's clinical condition was stable, the "worsening hypoxemia will be closely followed." Twenty minutes later,

FI_{O_2}	0.6	BP	122/94
pH	7.43	P	92/min
P_{CO_2}	39 mm Hg	RR	24/min
P_{O_2}	64 mm Hg	Temp	99°F

Four hours later,

FI_{O_2}	0.6	BP	130/96
pH	7.45	P	100/min
P_{CO_2}	33 mm Hg	RR	28/min
P_{O_2}	46 mm Hg	Temp	99°F

There was no significant change in the patient's clinical status. A chest x-ray revealed increased right middle and lower lobe infiltrates. The FI_{O_2} was increased to 80%.

FI_{O_2}	0.8	BP	130/96
pH	7.47	P	98/min
P_{CO_2}	35 mm Hg	RR	28/min
P_{O_2}	59 mm Hg	Temp	99°F

Two hours later,

FI_{O_2}	0.8	BP	138/100
pH	7.48	P	108/min
P_{CO_2}	32 mm Hg	RR	30/min
P_{O_2}	45 mm Hg	Temp	99°F

The patient was placed on 100% oxygen and transferred to intensive care because of the "worsening pneumonia manifested by worsening hypoxemia at 80% oxygen." The patient was anxious but stated that she felt better than she had the day before.

FI_{O_2}	1.0	BP	130/100
pH	7.48	P	110/min
P_{CO_2}	33 mm Hg	RR	30/min
P_{O_2}	49 mm Hg	Temp	99°F

The following observations are important: (1) her clinical status has improved since admission; (2) the pneumonitis is clinically resolving; and

(3) the blood gases on 100% oxygen are similar to those on 40% oxygen 15 hours earlier (12:00 midnight).

Over the next 2 hours, the FI_{O_2} was incrementally decreased with careful monitoring until the FI_{O_2} was again 0.4.

FI_{O_2}	0.4	BP	126/94
pH	7.45	P	94/min
PCO_2	35 mm Hg	RR	24/min
PO_2	64 mm Hg	Temp	99°F

The fact that this patient manifested better arterial oxygenation at 40% than at 100% inspired oxygen is best explained as DAA—another factor limiting the therapeutic range of oxygen therapy to less than 50%.

PULMONARY OXYGEN TOXICITY

The inherent toxicity of oxygen to tissues was debated and demonstrated at the turn of the century.[76, 77] Oxygen has been applied routinely as a medical regimen for more than 60 years, but little clinical importance was attached to oxygen toxicity until the 1950s when ventilators made it possible to prolong life in the critically ill patient.[78] Keeping in mind that clinical tragedies from improper oxygen administration to chronic hypercarbic patients and premature infants still occur, we should be concerned presently about oxygen toxicity as pertaining to cellular damage and repair of lung parenchyma.

Intracellular Metabolism of Oxygen

Cellular metabolism involves the step-wise reduction of oxygen to water with the addition of an electron at each step:

- Step 1 produces a superoxide molecule (O_2^-).
- Step 2 produces hydrogen peroxide (H_2O_2).
- Step 3 produces an hydroxyl ion ($\cdot OH^-$).
- Step 4 produces water (H_2O).

The free radicals O_2^- and $\cdot OH^-$ are highly reactive molecules that tend to cause destructive and unregulated reactions of organic molecules. They are referred to as "toxic" oxygen radicals because they are capable of damaging cell membranes and mitochondria as well as inactivating many cytoplasmic and nuclear enzymes.[79] Mammalian cells contain enzyme systems that allow the stepwise reduction of oxygen to proceed quickly, thereby preventing accumulation of the toxic oxygen radicals. One such enzyme is superoxide dismutase (SOD) that rapidly inactivates the superoxide molecule.[80] Intracellular hyperoxia is known to increase the rate of oxygen metabolism independent of energy demand.[81]

Alveolar Oxygen Tensions

Small mammals exposed to 100% oxygen atmospheres for several days manifest severe lung injury. These animals are known to deplete enzymes involved in oxygen reduction rapidly and therefore accumulate toxic oxygen radicals when the cells are hyperoxic.[81] Lung endothelial cells are known to be affected earlier and to a greater extent than epithelial cells.[82–85]

Primates with normal lungs are known to have adequate enzyme reserves to avoid accumulation of toxic oxygen radicals in hyperoxic conditions. However, hyperoxia that appears innocuous in the normal lung may result in endothelial cell malfunction if the lung suffered previous insult. The epithelial cells are the last parenchymal cells to demonstrate abnormal function secondary to hyperoxia. Significant enzyme function variability is seen in primates and undoubtedly exists in man.[86]

In persons with normal lungs, alveolar oxygen tensions less than 350 mm Hg ($F_{I_{O_2}}$ < 0.6 ambient) do not result in clinically significant parenchymal abnormalities. However, previously damaged or stressed parenchyma may manifest significant abnormal function when confronted with alveolar oxygen tensions in excess of 250 mm Hg ($F_{I_{O_2}}$ > 0.5 ambient),[86] particularly when the process of acute lung injury is present.

Acute Lung Injury

This metabolic malfunction of lung parenchymal cells is believed to occur when normal defense and reparative processes dysfunction.[86] Acute lung injury (ALI) occurs most commonly in patients who have experienced overwhelming systemic insults. When severe, ALI is most commonly referred to as ARDS.[87] There must be no doubt that $F_{I_{O_2}}$ values > 0.5 in critically ill patients with ALI are potentially damaging to the lung. The unanswered questions pertain to the extent and relative importance of this process when compared to other life-threatening processes involved with the patient, and whether $F_{I_{O_2}}$ values < 0.5 may be damaging in some situations.

INDICATIONS FOR GREATER THAN 50% OXYGEN

High concentrations of inspired oxygen must never be withheld during resuscitation, periods of acute cardiopulmonary instability, or for patient transport. All measures possible must be instituted to allow minimal $F_{I_{O_2}}$ values for maintenance of adequate oxygenation. The avoidance of excessively high inspired oxygen concentrations is a common issue in critical care units. One must realize that appropriate tissue oxygenation is essential to the maintenance of life, especially in patients with multiorgan systems disease. There can be no dogmatic guidelines concerning appropriate degrees of arterial oxygenation to ensure tissue oxygenation. This must always be a clinical decision based on a thorough knowledge of cardiopulmonary homeostasis, careful monitoring, and physical examination.

SUMMARY

The therapeutic effectiveness of oxygen therapy is essentially limited to the dose range of 22% to 50%. This statement is justified because (1) hypoxemia due to shunt effect mechanisms usually is reversed with less than 50% inspired oxygen, (2) DAA tends to counteract improvements in arterial oxygenation from $F_{I_{O_2}}$ values > 0.5, and (3) pulmonary oxygen toxicity is a potential risk factor in many patients requiring oxygen therapy greater than 50%.

Pulmonary pathology can produce either true shunting ($V_A/Q = 0$) or shunt effect ($V_A/Q > 0$ and < 0.8). In general, the closer the V_A/Q is to zero, the lesser the alveolar P_{O_2}, thus the higher the $F_{I_{O_2}}$ required to saturate the capillary blood fully. The low V_A/Q alveoli will in all probability have small volumes. The smaller the alveolar volume, the more susceptible to collapse with any degree of denitrogenation.

Consideration must be given to improving V_A/Q relationships when responsive hypoxemia requires 50% oxygen or more. Bronchodilators, bronchial hygiene therapy, and diuretic therapy, when appropriate, will decrease the need for relatively high $F_{I_{O_2}}$ values. In our experience, 5 to 10 cm H_2O CPAP often allows the hypoxemia to be treated at $F_{I_{O_2}}$ values < 0.5.

Oxygen is a *drug*. When appropriately used it is extremely beneficial; when misused or abused it is potentially harmful. Unfortunately, the detrimental effects of oxygen are seldom recognized as such.

ALVEOLAR HYPERVENTILATION AND OXYGEN THERAPY

Alveolar hyperventilation (see chap. 4) may have three physiologic origins: (1) hypoxemia, (2) response to metabolic acidosis, or (3) central nervous system response. It is unusual to find significant hypoxemia when alveolar hyperventilation is due to the second or third cause. Therefore it is a reasonable assumption that *whenever alveolar hyperventilation with moderate or severe hypoxemia is present, the alveolar hyperventilation is probably secondary to the hypoxemic state.*

When alveolar hyperventilation is the result of arterial hypoxemia, both the cardiovascular and the pulmonary systems are working harder than normal to maintain that arterial oxygen tension at which the peripheral chemoreceptors (see chap. 5) are minimally stimulated.[88] When an increased oxygen atmosphere is breathed, the alveolar oxygen tensions will most likely be increased. *The increased $P_{A_{O_2}}$ means that the heart and the ventilatory muscles can do less work and still maintain the arterial oxygen tension at the level that preceded oxygen therapy.* The organism will not preferentially increase the arterial oxygen tension level if ventilatory work is great or if myocardial work is significantly increased. In essence, then, *the patient manifesting alveolar hyperventilation secondary to hypoxemia will preferentially decrease ventilatory and myocardial work in response to oxygen therapy, rather than increase arterial oxygen tensions to nonhypoxemic levels.*

Below are the blood gas measurements and the vital signs of a 35-year-old man with bilateral pneumonia (MV = minute ventilation):

pH	7.52	BP	150/100
P_{CO_2}	28 mm Hg	P	130/minute
P_{O_2}	60 mm Hg	RR	32/minute
		V_T	500 ml
		MV	16 L

Physical examination showed the patient to be sweating, anxious, and complaining of difficulty in breathing. Note the hypertension, tachycardia, and tachypnea. His blood gas measurements reveal an acute alveolar hyperventilation with mild to moderate arterial hypoxemia.

An oxygen mask that delivered approximately 50% oxygen was placed and 30 minutes later the patient was comfortable and had no subjective complaints. Repeat studies revealed:

pH	7.45	BP	120/80
P_{CO_2}	35 mm Hg	P	100/minute
P_{O_2}	70 mm Hg	RR	22/minute
		V_T	450 ml
		MV	9.9 L

His blood pressure was normal, and the tachycardia and tachypnea were significantly decreased. Arterial blood gas analysis revealed a marked decrease in alveolar ventilation and an increase in arterial oxygen tension. The most striking changes due to oxygen therapy were the decreases in ventilatory and myocardial work.

The need for oxygen therapy would not be fully appreciated if one judged the effect of oxygen therapy by the arterial oxygen tension alone. However, the value of oxygen therapy is obvious when one understands that the original purpose of delivering oxygen to this patient was to support the cardiovascular and ventilatory systems by decreasing their work. In other words, the oxygen therapy was not used primarily to treat the hypoxemia; rather, it was used to decrease the work of breathing and the myocardial work while maintaining a satisfactory oxygenation status.

Another example is a 55-year-old man admitted to the coronary care unit with a diagnosis of inferior wall infarct. He complained of severe chest pain, and his ECG showed ventricular arrhythmia. His blood gases were interpreted as being in an acceptable ventilatory range with a moderate hypoxemia:

pH	7.42	BP	140/90
P_{CO_2}	33 mm Hg	P	130/minute, irregular
P_{O_2}	55 mm Hg	RR	25/minute

Administration of 40% oxygen improved the alveolar ventilation and improved the hypoxemia somewhat:

pH	7.40	BP	120/80
P_{CO_2}	37 mm Hg	P	110/minute, regular
P_{O_2}	60 mm Hg	RR	20/minute

Note that the pulse became regular and decreased to 110/minute, tachypnea was reduced, and the patient had far less chest pain. In this case, myocardial oxygenation was probably improved by decreasing the myocardial work that resulted from the hypoxemia. The reader must not get the impression that oxygen is an anti-arrhythmic drug; this example is meant to emphasize the importance of oxygen therapy for purposes other than dramatically increasing the arterial P_{O_2}.

ACUTE VENTILATORY FAILURE AND OXYGEN THERAPY

When the body is suddenly deprived of adequate alveolar ventilation, acidemia and hypoxemia inevitably follow. This combination rapidly leads to tissue hypoxia. *High arterial carbon dioxide tension with acidemia is defined as acute ventilatory failure.* The severity is judged on the degree of acidemia and the clinical situation. Until proved otherwise, acute ventilatory failure is a medical emergency! The ventilatory system must be immediately supported unless the precipitating cause can be rapidly reversed. Proper mechanical support of ventilation will usually reestablish normal alveolar ventilation, and this should reverse the acidemia and hypoxemia. *Oxygen therapy is secondary in the support of acute ventilatory failure, because oxygen therapy alone cannot improve the ventilatory status in this circumstance.*

CHRONIC VENTILATORY FAILURE AND OXYGEN THERAPY

This condition is usually secondary to chronic obstructive pulmonary disease. The patient has adjusted to his ventilatory failure and is not in acute distress; the arterial carbon dioxide tension is greater than 50 mm Hg and the arterial oxygen tension is less than 55 mm Hg. The disease has resulted in high airway resistance, deadspace, and shunting, which together have resulted in a high oxygen cost of breathing. The significant work of breathing has contributed to the patient's accommodating an inadequate alveolar ventilation and low arterial oxygen tension. He depends greatly on the heart's ability to maintain an adequate cardiac output, so he has little cardiopulmonary reserve to meet physiologic stress. His drive to breathe may be primarily from chemoreceptor stimulation.[89]

The typical patient is a 70-year-old man with a diagnosis of chronic obstructive pulmonary disease. At rest his vital signs and blood gases are:

pH	7.43	BP	160/120
P_{CO_2}	65 mm Hg	P	110/minute
P_{O_2}	43 mm Hg	RR	30/minute
		V_T	300 ml
		MV	9 L

It should be noted that the patient has a pH greater than 7.40. This is typical and is believed to be due to water and chloride ion shifts between intracellular and extracellular spaces, occurring as part of the metabolic compensation for the respiratory acidemia.[90]

It must be remembered that this patient may breathe primarily in response to chemoreceptor stimuli and *only* hard enough to retain his baseline hypoxemic state. Administering 40% oxygen to this patient may result in a *profound* decrease in the demand for ventilation; that is, the increased *alveolar* oxygen tension allows the usual arterial oxygen tension to be maintained at even less alveolar ventilation than before the oxygen was administered. *The organism may elect to breathe less rather than increase the Pa_{O_2}.* This results in an acute *decrease* in alveolar ventilation (increased Pa_{CO_2}) and acidemia.

The vital signs and blood gas measurements of this patient on 40% oxygen may be:

pH	7.20	BP	200/40
P_{CO_2}	90 mm Hg	P	140/minute
P_{O_2}	60 mm Hg	RR	45/minute, shallow
		V_T	200 ml
		MV	9 L

Oxygen therapy has produced an acute ventilatory failure! This acute decrease in alveolar ventilation is superimposed on the chronic ventilatory failure. Despite improved arterial oxygen tensions, the acute acidemia and general central nervous system obtundation now threaten tissue oxygenation to a greater degree than the preexisting hypoxemia.

The primary effect of oxygen therapy in patients with chronic ventilatory failure may be the change in ventilatory status. This is not true in persons with acute ventilatory failure or other conditions when the drive to breathe is *not* chemoreceptor stimulation from hypoxemia.

ACUTE-ON-CHRONIC VENTILATORY FAILURE: THE "LOW-CONCENTRATION OXYGEN" TECHNIQUE

The typical patient for the "low-concentration oxygen" technique is the "chronic lunger." He suffers from chronic ventilatory failure and has acquired an acute disease such as infectious pneumonia. In response to an acute shunt-producing disease, he attempts to increase his ventilatory and myocardial work to maintain the baseline Pa_{O_2}. However, he finds it detrimental to increase ventilatory work, because in doing so he consumes more oxygen than is gained with increased alveolar ventilation (see chap. 8). And so, in an attempt to meet the hypoxemic challenge of the increased shunt, he begins to breathe *less*. On room air, his blood measurements and vital signs might be:

pH	7.25	BP	200/140
Pco_2	90 mm Hg	P	140/minute
Po_2	30 mm Hg	RR	45/minute, labored
		V_T	200 ml
		MV	9 L

Tissue hypoxia ensues because of the combination of hypoxemia and acidemia, and in response the patient breathes less and less. This physiologic vicious cycle leads to death. If one were to judge the severity of ventilatory failure on Pa_{CO_2} alone, this patient would appear to be *in extremis*. However, the pH is *not* severely acidemic, which means the *acute* change in alveolar ventilation has not been as great as the 90 mm Hg Pa_{CO_2} would lead one to believe. *The severity of acute ventilatory failure is judged on the severity of acidemia.*

The patient has a great deal of venous admixture (shunt effect) because of his chronic obstructive pulmonary disease. Therefore, very small increases in inspired oxygen concentration will have profound effects on arterial oxygenation. Increased *alveolar* oxygen tensions will allow this patient to meet the *acute* hypoxemic challenge without the demand for changing ventilation; that is, he will be able to resume the baseline hypoventilatory state and still maintain his baseline hypoxemic state.

Thirty minutes after 24% oxygen, the readings might be:

pH	7.30	BP	200/140
Pco_2	80 mm Hg	P	130/minute
Po_2	40 mm Hg	RR	40/minute, labored

The paradox is that this patient's response to oxygen is to increase alveolar ventilation, maintaining arterial oxygen tensions at the highest possible level. *The oxygen therapy has allowed the patient to increase alveolar ventilation back to his baseline level without sacrificing tissue oxygenation.* This leads to decreases in the acidemia and in the tissue hypoxia. The increased tissue oxygenation state allows even better alveolar ventilation, and by increasing the Fi_{O_2} to 28%, the following measurements are obtained after several hours:

pH	7.35	BP	170/120
P_{CO_2}	70 mm Hg	P	120/minute
P_{O_2}	45 mm Hg	RR	35/minute

The oxygen therapy has manipulated the ventilatory status so that the acute acidemia, and therefore the acute tissue hypoxia, are gone. In addition, the improved arterial P_{O_2} and pH have decreased pulmonary artery pressures and thereby improved right ventricular function. This allows the patient to maintain a good cardiopulmonary status for the next 24–36 hours, while the acute infectious pneumonia is being treated.

Proper oxygen therapy allows this patient to maintain his normal tissue oxygenation state *without* increased demands on his ventilatory work. He is thus able to tolerate the acute increase in shunting without requiring ventilator support. If this patient's response to low concentrations of oxygen had not resulted in an improvement in alveolar ventilation and pH, it might have been necessary to institute ventilatory support. Blood gas analysis documents the patient's response within hours following the onset of the acute problem, and the decision whether or not mechanical support of ventilation will be needed is usually quite evident at this time.

High-flow oxygen delivery systems should be used when feasible, because these patients often have irregular and shallow breathing patterns.

ACUTE ALVEOLAR HYPERVENTILATION SUPERIMPOSED ON CHRONIC VENTILATORY FAILURE

Not all chronic ventilatory failure patients with acute shunting disease have acute ventilatory failure superimposed on a chronic ventilatory failure. Some patients have the mechanical reserves to increase alveolar ventilation and have acute alveolar hyperventilation superimposed on a chronic ventilatory failure, as the following blood gas measurements show:

pH	7.52
P_{CO_2}	55 mm Hg
P_{O_2}	38 mm Hg

These measurements could be initially interpreted as partially compensated metabolic alkalosis *with hypoxemia* (see Chapter 6). Whenever such an interpretation is made, the presence of a marked hypoxemia should alert one to the possibility that this may be acute alveolar hyperventilation superimposed on chronic ventilatory failure.

The chronic ventilatory failure patient who responds to an acute disease by increasing alveolar ventilation responds to supportive oxygen therapy in the same way as any patient with an alveolar hyperventilation secondary to hypoxemia. Thus, 24% oxygen in this patient results in an increase in alveolar oxygen tension and a decrease in alveolar ventilation to the baseline state:

pH	7.45
P_{CO_2}	65 mm Hg
P_{O_2}	50 mm Hg

Great care must be taken to prevent the administration of too much oxygen.

8

Arterial-Mixed Venous Oxygen Content Difference

Although the initial purpose for developing pulmonary artery catheters was the need to monitor left ventricular filling pressures, these catheters also provide access to pulmonary artery blood for blood gas measurement. Repeated clinical observations determined that when these pulmonary artery blood gases are used in conjunction with arterial blood gas measurements, the results frequently clarify the cardiopulmonary status and allow appropriate therapeutic procedures to be instituted and monitored. In some circumstances the need for pulmonary arterial oxygenation measurements can be considered justification for placement of a pulmonary artery catheter.

PULMONARY ARTERY CATHETERS

Development of the pulmonary artery balloon-tipped flotation catheter has made right ventricular and pulmonary artery catheterization technically feasible and relatively safe to perform at the bedside of the patient in intensive care. The basic double-channel catheter has a fluid channel that opens at the distal tip and a second air channel connected to a balloon located close to the end of the catheter. The balloon may be repeatedly inflated and deflated with small amounts of air.

The catheter is introduced into the systemic thoracic venous system where the balloon is appropriately inflated allowing the blood flow to move the balloon tip in a manner similar to an embolus. In essence, the blood flow "carries" the tip of the catheter through the right ventricle and pulmonary artery and pulmonic valve into the pulmonary artery. Prior to introduction of the catheter, the fluid channel is filled with heparinized saline and con-

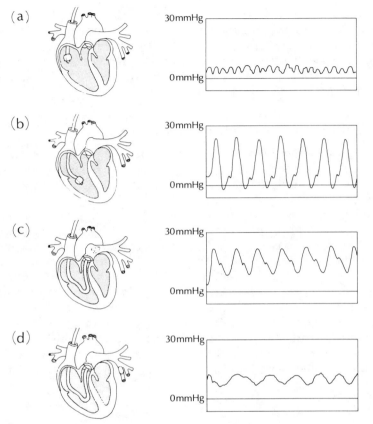

FIG 8–1.
Typical pressure patterns as the tip of the Swan-Ganz catheter traverses the right side of the heart and pulmonary artery. **a,** right atrial pressure; **b,** right ventricular pressure—note that diastolic pressure is zero baseline or below; **c,** pulmonary artery pressure—note that diastolic pressure is significantly above zero baseline; **d,** pulmonary wedge pressure—catheter tip senses only pulmonary capillary back pressure since balloon obstructs arterial flow. Deflation of the balloon should result in immediate return of the pulmonary artery pressure pattern (see text).

nected to a pressure transducer that allows for instantaneous display of the various pressure patterns on an oscilloscope.

Figure 8–1 illustrates the pressure patterns displayed as the catheter tip traverses the right atrium, right ventricle, and main pulmonary artery and eventually lodges in a pulmonary artery branch. With the balloon deflated, there must be free flow of pulmonary artery blood around the tip of the catheter. With the balloon properly inflated, the pressure reading just beyond the catheter tip will reflect the back pressure through the pulmonary circulation. These "wedged" pressure readings relate to the filling pressure of the left ventricle in a manner similar to the way central venous pressure readings relate to right ventricular filling pressures. With the balloon deflated, the pressure reading represents the phasic (systolic/diastolic) pulmonary artery pressures. Under these circumstances, a blood sample properly drawn through the fluid channel (see chap. 20) is obviously pulmonary artery blood.

Thermodilution Cardiac Output Measurements

A triple-channel pulmonary artery catheter contains a second fluid-filled channel that ends approximately 30 cm from the tip of the catheter. This opening is designed to lie in the right atrium or superior vena cava and is used as a central venous pressure monitor.

The four-channel pulmonary artery catheter (Fig 8–2) has a thermistor near the tip of the catheter and an electric circuit leading from the thermistor to a calculator. A known quantity of a cold solution of known temperature may be injected into the channel, whose outlet is in the area of the right atrium. The injected solution mixes with blood in the right ventricle and is ejected into the pulmonary artery over several ventricular contractions. The net effect of this mixing is to temporarily decrease the temperature of the blood passing through the pulmonary artery during this short interval of time. The temperature change is measured by the thermistor at the end of the catheter. Cardiac output is then calculated from knowing the amount of cold injected and the

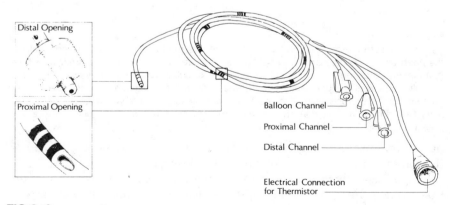

FIG 8–2.
The four-channel pulmonary artery catheter. The distal channel and balloon channel comprise the basic two-channel catheter. Addition of the proximal channel that opens in the right atrium results in the triple-channel catheter, usually 7 F in diameter. Addition of the thermistor channel results in the four-channel catheter used for thermodilution cardiac output measurements, usually 7 F in diameter.

average concentration of cold during the time required for total ejection of the cold solution from the right ventricle.

Central Venous Blood Gases

The superior and inferior vena cava represent a composite of several different organ systems. However, the coronary blood flow has an extremely high degree of oxygen extraction and is not represented by a blood sample taken from either vena cava because the coronary sinus empties directly into the right atrium. Blood taken from catheters with the tip placed in the right atrium shows tremendous variation from sample to sample because of channeling of the blood flow through the atrium from the various venous sources. Samples from a catheter tip in the right ventricle are also highly variable, and the catheter tip acts as a source of ventricular ectopic activity.

In healthy human subjects at rest, venous samples taken simultaneously from a catheter in the superior vena cava and pulmonary artery give reasonably close values. In critically ill patients, this close relationship does not exist.

Mixed Venous Blood Gases

A mixed venous oxygen tension may be measured only in the outflow tract of the right ventricle—the pulmonary artery. Several studies of pulmonary artery blood from healthy human volunteers have revealed a mixed venous oxygen tension of 40 mm Hg and an average arterial-venous oxygen content difference of approximately 5 vol%. These same subjects had normal systemic arterial blood gases, with their pulmonary artery blood revealing a carbon dioxide tension range of 44 to 46 mm Hg and a pH range of 7.34 to 7.36.

As shown in Table 8–1, these traditional values relating to normal healthy volunteers cannot be applied to critically ill patients. It has been repeatedly demonstrated that critically ill patients with adequate cardiovascular reserves increase their cardiac output above their normal resting value in response to their increased physiologic demands. The net effect is a decrease in the amount of oxygen extracted from each aliquot of blood (a decreased arterial-venous oxygen content difference). The critically ill patient who begins to decompensate will often have a "normal" cardiac output for a time before complete decompensation occurs. Simultaneously there is an increased arterial-venous oxygen extraction and a decreased mixed venous oxygen tension. These findings are often observed before significant changes in arterial oxygen tension occur.

TABLE 8–1.

Predicted Oxygenation Values in Health and Disease for Pulmonary Artery Blood

Condition	$P\bar{v}_{O_2}$		% Hb SAT.		$[Ca_{O_2} - C\bar{v}_{O_2}]$ (vol%)	
	Range	Average	Range	Average	Range	Average
Healthy resting human volunteer	37–43	40	70–76	75	4.5–6.0	5.0
Critically ill patient, cardiovascular reserves excellent	35–40	37	68–75	70	2.5–4.5	3.5
Critically ill patient, cardiovascular stable, limited cardiovascular reserves	30–35	32	56–68	60	4.5–6.0	5.0
Critically ill patient, cardiovascular decompensation	<30	<30	<56	<56	>6.0	>6.0

OXYGEN CONSUMPTION VS. OXYGEN EXTRACTION

Oxygen consumption ($\dot{V}_{O_2}$) is defined as the milliliters (ml) of oxygen consumed by the body in one minute. A 70-kg individual at basal metabolic rate will consume approximately 250 ml of oxygen per minute. The oxygen consumption is measured by analysis of the oxygen difference between the inhaled and exhaled gases over one minute.

Oxygen extraction is defined as the milliliters (ml) of oxygen extracted from 100 ml of systemic blood flow. This is expressed as ml/dl (milliliters per deciliter) or vol% (volume percent). Oxygen extraction is measured by analysis of the oxygen difference between the arterial and mixed venous blood. This measurement is referred to as the arterial to mixed venous oxygen content difference [$C_{(a-v)}O_2$] and is normally 5 vol% (4.5 to 6 vol%) at rest.

Theoretically the oxygen consumption (ml/min) could be calculated by multiplying oxygen extraction (ml/dl) times the cardiac output (Q_T) (L/min) times 10:

$$\dot{V}_{O_2} = C_{(a-v)}O_2 \times Q_T \times 10$$

This emphasizes the fact that oxygen extraction [$C_{(a-v)}O_2$] and oxygen consumption ($\dot{V}_{O_2}$) are not the same! As shown in Table 8–2, for any given oxygen consumption the $C_{(a-v)}O_2$ will vary inversely with the cardiac output. In other words, the $C_{(a-v)}O_2$ may be utilized to reflect the adequacy with which the cardiac output is responding to oxygen requirements.

CLINICAL USE OF THE $C_{(a-v)}O_2$

Reference values relating to pulmonary artery blood gas samples and the derived values have been listed (see Table 8–1). The clinical application of these values also requires a simultaneous measurement of an arterial blood gas. These values should be considered only as guidelines and they assume a normal oxygen-carrying capacity, clinical evidence of adequate peripheral perfusion, adequate alveolar ventilation, and normal acid-base status with the patient either breathing spontaneously or being supported on the ventilator.

When other factors such as severe anemia, lack of peripheral perfusion, severe hypercarbia, and acidemia are superimposed, these guidelines begin to lose their clinical usefulness. These physiologic measurements should be used as an early warning of impending or early cardiovascular decompensation. Their clinical value lies in the fact that changes in venous (pulmonary artery) blood gases often occur earlier than changes in routine arterial blood gases, thus allowing for the initiation of corrective therapeutic maneuvers to reverse the pathophysiology at an earlier stage.

In nonseptic critically ill patients with no excessive skeletal muscle activity (e.g., shivering, seizures, constant struggling against restraints) and with a stable temperature, it is often clinically reasonable to assume a constant oxygen consumption. Therefore, in these patients, changes in arterial-mixed venous oxygen content differences directly reflect changes in cardiac output.

$C_{(a-v)}O_2$ AND HYPOXEMIA

The oxygenation status of the mixed venous blood will have an effect on the arterial oxygenation because the lung always has some degree of intrapulmonary shunting (see chaps. 5 and 9). The greater the $C_{(a-v)}O_2$, the lesser will be the $C\bar{v}_{O_2}$. As illustrated in Table 8–3, a major way the body compensates for the hypoxemia resulting from intrapulmonary shunting is to increase cardiac output; thereby decreasing the $C_{(a-v)}O_2$; thereby increasing the $C\bar{v}_{O_2}$. The increased pulmonary arterial oxygen content means that the shunted blood has more oxygen and

TABLE 8–2.

Relationship of Cardiac Output to Oxygen Extraction

Condition	Oxygen Consumption (cc/min)	Cardiac Output ($\dot{Q}_T$) (L/min)	Oxygen Extraction $(Ca_{O_2} - C\bar{v}_{O_2})$ [vol% (cc/L)]	
Normal cardiac output	250	5	5	(50)
Increased cardiac output	250	10	2.5	(25)
Decreased cardiac output	250	2.5	10	(100)

thereby will have a lesser hypoxemic effect on the arterial blood (see chap. 9).

REFLECTING THE $C_{(a-v)}O_2$

Thus far we have discussed the factors that make the measurement of $C_{(a-v)}O_2$ clinically useful in determining the adequacy or inadequacy of the cardiovascular system's role in assuring tissue oxygenation. Many alternative methods have been suggested to gain similar information.

The Oxygen Extraction Ratio

The interpretation of a given $C_{(a-v)}O_2$ must include the level of hemoglobin content that is present. The oxygen extraction ratio [$C_{(a-v)}O_2$/ Ca_{O_2}] has been suggested as a means of reflecting the degree of oxygen extraction with the arterial content automatically considered. Since the tissues normally extract 25% of the arterial oxygen content, it would be reasonable to assume that an oxygen extraction ratio greater than 25% might reflect either an inadequate arterial oxygen content or an inadequate cardiac output to meet tissue oxygen demands.

TABLE 8–3.

Comparison Effect of Cardiac Output on the Arterial Oxygen Tension

$\dot{Q}s/\dot{Q}_T$ (%)	$\dot{V}_{O_2}$ (cc)	$\dot{Q}_T$ (L/min)	$(Ca_{O_2} - C\bar{v}_{O_2})$ (vol%)	Pa_{O_2} (mm Hg)
25	250	10	2.5	127
25	250	5	5.0	84
25	250	2.5	10.0	55

$P_{A_{O_2}}$ = 355 mm Hg, $F_{I_{O_2}}$ = 50%, Hb = 15 gm%, Cc_{O_2} = 21.17 vol%.

Oxygen Delivery

Oxygen delivery (O_2DEL) is:

$$Ca_{O_2} \times Q_T \times 10$$

representing the total milliliters of oxygen delivered to the tissues per minute. The normal O_2DEL is 1,000 ml, assuming Ca_{O_2} is 20 vol% and Q_T is 5 L. Once the arterial P_{O_2} is greater than 60 mm Hg ($Sa_{O_2} > 90\%$), the O_2DEL is almost entirely a function of cardiac output.

Mixed Venous Oxygen Tension or Saturation

Oxygen delivery minus oxygen extraction will determine the mixed venous oxygenation. The mixed venous oxygen tension ($P\bar{v}_{O_2}$) or saturation ($S\bar{v}_{O_2}$) can be used to reflect oxygen extraction since tissues should be able to extract oxygen until the hemoglobin saturation approaches 50%. In other words, assuming perfusion is adequate, it is reasonable to assume that tissue oxygen needs have been met when the $P\bar{v}_{O_2}$ is > 28 mm Hg or the $S\bar{v}_{O_2} > 60\%$, since more could have been extracted if required. On the other hand, $S\bar{v}_{O_2} < 60\%$ or $P\bar{v}_{O_2} < 28$ mm Hg suggests that the tissues may not have been able to extract all the oxygen required due to increased hemoglobin-oxygen affinity (see chap. 5).

SUMMARY

The most direct measurement of blood oxygen extraction is the arterial-mixed venous oxygen content difference. Appropriate interpretation of the $C_{(a-v)}O_2$ allows for cardiovascular components of oxygenation to be assessed in reference to oxygen demands. Special attention must be paid to the presence of anemia, and the concept of oxygen extraction ratio has been suggested as a means of automatically making this assumption. In our opinion, the $C_{(a-v)}O_2$ is the most direct and useful tool for assessing the cardiac/metabolic factors affecting arterial oxygenation.

The calculation of oxygen delivery may be utilized to assess the adequacy of cardiac function in meeting tissue oxygen demands as long as Sa_{O_2} is greater than 90% and the Hb content is adequate. $P\bar{v}_{O_2}$ or $S\bar{v}_{O_2}$ can be utilized to reflect the result of oxygen delivery minus oxygen extraction. The introduction of technology allowing continuous monitoring of $S\bar{v}_{O_2}$ has brought great attention to this approach (see chap. 16).

9

Applying the Physiologic Shunt

Most clinicians tend to assume that hypoxemia is directly attributable to intrapulmonary shunting. It can be unequivocally stated that when hypoxemia is present there must be some degree of intrapulmonary shunting; however, the effect of that shunt on arterial oxygen tension depends on cardiac function and metabolic rate. Calculation of the physiologic shunt (Qsp/QT) represents the best available means of delineating the extent to which the pulmonary system contributes to hypoxemia. For this reason it is essential to completely comprehend this calculation and its clinical application.

Prior to the widespread availability of pulmonary artery catheterization, intrapulmonary shunting was traditionally measured in the diagnostic or research laboratory while the patient was breathing 100% oxygen. This measurement of intrapulmonary shunting at an $F_{I_{O_2}}$ of 1.0 was noted as Qs/QT. As measurement of the intrapulmonary shunt became clinically popular, it was convenient to make the measurements at $F_{I_{O_2}}$ values less than 1.0. This so-called Physiologic Shunt was symbolized Qsp/QT to denote that the measurements were made at an $F_{I_{O_2}}$ below 1.0. The Qsp/QT (physiologic shunt) is often symbolized as Qva/QT (venous admixture). These both denote the measurements made at less than 100% inspired oxygen. This text shall consistently use Qsp/QT to denote the clinical measurement of intrapulmonary shunting with the patient breathing less than 100% oxygen.

THE CONCEPT OF INTRAPULMONARY SHUNTING

The *physiologic shunt (Q̇sp/Q̇T)* is defined as that portion of the cardiac

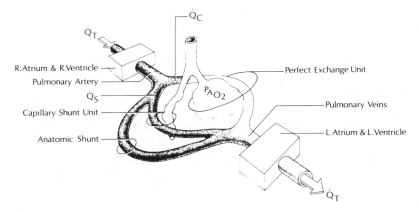

FIG 9–1.
Mathematical concept of physiologic shunting (see text). $\dot{Q}_T$ is cardiac output per unit time; $\dot{Q}_C$ is the portion of the cardiac output that exchanges perfectly with alveolar air; $\dot{Q}_S$ is the portion of the cardiac output that does not exchange with alveolar air; $P_{A_{O_2}}$ is the alveolar oxygen tension.

output entering the left side of the heart without perfectly respiring with perfect alveoli. In reference to oxygenation, a "perfect alveolus" would contain the oxygen tension predicted by the ideal alveolar gas equation (see Equation No. 10). This ideal alveolar P_{O_2} at sea level and room air is 101 mm Hg. If we assume perfect diffusion, then the end pulmonary capillary blood would have an oxygen tension equal to the alveolar tension. Thus, ideal end pulmonary capillary oxygen tension ($C\acute{c}_{O_2}$) can be calculated.

If all blood is perfectly exchanged with perfect alveoli, the arterial oxygen tension at room air would always be 101 mm Hg. Thus, in the absence of intrapulmonary shunting, there can be no hypoxemia.

In reference to oxygenation, intrapulmonary shunting can be due to blood going from the right to the left side of the heart without respiring with alveolar gas (*true shunt mechanisms*) or blood that respires but achieves a P_{O_2} less than the ideal (*shunt effect mechanisms*).

Figure 9–1 should be helpful in understanding the following mathematical derivation of the shunt equation.

THE FICK EQUATION

In 1870, Adolph Fick introduced the principle of dilution methods for measuring cardiac output, with the initial example involving oxygen transport by the blood. This concept has become known as the *Fick principle* and its initial application as the *Fick equation.*

The total quantity of oxygen potentially available for tissue utilization per unit time includes the arterial oxygen content (Ca_{O_2}) multiplied by the quantity of arterial blood presented to the tissues per unit time, the total cardiac output ($\dot{Q}T$):

$$\text{Oxygen available} = [\dot{Q}T][Ca_{O_2}] \tag{1}$$

The quantity of oxygen returned to the lungs is expressed as the product of total cardiac output ($\dot{Q}T$) and the mixed venous oxygen content ($C\bar{v}_{O_2}$):

$$\text{Oxygen returned} = [\dot{Q}T][C\bar{v}_{O_2}] \tag{2}$$

Oxygen consumption per unit time ($\dot{V}_{O_2}$) should reflect the oxygen that has been extracted from the blood in that time period—that is, the difference between the oxygen available [equation (1)] and the oxygen returned [equation (2)]:

$$\dot{V}_{O_2} = [\dot{Q}T][Ca_{O_2}] - [\dot{Q}T][C\bar{v}_{O_2}] \tag{3}$$

Equation (3) may be rewritten as:

$$\dot{V}_{O_2} = [\dot{Q}T][Ca_{O_2} - C\bar{v}_{O_2}] \tag{4}$$

Equation (4) is one way of writing the Fick equation; however, it is more commonly written as:

$$\dot{Q}T = \frac{\dot{V}_{O_2}}{[Ca_{O_2} - C\bar{v}_{O_2}](10)} \tag{5}$$

$\dot{Q}T$ cardiac output in liters per minute; $\dot{V}_{O_2}$ is oxygen consumption in milliliters per minute. $[Ca_{O_2}-C\bar{v}_{O_2}]$ is the oxygen content difference between the arterial and mixed venous blood in milliliters of oxygen per 100 ml of blood (vol% or ml/dl). To express the cardiac output in liters per minute, the oxygen content difference must be multiplied by a factor of 10.

The total cardiac output ($\dot{Q}T$) can be divided arbitrarily into two major components:

$$\dot{Q}T = \dot{Q}\acute{c} + \dot{Q}s \tag{6}$$

$\dot{Q}\acute{c}$ is the portion of the cardiac output that *exchanges perfectly* with alveolar air. $\dot{Q}s$ is the portion of the cardiac output that *does not exchange at all* with alveolar air.

$\dot{Q}\acute{c}$ mathematically represents all the blood to which oxygen is being added as it traverses through the lung. The blood leaving these perfectly exchanging alveolar–capillary units may theoretically be said to contain an end-pulmonary capillary oxygen content ($C\acute{c}_{O_2}$). This value is based in part on the assumption that complete equilibration between the idealized alveolar gas tension and end-pulmonary capillary gas tension exists. In those alveolar–capillary units with capillary transit times within normal ranges (0.3–0.7 sec) and alveolar oxygen tensions (PA_{O_2}) greater than 100 mm Hg, the assumption is clinically valid.[91] The "calculated" alveolar oxygen tension does not represent a real tension in any specific alveoli but represents an average value that is dependent on the physical laws of gas exchange and the respiratory exchange ratio.*

The mixed venous oxygen content represents the averaged oxygen content being returned to the lungs, and its value can be measured only in pulmonary artery blood. The oxygen content of shunted blood ($\dot{Q}s$) reaching the systemic arterial circulation is unchanged from its value in the pulmonary artery. The exchanging portion of the cardiac output ($\dot{Q}\acute{c}$) represents the only blood to which oxygen is added. Its oxygen content is referred to as *end-pulmonary capillary oxygen content* ($C\acute{c}_{O_2}$). Therefore, the organism's oxygen consumption also may be derived from an expression written as equation (7) instead of equation (4). Because equations (4) and (7) both equal the oxygen consumption value ($\dot{V}O_2$), they are equal to each other:

$$\dot{V}O_2 = \dot{Q}\acute{c}[C\acute{c}_{O_2} - C\bar{v}_{O_2}] \tag{7}$$

$$\dot{Q}T[Ca_{O_2} - C\bar{v}_{O_2}] = \dot{Q}\acute{c}[C\acute{c}_{O_2} - C\bar{v}_{O_2}] \tag{8}$$

*The validity of these assumptions depends to a large extent on the presence of steady-state conditions while the assessment is being undertaken.

Pulmonary Capillary Oxygen Content

As stated earlier, the pulmonary capillary oxygen content is in reality a theoretical entity; its mathematical calculation is based on theoretical concepts. The calculation of the pulmonary capillary oxygen content depends in part on the calculation of an idealized alveolar oxygen tension. This value represents a hypothetical average alveolar oxygen tension and does not represent the actual alveolar oxygen tension of any particular alveolus. Because alveolar oxygen tensions vary throughout the lung, it is convenient to deal mathematically with the concept of an *ideal alveolar oxygen tension.*

The calculation of an ideal alveolar oxygen tension is obtained from the ideal alveolar gas equation. This equation corrects for changes in oxygen tension owing to the fact that the respiratory exchange ratio is less than 1.0 (approximately 0.8). This means that less carbon dioxide is transferred into the alveoli than the amount of oxygen removed from the alveoli. The arterial carbon dioxide tension can be used to replace the alveolar carbon dioxide tension, since it is a very close approximation. A useful approximation of the exact ideal alveolar gas equation is:

$$P_{A_{O_2}} = [P_B - P_{H_2O}]F_{I_{O_2}} - P_{a_{CO_2}}(1.25) \qquad (9)$$

Under clinical circumstances in which the arterial carbon dioxide tension is less than 60 mm Hg, and especially when oxygen therapy is administered, it is acceptable to use an even more simplified version of the alveolar gas equation:

$$P_{A_{O_2}} = [P_B - P_{H_2O}]F_{I_{O_2}} - P_{a_{CO_2}} \qquad (10)$$

THE CLASSIC PHYSIOLOGIC SHUNT EQUATION

The physiologic shunt equation expresses the relationship between the $\dot{Q}_T$ and the shunted cardiac output. Therefore, equation (6) is solved in terms of $\dot{Q}_C$:

$$\dot{Q}_C' = [\dot{Q}_T - \dot{Q}_S] \qquad (11)$$

Substituting equation (11) for $\dot{Q}_C'$ in equation (8) results in the following equation:

$$\dot{Q}_T[C_{a_{O_2}} - C\bar{v}_{O_2}] = [\dot{Q}_T - \dot{Q}_S][C_{c_{O_2}}' - C\bar{v}_{O_2}] \qquad (12)$$

Expanding equation (12) algebraically:

$$\dot{Q}TCa_{O_2} - \dot{Q}TC\bar{v}_{O_2} = \dot{Q}TCc'_{O_2} - \dot{Q}TC\bar{v}_{O_2} - \dot{Q}sCc'_{O_2} + \dot{Q}sC\bar{v}_{O_2} \quad (13)$$

Note that two of the six terms ($\dot{Q}TC\bar{v}_{O_2}$) are identical and common to both sides of the equation and therefore can be removed from the equation.

The collection and factoring of all $\dot{Q}s$ terms on the left side and all $\dot{Q}T$ terms on the right side of the equation result in:

$$\dot{Q}s[Cc'_{O_2} - C\bar{v}_{O_2}] = \dot{Q}T[Cc'_{O_2} - Ca_{O_2}] \quad (14)$$

This relationship can now be written as a ratio of *shunted* cardiac output to *total* cardiac output:

$$\frac{\dot{Q}s}{\dot{Q}T} = \frac{[Cc'_{O_2} - Ca_{O_2}]}{[Cc'_{O_2} - C\bar{v}_{O_2}]} \quad (15)$$

$\dot{Q}s$ may be considered equivalent to true shunting (anatomic plus capillary). Where shunt effect exists, that blood component will be incompletely oxygenated; therefore, that portion of the cardiac output is divided into two subcomponents: $\dot{Q}c'$ and $\dot{Q}s$. In other words, shunt effect is divided mathematically as though a portion of that blood exchanged perfectly and the remainder did not exchange at all. The shunt calculation usually contains some element of shunt effect. *The term $\dot{Q}sp$ denotes the physiologic shunt, that is, the sum of the true shunt and shunt effect.* Therefore, equation (15) is most commonly expressed as:

$$\frac{\dot{Q}sp}{\dot{Q}T} = \frac{[Cc'_{O_2} - Ca_{O_2}]}{[Cc'_{O_2} - C\bar{v}_{O_2}]} \quad (16)$$

Equation (16) is the *classic physiologic shunt equation*.[92] It has the advantage of being derived as a ratio so that no absolute measure of cardiac output is required. In this form, the equation very clearly demonstrates that as the shunted cardiac output ($\dot{Q}sp$) approaches zero, the arterial oxygen content must approach the theoretical end-pulmonary capillary oxygen content. As long as a portion of the cardiac output exists as shunted blood, the arterial oxygen content always will be less than the theoretical end-pulmonary capillary oxygen content. In other words, because shunted blood has the same oxygen content as mixed venous blood ($C\bar{v}_{O_2}$), when this blood mixes with blood from perfectly exchanging cardiac output ($\dot{Q}\dot{c}$), a lowered oxygen content equilibrium must be established. The end result is always an arterial oxygen content somewhere between the end-pulmonary capillary oxygen content and the mixed venous oxygen content.

The Clinical Shunt Equation

The classic physiologic shunt equation [equation (16)] may be mathematically manipulated by adding and subtracting an arterial oxygen content to the denominator of the term on the right. The new form of the equation can then be written:

$$\frac{\dot{Q}sp}{\dot{Q}T} = \frac{[Cc'_{O_2} - Ca_{O_2}]}{[Ca_{O_2} - C\bar{v}_{O_2}] + [Cc'_{O_2} - Ca_{O_2}]} \tag{17}$$

This represents the most useful clinical form of the physiologic shunt equation because it expresses in a clearer manner the concepts and measurements applied to the clinical setting. The appearance of an arterial-mixed venous content difference in the denominator makes it quite apparent that cardiac output plays an important role in altering the result of shunted cardiac output (namely, arterial hypoxemia).

CONCEPTUALIZING THE SHUNT EQUATION

The implications of the physiologic shunt equation [equation (16)] may be conceptualized by considering the oxygen content terms (Cc'_{O_2}, Ca_{O_2}, $C\bar{v}_{O_2}$) as entities that can be extracted from the blood and poured into a container. Figure 9–2 represents such a container with the oxygen content levels of blood from three sites: (1) level C is from the end pulmonary capillaries (Cc'_{O_2}), which have the highest oxygen content in the body; (2) level V is from the pulmonary artery and represents the mixed venous content ($C\bar{v}_{O_2}$);* and (3) level A is from the systemic arterial system (Ca_{O_2}).

Certain factors such as hemoglobin concentration can affect all three levels, whereas other factors primarily affect individual sites. The most

---

*Although coronary sinus blood is normally the most desaturated blood in the body, pulmonary artery (mixed venous) blood is appropriately used to reflect the lowest oxygen content in terms of total body homeostasis.

important clinical variable affecting level C ($C\acute{c}_{O_2}$) is $F_{I_{O_2}}$, whereas both total cardiac output ($\dot{Q}T$) and oxygen consumption ($\dot{V}O_2$) affect level V ($C\bar{v}_{O_2}$). Changes in the physiologic shunt ($\dot{Q}sp$) specifically affect level A (Ca_{O_2}).

As illustrated in Figure 9–3, the numerator of the shunt equation is represented by the difference between levels C and A—specified as Diff N. The denominator of the equation is represented by the difference between levels C and V—specified as Diff D. Therefore, the shunt equation is represented visually by the ratio Diff N/Diff D. Changes of unequal magnitude among these three levels will change the Diff N/Diff D ratio, which is equivalent to changes in the physiologic shunt calculation.

Figure 9–4 lists the important values and graphically represents the oxygen content "levels" in a healthy person with a hemoglobin concentration of 15 gm%. Presume this individual develops fulminant right middle and lower lobe consolidated pneumonitis. If arterial and pulmonary artery blood gas measurements were obtained, they could very likely reveal the circumstances represented in Figure 9–5,I. The arterial oxygen tension and content have significantly decreased due to the large intrapulmonary shunt. In this example, the cardiac function has not appropriately responded (cardiac output has not increased), meaning that the arterial-venous oxygen content difference ($C_{(a-\bar{v})}O_2$) has not

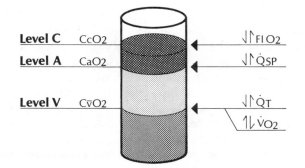

FIG 9–2.
Schematic representation of blood oxygen levels that could theoretically be obtained from three separate sites in the cardiovascular system: *Level C* represents the end pulmonary capillary blood oxygen content ($C\acute{c}_{O_2}$), *Level A* represents the systemic arterial blood oxygen content (Ca_{O_2}), and *Level V* represents the mixed venous (pulmonary artery) blood oxygen content ($C\bar{v}_{O_2}$). The most common clinical variables that specifically affect these various levels is shown: *Level C* is most commonly affected by changes in $F_{I_{O_2}}$ (inspired oxygen fraction), *Level A* is specifically affected by changes in the physiological shunt ($\dot{Q}sp$), *Level V* is specifically affected by both the total cardiac output ($\dot{Q}T$) and the rate of oxygen consumption ($\dot{V}_{O_2}$).

$$\frac{\dot{Q}_{SP}}{\dot{Q}_T} = \frac{C_cO_2 - C_aO_2}{C_cO_2 - C\bar{v}O_2} = \frac{\text{DIFF N}}{\text{DIFF D}}$$

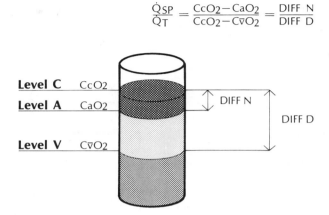

FIG 9–3.
Oxygen content levels as they relate to the physiologic shunt equation. $\dot{Q}sp$ = physiologic shunt, $\dot{Q}_T$ = total cardiac output, $C\acute{c}_{O_2}$ = ideal end pulmonary capillary oxygen content, Ca_{O_2} = systemic arterial oxygen content, $C\bar{v}_{O_2}$ = pulmonary arterial oxygen content. Levels *C, A,* and *V* are explained in legend for Figure 9–2. The numerator of the physiologic shunt equation [Eq. (6); see text] is represented as *Diff N* (difference in the numerator); the denominator of the shunt equation is represented as *Diff D* (difference in the denominator). Changes of *unequal magnitude* between *Diff N* and *Diff D* will result in variations in the calculated physiologic shunt.

changed. A decreased level A with an unchanged AV content difference dictates that level V must decrease. Because of the greater increase in Diff N compared with the increase in Diff D, the physiologic shunt has greatly increased and is the primary cause of the hypoxemia (the decreased arterial oxygen content and tension).

Under normal conditions, the severe hypoxemia would lead to an increased cardiac output. This would result in a decrease in the arterial-venous oxygen, i.e., an increased level V (see Fig 9–5,I). A new steady state would result in an increase in level A without a significant change in the Diff N/Diff D ratio. In other words, the arterial PO_2 improves greatly without a significant change in the physiologic shunt. The improved arterial PO_2 is secondary to cardiovascular compensation. The underlying pulmonary disease has not changed.

The previous illustration assumes that supplemental oxygen (FI_{O_2} 0.5) is administered while the cardiac output remains unchanged (see Fig 9–5,II). Level C is increased secondary to the increased alveolar PO_2. Since the physiologic shunt remains the same and the arterial-venous oxygen remains the same, a new steady state results in levels A and V also increasing. In other words, the oxygen therapy has improved the arterial PO_2 while the physiologic shunt (note that the Diff N/Diff D ratio is unchanged) and the $C_{(a-\bar{v})}O_2$ remain essentially unchanged.

A more realistic circumstance is depicted in the changes shown in section III (see Fig 9–5). The patient has been given oxygen therapy *and* his cardiac output has increased. Note that in the new steady state, level A has increased because both levels C and V were increased. Thus, the hypoxemia is dramatically improved while the ratio Diff N/Diff D has not significantly changed. *The arterial PO_2 has improved while the physiologic shunt has remained essentially unchanged!*

Suppose this patient, with acute pneumonia, increased cardiac output, and increased FI_{O_2} (Fig 9–6,C), sustains an acute myocardial injury and the cardiac output decreases significantly below the normal resting value. The increase in the $C_{(a-\bar{v})}O_2$ would lead to a new steady state in which both levels A and V are decreased while the Diff N/Diff D ratio is not significantly changed (see Fig 9–6,D). *The decrease in arterial PO_2 has occurred without a significant change in the physiologic shunt!* Note that the blood gases give two essential pieces of information: the physiologic shunt is unchanged and the $C_{(a-\bar{v})}O_2$ is increased.

NORMAL

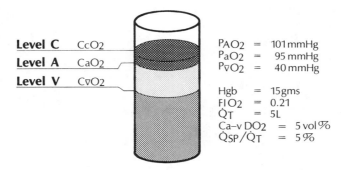

Level C	$CcO2$		$PAO2$	=	$101\,mmHg$
Level A	$CaO2$		$PaO2$	=	$95\,mmHg$
Level V	$CvO2$		$P\bar{v}O2$	=	$40\,mmHg$
			Hgb	=	$15\,gms$
			$FIO2$	=	0.21
			$\dot{Q}_T$	=	$5L$
			$Ca{-}v\,DO2$	=	$5\,vol\%$
			$\dot{Q}_{SP}/\dot{Q}_T$	=	5%

FIG 9–4.
Schematic representation of the blood oxygen content levels in a normal individual. Representative normal values are listed for the major factors commonly affected in pathologic states. *Level C:* end pulmonary capillary blood oxygen content level ($C\acute{c}_{O_2}$). *Level A:* systemic arterial blood oxygen content level (Ca_{O_2}). *Level V:* pulmonary arterial blood oxygen content level ($C\bar{v}_{O_2}$); PA_{O_2}, alveolar oxygen tension; Pa_{O_2}, systemic arterial oxygen tension; $P\bar{v}_{O_2}$, pulmonary arterial oxygen tension; Hgb, hemoglobin content; FI_{O_2}, inspired oxygen fraction; $\dot{Q}_T$, total cardiac output; $Ca{-}\bar{v}D_{O_2}$, arterial venous oxygen content difference [$C_{(a-\bar{v})}O_2$]; $\dot{Q}sp/\dot{Q}_T$, calculated physiologic shunt.

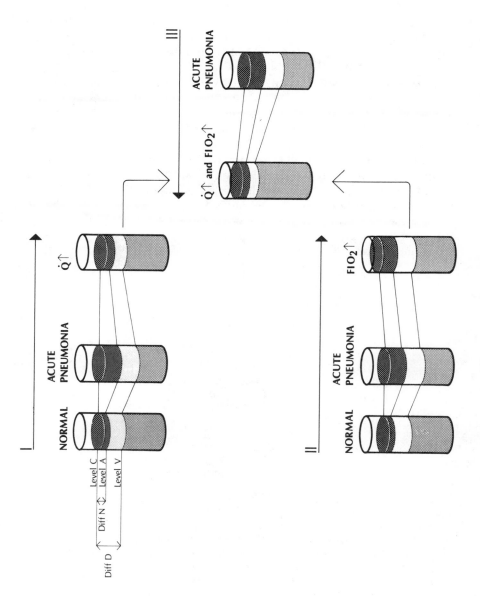

FIG 9–5.
Schematic representation of changes in blood oxygen levels under various conditions. The purpose of this illustration is to conceptualize the difference between physiologic shunting and the hypoxemic effect of physiologic shunting. *I*, *II*, and *III* illustrate changes in a normal individual who contracts pneumonitis that causes a significant increase in intrapulmonary shunting without any compensatory physiologic change. The status from normal to *acute pneumonia* shows: no change in *Level C* because ventilation and F_{IO_2} are unchanged, a significant drop in *Level A* due to increased shunting created by the pneumonia, and a drop in *Level V* because the AV content difference is unchanged (cardiac output and oxygen consumption unchanged). Since *Diff N* has increased to a greater degree than *Diff D*, the calculated shunt increases (see Fig 9–3 and text). *Condition I* shows an increased cardiac output ($\dot{Q}$ ↑) in response to the acute hypoxemia. *Level C* remains unchanged since neither ventilation nor F_{IO_2} has been altered. The AV content difference has narrowed because the cardiac output has increased, while oxygen consumption remains unchanged. The increase in *Level V* results in a new dynamic equilibrium in which *Level A* is also increased. Note that the relationship between *Diff N* and *Diff D* is only slightly altered. Thus, *Level A* (and therefore the Pa_{O_2} ↑) has increased with little change in the calculated shunt. In this instance the compensation for hypoxemia is cardiovascular; the intrapulmonary shunt has not changed. *Condition II* shows an increased inspired oxygen concentration (F_{IO_2} ↑). *Level C* increases, while AV content difference remains unchanged (cardiac output and oxygen consumption unchanged). A new dynamic equilibrium results in *Level A* (and therefore the Pa_{O_2} increasing). The relationship between *Diff N* and *Diff D* is only slightly altered. *Level A* (and therefore Pa_{O_2}) has increased with little change in the calculated shunt. In this instance, compensation for hypoxemia is via oxygen therapy; the intrapulmonary shunt is essentially unchanged. *Condition III* shows both cardiac output and inspired oxygen concentration changes ($\dot{Q}$ ↑ and F_{IO_2} ↑). Note the profound increase in *Level A* (and therefore Pa_{O_2} ↑) with little alteration in the *Diff N/ Diff D*.

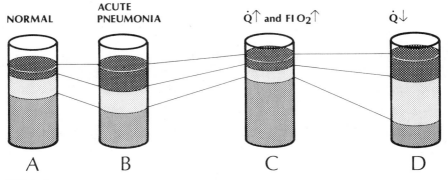

FIG 9–6.

A, B, and C represent changes described in Figure 9–5 *(Condition III)*, where both increased cardiac output and oxygen therapy have significantly raised the Pa_{O_2} in a patient with acute pneumonia. A sudden drop in cardiac output ($\dot{Q} \downarrow$) results in an increased AV content difference (decreased cardiac output with unchanged oxygen consumption). $C\dot{c}_{O_2}$ remains unchanged since the ventilation and FI_{O_2} are the same. The new dynamic equilibrium results in a significant drop in Ca_{O_2} (and therefore Pa_{O_2}). The *Diff N/Diff D* is essentially unchanged. In other words, the significant drop in Pa_{O_2} results primarily from an acute decrease in cardiac function and *not* from an increase in physiologic shunt.

The physiologic shunt calculation can reliably reflect the degree of gas exchange abnormality attributable to intrapulmonary disease (as well as right to left intracardiac shunt) regardless of the numerous other factors that may also play a role. Since multiple causes of hypoxemia are frequently encountered in critically ill patients, the ability to quantitate the degree of intrapulmonary pathophysiology is an extremely important clinical tool.

ACCOMPLISHING THE SHUNT CALCULATION

FI_{O_2}

Although alveolar oxygen tensions approach the ideal calculation in the normal state, most disease states tend to accentuate the FI_{O_2} to PA_{O_2} disparity. In an attempt to minimize this factor when calculating the physiologic shunt, it became traditional to obtain the blood sample with the patient breathing 100% oxygen. However, it has been repeatedly demonstrated that lung areas with low V/Q values tend to collapse with high concentrations of oxygen (see the section on denitrogenation absorption atelectasis in chap. 7). Nonetheless, the impression has persisted that shunt calculations are meaningful only when done at 100% oxygen. Overwhelming experimental and clinical evidence reveals that

clinically reliable shunt calculations accurately quantitating pulmonary pathol-
ogy can be accomplished at any consistent $F_{I_{O_2}}$. If a reference $F_{I_{O_2}}$ is desired,
we recommend 0.5; however, the shunt calculation at maintenance
$F_{I_{O_2}}$ provides clinically reliable information while being convenient and
practical.

Obtaining the Samples

The patient is placed supine between 0 and 45 degrees in a head-
up position. Tracheal suctioning and other nursing needs are addressed
so that the patient will not be disturbed for 5 minutes. The desired
$F_{I_{O_2}}$ is checked by an oxygen analyzer.

After 5 minutes, the arterial and pulmonary arterial samples are
obtained and immediately placed on ice and taken to the blood gas
laboratory. The blood gas machines are calibrated prior to the delivery
of the sample. The vital signs are recorded, hemodynamics measured,
$F_{I_{O_2}}$ analyzed, and tidal volumes measured.

Calculations

Analysis of both arterial and pulmonary arterial samples is accomplished for pH, P_{CO_2}, P_{O_2}, Hb, and HbO_2. It is recommended that carboxyhemoglobin (HbCO) and methemoglobin also be measured. The
Ca_{O_2} and $C\bar{v}_{O_2}$ are calculated. If HbCO is not directly measured, an
assumed HbCO value of 1.5% is recommended.[93]

The Cc'_{O_2} is calculated by first deriving the ideal alveolar oxygen
tension. Pulmonary capillary hemoglobin is assumed to be the same as
arterial hemoglobin. If the $P_{A_{O_2}}$ is greater than 150 mm Hg ($F_{I_{O_2}}$ greater
than 30% at sea level), all available hemoglobin is assumed to be completely saturated.* The $P_{C_{O_2}}$ is assumed equal to $P_{A_{O_2}}$. Therefore, the
end pulmonary capillary P_{O_2}, HbO_2, and Hb are derived and the Cc'_{O_2}
is calculated.

*The following correction factors are recommended for $P_{A_{O_2}}$ below 150 mm Hg:

1. If $P_{A_{O_2}} > 150$ mm Hg, $Cc'_{O_2} = Hb(1.0 - HbCO)(1.34) + 0.0031(P_{A_{O_2}})$.

2. If $P_{A_{O_2}} > 125$ and < 150 mm Hg, $Cc'_{O_2} = Hb[(1.0 - HbCO) - 0.01](1.34 + 0.0031(P_{A_{O_2}})$.

3. If $P_{A_{O_2}} > 100$ and < 125 mm Hg, $Cc'_{O_2} = Hb[(1.0 - HbCO) - 0.02](1.34) + 0.0031(P_{A_{O_2}})$.

With values now calculated for Ca_{O_2}, $C\bar{v}_{O_2}$, and Cc'_{O_2}, equation (16) can be solved.

GUIDELINES FOR INTERPRETATION OF SHUNT VALUES

1. A calculated shunt less than 10% is clinically compatible with normal lungs.

2. A calculated shunt of 10% to 19% denotes an intrapulmonary abnormality that is seldom of clinical significance in terms of maintaining respiratory homeostasis.

3. A calculated shunt of 20% to 29% reflects significant intrapulmonary disease. In a patient with limited cardiovascular or central nervous system function, this degree of shunt may be life-threatening.

4. A calculated shunt greater than 30% is potentially life-threatening and usually requires aggressive cardiopulmonary supportive therapy. Patients with shunt calculations in excess of 60% have survived.

5. Due to shunt effect mechanisms, the shunt calculation usually decreases as the $F_{I_{O_2}}$ is increased from 21% to 50%.[70, 72] Therefore, changes in $F_{I_{O_2}}$ should be considered when serial shunt calculations are interpreted.

6. Changes in cardiac output alone may affect the intrapulmonary shunt calculation. Although the factors that cause this phenomenon are not clear, the observation is undeniable. As cardiac output increases, the Qsp may increase, and vice versa. In our experience, cardiac output changes alone seldom account for more than a 5% variation in Qsp. However, changes in cardiac output often effect $P\bar{v}O_2$ which may dramatically alter hypoxic pulmonary vasoconstriction (see chap. 7). In diseased lungs a change in $P\bar{v}O_2$ can create large changes in Qsp.

ALTERNATIVES TO MEASURING THE SHUNT

The arterial oxygen tension measurement quantitates hypoxemia. Since several factors contribute to hypoxemia, it is clinically desirable to differentiate and quantitate cardiovascular from pulmonary factors. In the absence of right-to-left intracardiac shunting, the shunt calculation provides a quantification of the *intrapulmonary component* of hypoxemia. However, most patients do not have (or require) a pulmonary artery catheter. Thus, there is a realistic need for alternative methods that *reflect* changes in the physiologic shunt without benefit of pulmonary artery blood gases.

Such alternatives to the shunt calculation are not shortcuts or simpler techniques; there is no shortcut to comprehending the complexity of pulmonary physiology! For proper clinical interpretation, these alternatives usually require a more thorough understanding of physiologic shunting than when the shunt is actually calculated. It is imperative to understand the limitations of these alternative methods so they are not *misused* to the patient's detriment.

Equation (17) indicates that $\dot{Q}sp$ can be calculated without pulmonary artery blood analysis if the arterial-venous oxygen content difference $[C_{(a-\bar{v})}O_2]$ is known. As discussed in chapter 8, a patient with an adequately functioning and stable cardiovascular system as well as a stable metabolic rate will have a *consistent* $C_{(a-\bar{v})}O_2$. Therefore, *alternative methods for calculating the physiologic shunt can only be applied to patients with good cardiovascular function and stable metabolic rate.* Since most acutely hypoxemic patients with poor cardiovascular function are candidates for pulmonary artery catheter monitoring, this first limitation is compatible with good clinical care and judgment.

The Estimated Shunt Equation

In our opinion, the best alternative method for reflecting changes in the physiologic shunt is the *estimated shunt equation:*

$$\frac{\dot{Q}sp}{\dot{Q}_T} = \frac{Cc'_{O_2} - Ca_{O_2}}{3.5 + Cc'_{O_2} - Ca_{O_2}} \tag{18}$$

The $[C_{(a-\bar{v})}O_2]$ is assumed to be 3.5 vol%, since the clinical circumstances in which the application of this form of the equation is reasonable assume an adequate cardiovascular reserve. It has been noted that in resting, healthy human volunteers, the normal $C_{(a-\bar{v})}O_2$ ranges between 4.5 and 6.0 vol%.[94] However, it has been documented that most critically ill patients who are maintaining cardiovascular stability have $C_{(a-\bar{v})}O_2$ values below normal—i.e., ranging between 2.5 and 4.5 vol%.[95] On this basis, an assumed value of 3.5 vol% is more representative in the critically ill patient with adequate cardiovascular reserves. The estimated shunt equation is applicable to most hypoxemic patients with cardiovascular stability.

Alveolar to Arterial Oxygen Tension Gradient $[P_{(A-a)}O_2]$

When arterial oxygen tension is greater than 150 mm Hg, the arterial hemoglobin may be considered fully saturated with oxygen. In this situation, it is logical to assume that the hemoglobin in the portion of the cardiac output exchanging perfectly ($\dot{Q}c$) is also 100% saturated since it must always have as high or higher an oxygen content than arterial blood. Under these *limited* clinical conditions, the oxygen content difference in the numerator of the shunt equation (16) is based on the difference between oxygen tensions in the ideal end pulmonary capillary blood ($P\dot{c}O_2$) and in arterial blood (Pa_{O_2}). Since the ideal PA_{O_2} must equal $P\dot{c}O_2$, this difference in oxygen dissolved in the blood is clinically referred to as the *alveolar to arterial oxygen tension gradient*.

The alveolar to arterial oxygen tension gradient [$P_{(A-a)}O_2$] was the first index suggested for quantifying disruption of pulmonary oxygen transfer without requiring mixed venous blood sampling.[96] Although the $P_{(A-a)}O_2$ is a useful index in stable patients breathing room air, its appropriateness in acutely ill or anesthetized patients is questionable since the value varies independently with changes in FI_{O_2}, Sa_{O_2} and $S\bar{v}_{O_2}$.[97-100]

In clinical circumstances in which the cardiovascular reserve and the arterial-venous oxygen content difference may be reasonably assumed to be adequate, and the arterial oxygen tension is greater than 150 mm Hg, the $P_{(A-a)}O_2$ may be used clinically to reflect intrapulmonary shunting.

A major limitation to the clinical application of this gas exchange index is that we maintain and monitor patients who have a Pa_{O_2} much less than 150 mm Hg and in whom we vary FI_{O_2}. With an arterial PO_2 below 100 mm Hg, changes in the oxygen content increasingly become a function of changes in the hemoglobin saturation rather than in the dissolved oxygen.

To illustrate this point, we made shunt calculations at both 30% and 50% oxygen in hypoxemic patients who were cardiovascularly stable but had pulmonary artery catheters in place. Figure 9–7 compares the change in shunt calculation with change in FI_{O_2} with the change in the A-a gradient (see Fig 9–7,A) and the change in $C\dot{c}_{O_2} - Ca_{O_2}$ (see Fig 9–7,B). Note that the numerator of equation (17) ($C\dot{c}_{O_2} - Ca_{O_2}$) had a *positive* correlation with changes in the shunt, whereas the $P_{(A-a)}O_2$ had a *negative* correlation. The $C_{(a-\bar{v})}O_2$ of this group did not significantly change, while both the $\dot{Q}sp/\dot{Q}T$ and the $P_{(A-a)}O_2$ changes were statistically significant.

It is reasonable to conclude that in acutely ill patients, the $P_{(A-a)}O_2$ is a reliable reflection of changes in the physiologic shunt only when: (1) there is cardiovascular stability, (2) the FI_{O_2} is constant, and (3) the PO_2 is greater than 100 mm Hg. The latter two factors are *not* requisites for applying the estimated shunt equation.

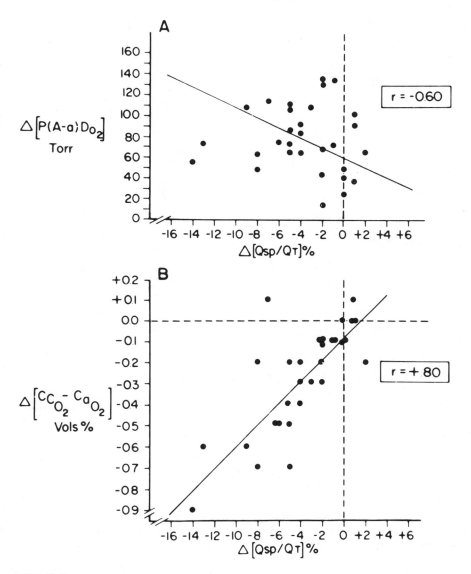

FIG 9–7.
Δ [Qsp/QT]% = difference in calculated shunt from FI_{O_2} 0.3 to 0.5; Δ [P(A − a)D_{O_2}] = difference in alveolar to arterial oxygen tension from FI_{O_2} 0.3 to 0.5; Δ [Co_{O_2} − Ca_{O_2}] = difference in end-pulmonary capillary minus arterial oxygen content from FI_{O_2} 0.3 to 0.5; *r* = correlation coefficient. **A,** the A − a gradient uniformly increases as the calculated physiologic shunt is decreased or unchanged. **B,** the end-pulmonary capillary-arterial oxygen content difference generally decreases as the calculated shunt decreases.

TABLE 9–1.

Comparison of Gas Exchange Indices (R)

Parameter	(Mean ± SD)	Range Min − Max	R Value
Qsp/QT	22.3 (11.2)	3.0–53.0	
Est Shunt	27.6 (11.3)	2.7–62.3	+0.94
RI	3.1 (2.6)	0.3–14.0	+0.74
Pa_{O_2}/PA_{O_2}	0.3 (0.2)	0.06–0.77	−0.72
Pa_{O_2}/FI_{O_2}	1.8 (0.9)	0.1–4.3	−0.71
$P_{(A-a)}O_2$	222.8 (141.7)	32–611	+0.62

Gas Exchange Indices

Many studies have been recently published assessing the reliability of newer oxygen-tension–based indices in reflecting Qsp/QT,[97–99, 101–107] including the alveolar to arterial oxygen tension gradient $[P_{(A-a)}O_2]$, the arterial to alveolar oxygen tension ratio (Pa_{O_2}/PA_{O_2}), the arterial oxygen tension to inspired oxygen concentration ratio (Pa_{O_2}/FI_{O_2}), and the Respiratory Index (RI) $[P_{(A-a)}O_2/Pa_{O_2}]$. We assessed the reliability of these four indices and the Estimated Shunt (Est Shunt) to reflect Qsp/QT in a heterogeneous group of critically ill patients.[108] The results are listed in Table 9–1.

In contrast to the $P_{(A-a)}O_2$, the arterial to alveolar oxygen tension ratio (Pa_{O_2}/PA_{O_2}) is relatively unaffected by changes in FI_{O_2}.[102, 104, 109, 110] This index has been shown to be more reliable at FI_{O_2} values below 0.55[109] or when Pa_{O_2} is less than 100 mm Hg with the patient on an FI_{O_2} greater than 0.3.[14] Gas exchange abnormalities secondary to true intrapulmonary shunting (V/Q = 0) are more accurately quantified by the Pa_{O_2}/PA_{O_2} than are those associated with low V/Q (<1 but >0).[98, 109, 110] Our data[108] show this index to be unreliable as an indicator of Qsp/QT.

To avoid the calculation of the alveolar P_{O_2}, the arterial oxygen tension to inspired oxygen fraction ratio (Pa_{O_2}/FI_{O_2}) was introduced.[111, 112] This index is affected by changes in Pa_{CO_2}[101] and has accumulated conflicting data on the accuracy with which it reflects Qsp/QT. Values for Pa_{O_2}/FI_{O_2} of less than 2 have been reported to correlate well with Qsp/QT values of > 20%.[113, 114] However, unacceptable correlations have been reported in burn patients, critically ill children, and adults with respiratory tract disease.[104, 115–117] Our data show this index comparable to the Pa_{O_2}/PA_{O_2} in terms of reflecting the Qsp/QT.

The Respiratory Index (RI) was introduced to minimize the inherent problems of the $P_{(A-a)}O_2$. Our data confirm that the RI is a distinct improvement upon the $P_{(A-a)}O_2$, but it falls short of being a reliable reflection of the Qsp/QT (R = 0.74).

SUMMARY

Qsp/QT is calculated using oxygen contents derived from measured values for P_{O_2}, hemoglobin concentration (Hb), and oxyhemoglobin saturation (S_{O_2}). The nonlinear nature of the oxyhemoglobin dissociation curve dictates that changes in oxygen tension must poorly correlate with changes in oxygen content. The Estimated Shunt was introduced to circumvent these inherent problems of indices based on oxygen tension by utilizing oxygen contents. An $C_{(a-\bar{v})}O_2$ of 3.5 vol% was placed in the denominator since this was found to be the mean value in patients in the intensive care unit with clinically adequate cardiac function. The most frequently voiced objection to the Est Shunt is that the calculation is not easily accomplished "in one's head" as are most of the oxygen-tension–based indices. It should be noted that no study has been published showing the Est Shunt to be an unreliable reflector of Qsp/QT. Our data demonstrate that the Est Shunt provides an excellent reflection of the Qsp/QT (R = 0.94) over a wide range of shunt values, inspired oxygen concentrations, and patient pathology. When contrasted with the correlation coefficients of the other four indices (see Table 9–1), the Est Shunt clearly stands out as superior.

We do not suggest that the Est Shunt is an adequate substitute for measurement of the Qsp/QT when the absolute value is of importance or when pulmonary artery blood samples are available. However, the excellent correlation between Qsp/QT and Est Shunt (R = 0.94) suggests that this variance will be consistent over a wide range and is far superior to oxygen-tension indices.

10

Assessment of Physiologic Deadspace

A primary advantage of blood gas measurement is the ability to differentiate and quantify degrees of cardiopulmonary pathology. Table 10–1 outlines the division of cardiopulmonary disease into shunt-producing and deadspace-producing components. "State of the art" technology allows the physiologic shunt to be clinically measured or reliably reflected in most patients (see chap. 9). Unfortunately, assessments of the physiologic deadspace are far less reliable and often impractical. At present, blood gas measurement does *not* routinely give reliable and quantitative reflections of deadspace-producing disease. Moreover, the indirect and imprecise methods available are fraught with numerous opportunities for misapplication.

This chapter discusses the clinical classification of deadspace-producing disease and the *limited* application of blood gas measurement in the identification and quantification of this pathology.

CLINICAL CLASSIFICATION

The minute ventilation (MV) is composed of gas that respires [alveolar ventilation (VA)] and gas that does not respire [deadspace ventilation (VD)]. Since VA is the only component that can transfer oxygen to the blood and remove carbon dioxide from the blood, any increase in VD requires an increase in MV to maintain the same VA. Therefore, to avoid ventilatory failure an increased VD demands an increased MV. This demand for an increased work of breathing is the primary reason why increases in physiologic deadspace are of clinical concern.

TABLE 10–1.

Physiologic Classification of Cardiopulmonary Disease

Deadspace-producing	Shunt-producing
A. Anatomic	A. Anatomic
1. Rapid, shallow breathing	1. Congenital heart disease
	2. Intrapulmonary fistula
	3. Vascular lung tumor
B. Alveolar deadspace	B. Capillary shunting
1. Acute pulmonary embolus	1. Acute atelectasis
2. Decreased pulmonary perfusion	2. Alveolar fluid
a. Decreased cardiac output	
b. Acute pulmonary hypertension	
C. Deadspace effect	C. Shunt effect
(ventilation in excess of perfusion)	(perfusion in excess of ventilation)
1. Alveolar septal destruction	1. Hypoventilation
2. Positive-pressure ventilation	2. Uneven distribution of ventilation
	3. Diffusion defect

Anatomic Deadspace

Anatomic deadspace is normally constant and predictable—approximately 1 ml/lb (2.2 ml/kg) of normal body weight. The major cause of increased anatomic deadspace is *rapid, shallow breathing,* which most often results from either of two pathophysiologic conditions: increased work of breathing or central nervous system malfunction (see chap. 4).

Alveolar Deadspace-Producing Disease

The two most common causes of acute increases in alveolar deadspace are pulmonary embolus and decreased pulmonary perfusion.

Acute Pulmonary Embolus.—This initially produces ventilated but unperfused alveoli. It is the classic example of alveolar deadspace disease.[118, 119] Some have classified this a shunting disease because it usually is *accompanied by arterial hypoxemia.*[120] The hypoxemia is due in part to concomitant low V/Q, increased work of breathing, decreased cardiac output, and other factors that are poorly understood.[121] There is no such thing as "typical" blood gases in acute pulmonary embolus.

Acutely Decreased Pulmonary Perfusion.—This is most commonly due to two factors in the critically ill patient:

1. Acutely Decreased Cardiac Output.—This results in decreased pulmonary arterial perfusion pressure so that less of the cardiac output flows through the non–gravity-dependent areas of the lung. This significantly increases the areas of ventilated but unperfused lung. *Clinically, this is perhaps the single most common cause of acutely increased deadspace ventilation.* Whenever there is clinical evidence of acutely decreased cardiac output, one must be concerned with increased work of breathing secondary to deadspace ventilation increase. The hypoxemia that accompanies decreased cardiac output is primarily due to decreased mixed venous oxygen content.

   2. Acute Pulmonary Hypertension.—Because of acutely increased pulmonary vascular resistance, the distribution of perfusion favors gravity-dependent lung; additionally, the right ventricular cardiac output tends to be somewhat diminished. Thus, acute pulmonary hypertension leads to increased deadspace ventilation. Acute pulmonary hypertension is most commonly caused by acidemia, low alveolar oxygen tensions, and severe arterial hypoxemia.

Ventilation in Excess of Perfusion

   Two possible circumstances may occur in alveoli that have ventilation in excess of perfusion. First, there may be increased exchange of gases, which results in an increase in alveolar ventilation (a decreased arterial carbon dioxide tension). Second, the excessive ventilation may not exchange with blood, and this results in an increase in deadspace ventilation. The outcome of any given circumstance of ventilation in excess of perfusion is unpredictable, infinitely complex, and everchanging. There are three common clinical situations in which ventilation in excess of perfusion is believed to be significant: alveolar septal destruction, positive-pressure ventilation, and positive end-expiratory pressure.

   Alveolar Septal Destruction.—This is most commonly found in the septal alveolar wall degeneration of emphysema where large single air sacs replace several alveoli. Due to the loss of surface area for gas exchange, much of the ventilation is believed to poorly exchange with blood.

   Positive-Pressure Ventilation.—This is most commonly encountered with the use of a mechanical ventilator or during general anesthesia, when significantly increasing minute ventilation is not accompanied by corresponding increases in cardiac output.[49, 122] In addition, there is a preference for the delivered gas to be distributed to the more poorly perfused lung areas.[123] Therefore, much of the increased total ventilation is deadspace because there has been no concomitant increase in pulmonary blood flow.[124]

Positive End-Expiratory Pressure.—This airway pressure maneuver is believed to increase alveolar size.[125] Varying effects on perfusion have been demonstrated, depending on the pathology present.[126, 127] However, it is a fair generalization that this therapy often produces lung units that have improved ventilation/perfusion.

ASSESSMENT OF THE PHYSIOLOGIC DEADSPACE

Three analytic methods are clinically available for assessing abnormal increases in physiologic deadspace: (1) minute ventilation to arterial P_{CO_2} disparity (MV-Pa_{CO_2}), (2) the arterial to alveolar CO_2 tension gradient (a-A P_{CO_2}), and (3) the deadspace to tidal volume ratio (V_D/V_T).

MV-Pa_{CO_2} Disparity

The normal pulmonary system increases the minute ventilation (MV) in response to increased physiologic deadspace. Where pulmonary reserves are adequate, the minute ventilation will increase to maintain an adequate arterial P_{CO_2}. Minute ventilation is the sum of alveolar and deadspace ventilation:

$$MV = \dot{V}_A + \dot{V}_D$$

To maintain baseline alveolar ventilation, minute ventilation must be increased in the presence of increased deadspace ventilation.

In the absence of increased metabolic rate, clinical observation that minute ventilation is increased with no expected decreases in arterial P_{CO_2} raises the possibility of increased physiologic deadspace. The basis for this concept of a *minute ventilation to Pa_{CO_2} disparity* is illustrated in Table 10–2 and Figure 10–1. Assuming a CO_2 production of 200 ml/min, the ideal relationship of MV, alveolar ventilation, and arterial P_{CO_2} is shown when minute ventilation is doubled, redoubled, and halved (see Table 10–2). This is graphically illustrated as a hyperbolic relationship between alveolar P_{CO_2} and alveolar ventilation (see Fig 10–1).

Although the arterial P_{CO_2} measurement is both a reflection of alveolar CO_2 tension and a reliable qualitative reflection of the adequacy

TABLE 10–2.

Ideal Minute Ventilation, Alveolar Ventilation,
and Arterial Carbon Dioxide Tension
Relationships

MV (L)	VA (L)	Pa_{CO_2} (mm Hg)
3	2	80
6	4	40
12	8	30
24	16	20

of alveolar ventilation, *the Pa_{CO_2} is not a quantitative measure of alveolar ventilation.* Therefore, in the absence of a quantitative measurement of alveolar ventilation, minute ventilation is used because it is clinically available and reliable. This substitution of minute ventilation for alveolar ventilation assumes that: (1) anatomic deadspace is normal and changes proportionately in response to increases in minute ventilation; (2) arterial P_{CO_2} values are not significantly greater than 40 mm Hg; and (3) CO_2 production is normal. Under these circumstances, the MV-Pa_{CO_2} relationship can be equated to the VA-Pa_{CO_2} relationship shown (see Fig 10–1). Thus, under the best of circumstances, an MV-Pa_{CO_2} disparity detects in a qualitative fashion the presence of *acute* deadspace-producing disease.

Arterial-Alveolar P_{CO_2} Gradient (a-A P_{CO_2})

Figure 10–2 shows a normal carbon dioxide exhalation curve in a healthy young person. In the absence of significant pulmonary disease, the final portion of phase III—the end tidal P_{CO_2}—is no more than 2 mm Hg less than the arterial P_{CO_2}. Acute increases in this a-A P_{CO_2} gradient reflect increases in physiologic deadspace.

This methodology can be useful as a monitoring tool provided baseline values are available for comparison (for further discussion, see chap. 15).

VD/VT

The clinical usefulness and application of the deadspace to tidal volume ratio depend on four factors that must be carefully noted.

1. Both anatomic and alveolar deadspace are being measured; thus, it is important to observe that the patient has a reasonably normal ven-

tilatory pattern. This observation rules out significant increases in dead-space ventilation due solely to increases in anatomic deadspace.

2. The metabolic rate must be within normal limits to the extent determinable by clinical observation—i.e., normal temperature, normal muscle activity, etc.

3. Cardiovascular function must be reasonably adequate to reflect the patient's total body tissue production of carbon dioxide.

4. The technical procedures for measuring deadspace to tidal volume ratios must be extremely exact; that is, the entire expired air sample must be collected and care must be taken to prevent any intermittent leak from the expired volume. In the spontaneously breathing patient, a long enough time must be allowed for the tidal volume variability to no longer affect the mean expired carbon dioxide tension. This time and variability factor makes the measurement far more practical and accurate for patients controlled on positive-pressure volume ventilators than for spontaneously breathing patients. The values of deadspace to tidal volume ratios in normal spontaneously breathing patients range from 0.2 to 0.4 (20% to 40%).

Development of the V_D/V_T

The basic premise for quantitating the deadspace to tidal volume

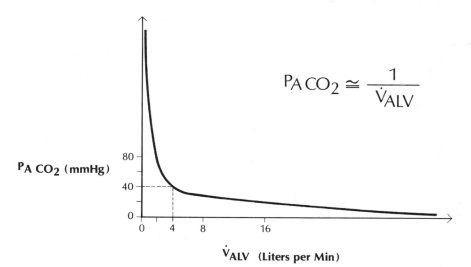

$$P_A CO_2 \cong \frac{1}{\dot{V}_{ALV}}$$

$P_A CO_2$ (mmHg)

$\dot{V}_{ALV}$ (Liters per Min)

FIG 10–1.
Theoretical relationship between $P_{A_{CO_2}}$ (alveolar carbon dioxide tension) and V_{ALV} (alveolar ventilation), assuming normal lungs and a normal metabolic rate.

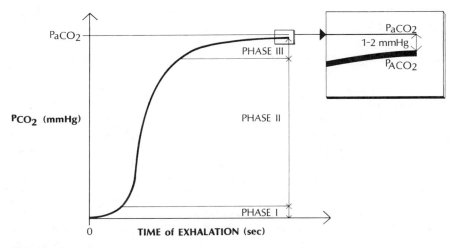

FIG 10–2.
A normal exhaled CO_2 curve. *Phase I* represents the low CO_2 tension in gas expelled from the anatomic deadspace. *Phase II* represents the increasing CO_2 tension as the exhaled gas becomes composed of increasingly more alveolar gas. *Phase III* represents the CO_2 plateau where the exhaled gas is composed primarily of gas from the alveoli. The inset shows the normal relationship between the Pa_{CO_2} (arterial carbon dioxide tension) and the carbon dioxide tension of end exhalation (end tidal) gas. The normal disparity is less than 3 mm Hg. Increases in this disparity most probably reflect increases in alveolar deadspace ventilation.

ratio is that the total gas volume expired is equal to the sum of the alveolar volume expired and the deadspace volume expired:

$$\dot{V}E = \dot{V}A + \dot{V}D \qquad (1)$$

$\dot{V}E$ is the total gas volume expired; $\dot{V}A$ represents the alveolar ventilation volume expired, and $\dot{V}D$ represents the alveolar deadspace volume expired.

A fraction of the expired gas is carbon dioxide. Over time, the collected CO_2 mixes uniformly with the total expired gas. The volume of CO_2 collected compared with the total gas volume collected is expressed as the mean expired fraction of carbon dioxide ($F\bar{E}CO_2$):

$$F\bar{E}CO_2 = \frac{CO_2 \text{ volume collected}}{\text{Total volume collected}} \qquad (2)$$

The carbon dioxide expired must come from either alveolar or deadspace volume:

$$\dot{V}E \times F\bar{E}CO_2 = (\dot{V}A \times FACO_2) + (\dot{V}D \times FDCO_2) \tag{3}$$

However, the fraction of carbon dioxide in deadspace air approaches that of inspired air (essentially zero). Therefore, equation (3) may be expressed as:

$$\dot{V}E \times F\bar{E}CO_2 = \dot{V}A \times FACO_2 \tag{4}$$

The volume of alveolar ventilation must be equal to the total expired volume minus the deadspace volume:

$$\dot{V}A = (\dot{V}E - \dot{V}D) \tag{5}$$

Inserting this equivalent term for alveolar ventilation into equation (4), multiplying, and collecting all similar volume terms on each side of the equation, we get the following mathematical relationships:

$$\dot{V}E \times F\bar{E}CO_2 = (\dot{V}E - \dot{V}D)FACO_2 \tag{6}$$

$$\dot{V}D \times FACO_2 = \dot{V}E \times FACO_2 - \dot{V}E \times F\bar{E}CO_2 \tag{7}$$

Dividing both sides of equation (7) by the fraction of alveolar carbon dioxide ($FACO_2$) and by the volume expired ($\dot{V}E$), we get:

$$\frac{\dot{V}D}{\dot{V}E} = \frac{FACO_2 - F\bar{E}CO_2}{FACO_2} \tag{8}$$

Two basic relationships are used to further simplify the equation: (1) the fraction of a gas (FCO_2) is proportional to the partial pressure of the gas (PCO_2); and (2) the alveolar carbon dioxide tensions can be very closely approximated by arterial carbon dioxide tension measurement. The term *expired volume* ($\dot{V}E$) is used interchangeably with the term *tidal volume* ($\dot{V}T$). Incorporating these basic relationships into equation (8) gives the *clinical deadspace equation:*

$$\frac{\dot{V}D}{\dot{V}T} = \frac{Pa_{CO_2} - P\bar{E}_{CO_2}}{Pa_{CO_2}} \tag{9}$$

Equation (9) is the form most commonly used to measure deadspace to tidal volume ratios. In a simplified concept, it can be visualized that the degree of dilution of alveolar carbon dioxide tension in expired air will increase as the size of the deadspace increases. In other words, the greater the portion of the tidal volume that is deadspace, the less will be the partial pressure of carbon dioxide in the expired air.

Sample Collection

Collection of a representative expired sample ($P\bar{E}_{CO_2}$) is essential and must be a collection of *total* expired gas. In the spontaneously breathing patient, this involves collecting expired gas through a one-way valve system into a large collecting balloon for 5 to 10 minutes. When applied to the unintubated patient, the system itself often alters the ventilatory pattern.

Experience has shown that in patients on volume ventilators in which only exhaled gases enter the exhalation tubing,* a 5-L sample of expired gas taken from the expiratory port of a volume ventilator gives the same $P\bar{E}_{CO_2}$ as a 5-minute collection in a large balloon. This is undoubtedly due to the regularity of the ventilatory pattern with positive pressure ventilation rates greater than 8/minute.

Interpretation of VD/VT

With positive-pressure ventilation, the deadspace ventilation is increased because the distribution of air to the non–gravity-dependent areas of the lung is increased. These factors are the reason a VD/VT less than 0.4 is rare in a patient on positive-pressure ventilation and a range of deadspace to tidal volume ratios between 0.4 and 0.6 is considered acceptable. In other words, a patient on the positive-pressure ventilator with a VD/VT of less than 0.6 is very likely to have a normal VD/VT ratio when spontaneously breathing.

In the absence of chronic obstructive pulmonary disease, a VD/VT

---

*Intermittent mandatory ventilation (IMV) systems allow fresh gas to flow to the exhalation tubing.

ratio greater than 0.8 on a volume ventilator represents a significant increase in deadspace ventilation. It would mean that the patient would have to significantly increase his spontaneous ventilation above normal to overcome the increased deadspace. This may necessitate excessive physiologic demands due to the increased work of breathing. V_D/V_T measurements between 0.6 and 0.8 on the positive-pressure ventilator are significant and must be evaluated in relation to the other system reserves and the general clinical status of the patient.

DEADSPACE VS. SHUNTING DISEASE

Although we are unable to measure physiologic deadspace reliably in most circumstances, the principles in this chapter are essential to the appropriate interpretation of blood gas measurements. Often, blood gas analysis may be helpful in ruling out certain disease categories by differentiating shunt-producing disease from deadspace-producing disease. To illustrate this point, consider the following case studies.

A 40-year-old, 110-lb woman with thrombophlebitis of the right leg for two days suddenly complains of chest pain and shortness of breath:

$F_{I_{O_2}}$ 0.21

pH	7.52	V_T	400 ml	BP	140/70
P_{CO_2}	27 mm Hg	RR	30/minute	P	110/minute
P_{O_2}	60 mm Hg	MV	12 L	T	100°F

The interpretation is "acute alveolar hyperventilation (acute respiratory alkalosis) with mild hypoxemia." The more than twice normal minute volume is reflected in the greatly increased alveolar ventilation. This *tends to rule out* acute deadspace disease.*

Now consider the following data in the same patient after 20 minutes of oxygen therapy:

$F_{I_{O_2}}$ 0.50

pH	7.48	V_T	400 ml	BP	120/80
P_{CO_2}	33 mm Hg	RR	20/minute	P	90/minute
P_{O_2}	90 mm Hg	MV	8 L	T	100°F

*Of course, multiple small pulmonary emboli may occur over a period of days without producing clinically detectable deadspace ventilation increases.

At 50% inspired oxygen, the ventilatory and myocardial work have been decreased. This is typical of acute alveolar hyperventilation due to hypoxemia (see chap. 6); i.e., it is more commonly the result of a shunt-producing disease. In fact, this woman had a pneumonia in the left lower lobe. Of course, blood gas measurements *alone* did not rule out pulmonary embolus, but they were *consistent* with that conclusion.

If the diagnosis were pulmonary embolus, the following data would have been more typical:

FI_{O_2} 0.21

pH	7.48	V_T	600 ml	BP	140/70
PCO_2	33 mm Hg	RR	25/minute	P	110/minute
PO_2	60 mm Hg	VM	15 L	T	100°F

FI_{O_2} 0.50

pH	7.45	V_T	600 ml	BP	120/70
PCO_2	35 mm Hg	RR	25/minute	P	100/minute
PO_2	110 mm Hg	MV	15 L	T	100°F

The minute volume is about three times normal and yet the alveolar ventilation is in the low normal range. This suggests increased deadspace ventilation. At 50% inspired oxygen, the significant increase in arterial oxygenation without significant changes in the ventilatory status is *suggestive* of deadspace-producing disease and *tends to rule out* shunt-producing disease.

These examples are clear-cut for teaching purposes. Clinically, the situation may be extremely complex and many factors may be involved. The following guidelines will prove beneficial in the vast majority of clinical circumstances; however, the reader should keep in mind that exceptions are not uncommon.

Guidelines for Acute Deadspace-Producing Diseases

1. Minute volume increases greatly with little or no response in alveolar ventilation (MV − MVA = MVD).
2. Changes in total ventilation are minimal in response to oxygen therapy, whereas increases in arterial oxygen tensions may be dramatic.
3. Accurate deadspace/tidal volume ratio measurements are technically difficult to obtain and of relatively little value in the presence of tachypnea.

Guidelines for Acute Shunt-Producing Diseases

1. Increased minute ventilation is directly reflected in alveolar ventilation.
2. When cardiopulmonary reserves are adequate to meet the stress:
   a. The blood gas measurements usually show an acute alveolar hyperventilation with hypoxemia.
   b. Clinical evidence of increased cardiovascular work is present—e.g., hypertension and tachycardia.
3. Assuming the hypoxemia is at least partially responsive to oxygen therapy (i.e., at least some shunt effect mechanisms are present), appropriate oxygen therapy results in:
   a. Decreased work of breathing as reflected in decreased ventilatory rate, decreased use of accessory muscles of ventilation, a subjective feeling of improvement, and Pa_{CO_2} level increased toward normal.
   b. Decreased myocardial work as reflected in a decrease of hypertension, a decrease in tachycardia, and the disappearance or diminishment in frequency of ventricular premature beats when present.
   c. *Significantly improved arterial oxygen tensions,* but only after the work of breathing and the myocardial work have been reduced significantly.

11

Temperature Correction of Blood Gases*

Arterial pH and blood gas values often have a central importance in the care of the critically ill patient. Since abnormal body temperatures are common in the critically ill, the practice of "temperature correcting" pH, P_{CO_2} and P_{O_2} values is widespread. There are few aspects of blood gas analysis that have provoked as much controversy as temperature correction. The root of this controversy lies in the fact that blood transport of carbon dioxide and oxygen involves both gas solution and complex chemical reactions that are affected by temperature variation. Simply stated, a blood sample of given O_2 and CO_2 contents will manifest different gas tensions when analyzed at various temperatures. Table 11–1 lists the temperature correction values for normal blood.

Despite the present popularity for temperature correction of blood gases, important questions have always existed concerning both the theoretic and clinical usefulness of this procedure. The objectives of this chapter are: (1) to define the process of temperature correction; (2) to review the physiologic significance of temperature induced in vivo changes; (3) to review the clinical relevance of blood gas temperature correction; and (4) to propose rational guidelines for the interpretation of blood gas values when abnormal patient temperatures exist.

DEFINING TEMPERATURE CORRECTION

An *open system* allows for gas exchange with the adjacent environment, e.g., capillary blood or a blood sample exposed to the air. A *closed*

*This chapter was co-authored by Dr. Hak Yui Wong.

TABLE 11–1.

Temperature Correction Values for Normal Blood

°C	°F	pH	P_{CO_2}	P_{O_2}
20	68	7.65	19	27
25	77	7.58	24	37
30	86	7.50	30	51
35	95	7.43	37	70
36	97	7.41	38	75
37	99	7.40	40	80
38	100	7.39	42	85
39	102	7.37	44	91
40	104	7.36	45	97

system does not allow mass exchange of gas content; a circumstance that exists in arterial blood as well as blood in a gas-tight syringe or in a gas analyzer. *In vitro* temperature-induced blood gas changes occur in a closed system where gas contents remain unchanged, whereas *in vivo* blood gas changes due to temperature variation occur in an open system.

To directly obtain in vivo pH and gas tensions, the measuring electrode's temperature would have to be adjusted to that of the patient, a process that would add at least 30 minutes to each measurement as well as complicate quality assurance (see chaps. 21 and 22). To avoid these undesirable factors, the pH, P_{CO_2} and P_{O_2} electrodes are encased in a constant 37°C environment to which the blood sample chamber is also exposed. Thus, despite the patient's temperature, the pH, P_{CO_2}, and P_{O_2} are analyzed in a closed system at 37°C.

The term "temperature correction" refers to applying mathematical adjustments to the measured 37°C values for the purpose of obtaining a more accurate reflection of the in vivo gas tensions. Commonly applied formulas have been extensively reviewed in relation to the numerous factors confounding their applicability.[128, 129] Although the derivation of temperature correction formulas is quite empirical in reference to in vitro changes in a closed system, it is generally agreed that they are reasonably accurate within the clinically relevant ranges. The increased availability of microprocessor technology that can readily perform the temperature correction process has further popularized this practice.

PHYSIOLOGIC CONSIDERATIONS

Interpretation of a biologic measurement depends upon identification of a "normal" range. Therefore, prior to judging the clinical relevance of temperature correction, it is necessary to examine the depth to which we understand and can identify physiologic variations induced by temperature change.

Oxygenation

A normothermic adult is capable of maintaining adequate oxygen delivery to tissues with an arterial Po_2 of 60 mm Hg or greater as long as hemoglobin content and cardiovascular function are adequate (see chap. 5). Since oxygen homeostasis at 37°C has been extensively studied, we are capable of defining minimal levels of arterial Po_2 that should adequately oxygenate tissues at that temperature. In contrast, identification of such minimal levels of Po_2 at various body temperatures are poorly documented because most of the data are confounded by concomitant pathophysiology and therapeutic intervention.

Hyperthermia

The effect of temperature change on adult oxygen consumption is well documented to be approximately 10% per degree centigrade or 7% per degree Fahrenheit. Thus, hyperthermia necessitates an increased oxygen consumption that is generally associated with an increased cardiac output and minute ventilation. As schematically depicted previously (see Fig 5–5), when initial Po_2 values are in the normoxic range, increasing temperature increases Po_2 while hemoglobin-oxygen affinity decreases (shift to right). The percent oxyhemoglobin saturation (So_2) changes little or not at all because of initial near total saturation. The increased Po_2 and decreased affinity both potentially facilitate oxygen unloading, a theoretically advantageous circumstance. However, when the initial Po_2 is in the hypoxemic range, the shift to the right due to hyperthermia will decrease arterial oxygen content for any Po_2 and theoretically threaten tissue oxygenation.

Available data do not help to clarify the appropriate clinical conclusions that should be drawn from this confusing physiology. For example, the assumption that the arterial Po_2 rises when body temperature increases has been shown to be true in sheep models subjected to controlled warming and cooling,[130] whereas studies of heat stroke victims fail to show temperature corrected arterial hypoxemia despite the patient's severe condition.[131] The net physiologic advantage or disadvantage of these changes is completely unknown.

Hypothermia

During hypothermia the arterial Po_2 can be expected to decrease predictably while oxygen unloading is potentially impeded by both an increased hemoglobin-oxygen affinity and the lower Po_2. However, data from accidental hypothermia in humans illustrate that a number of cardiopulmonary factors may contribute to the observed arterial hypoxemia in addition to those directly attributable to temperature change.[132] On one hand, physiologic principles dictate that as oxygen consumption falls with temperature the changes in gas solubility result in an increasing amount of dissolved oxygen. On the other hand, pathophysiologic factors like hypoventilation, vasoconstriction, and uneven tissue temperatures predispose toward inadequate oxygen delivery. There are no data to determine the minimal arterial Po_2 required to prevent tissue hypoxia under hypothermic conditions.

Summary

Although theoretical and empirical considerations suggest that the normal in vivo arterial Po_2 varies with temperature, the significance of this variation on oxygen delivery is modulated by many other factors. It is not feasible to infer a minimum safe range of arterial Po_2 for body temperatures other than 37°C. Thus, temperature corrected Po_2 values provide less useful clinical information concerning oxygenation homeostasis than the measured values at 37°C.

Acid-Base Balance

Arterial pH rises and Pco_2 falls during hypothermia when the analysis is made at actual body temperature. However, this "alkalotic" change with hypothermia does not occur when the measurements are made at 37°C. This calls into question the definition of "normal" acid-base balance at varying temperatures and how acid-base data should be analyzed and interpreted.[133] Although some hibernating animal data suggest that normal acid-base ranges are constant at differing temperatures,[134] the preponderance of evidence from comparative physiology and human data indicate that normal acid-base ranges vary with body temperature.[135, 136]

In warm-blooded animals the pH of intracellular and extracellular water, as well as the neutral pH of water, undergoes parallel changes with temperature variation.[133, 137] This indicates that these observed pH changes with temperature do not represent deviation from "normal" acid-base balance. Likewise, the coincident changes in Pco_2 with temperature variation are assumed to be an integral part of the process of maintaining electrochemical neutrality, and therefore do not represent deviation from "normal" carbon dioxide homeostasis. Similar changes in blood pH and P_{CO_2} in various parts of the peripheral circulation having different temperatures have been demonstrated.[138] Furthermore, blood subjected to in vitro temperature variation demonstrates no evidence of change in acid-base and electrolyte equilibrium despite significant pH and P_{CO_2} changes.[139]

Reasonable interpretation of this complex data establishes that the "normal" pH is not constant with temperature variation but varies in a predictable fashion. This concept further suggests that if the acid-base status is normal at any in vivo temperature, the in vitro pH and P_{CO_2} at 37°C should approach 7.40 and 40 mm Hg. Conversely, in vivo acid-base abnormalities should be appropriately reflected in the 37°C measurements.[133, 140, 141]

Clinical verification of the above hypothesis is reasonably provided by the historical fact that it was once common practice during hypothermic anesthesia to add CO_2 to the inspired gas to maintain a "temperature corrected" P_{CO_2} near 40 mm Hg.[142, 143] Subsequent dog studies demonstrated that mean arterial pressure and heart rate were better when CO_2 was not added to the inspired gas and 37°C P_{CO_2} values were maintained near 40 mm Hg.[144–147] These findings were substantiated in infants undergoing open heart surgery.[148]

It is reasonable to conclude that available human and animal data pertaining to biochemical and physiologic changes coincident with temperature variation demonstrate that pH and P_{CO_2} values measured at 37°C will best reflect the in vivo acid-base status regardless of body temperature.

P_{CO_2} and the Brain

Variation of arterial P_{CO_2} has profound effects on cerebral vascular smooth muscle tone. The impact of a low in vivo P_{CO_2} during hypothermia is of concern because the hypocarbia-mediated vasoconstriction could result in cerebral hypoxia. However, mammalian studies show that despite decreased cerebral blood flow and vasoconstriction with hypothermia, there is no evidence of cerebral hypoxia.[149, 150] These studies suggest that hypothermically induced decreases in cerebral blood flow are in keeping with the reduction in total body metabolic requirements. There is also evidence to suggest that cerebral blood flow response to P_{CO_2} may be shifted during temperature change such that the response is most sensitive in the middle of the range predicted for the temperature.[140]

This information may be summarized to state that despite the hypocarbia induced by hypothermia, there is no evidence that cerebral hypoxia results from the hypocarbia-induced vasoconstriction. Further, although regulation of cerebral blood flow is altered during hypothermia, P_{CO_2} remains the major regulator of cerebral vascular tone. Since the vascular sensitivity occurs at the range predicted for the temperature, 37°C P_{CO_2} is a reliable monitor for such vascular manipulation at any body temperature.

CLINICAL RELEVANCE OF TEMPERATURE CORRECTION

Justification for temperature correction of pH and blood gas values is based on the belief that "knowing" the in vivo status is an advantage to patient care. Such a belief implies that either the normal ranges for pH, P_{CO_2}, and P_{O_2} remain constant regardless of temperature or that the normal ranges are well established for all temperatures. The information previously presented leaves no doubt that both of these alternatives are without validity.

Following is a discussion of the scientific basis for clinical interpretation of blood gas measurements when alterations in body temperature are present.

Acid-Base Interpretation

The pH and P_{CO_2} changes attributable to temperature variation do not affect the calculated bicarbonate value. Therefore, the 37°C values for pH and P_{CO_2} reliably reflect the in vivo acid-base status at the patient's actual temperature. Since temperature corrected pH and P_{CO_2} values have no established physiologic reference points, the clinical application of such values is without foundation.

P_{CO_2} and Ventilation

When the arterial P_{CO_2} is utilized to reflect the adequacy of alveolar ventilation, our established guidelines are predicated on a normal CO_2 production at 37°C. Since both CO_2 production and arterial P_{CO_2} undergo parallel changes with temperature variation, clinical assessment of alveolar ventilation is most reliably reflected by applying the well-established homeostatic reference points at 37°C.

Even in the circumstance in which hypocarbia is desired to minimize the intracranial blood volume by cerebral vasoconstriction, the P_{CO_2} measurement and reference points at 37°C are as clinically reliable as the temperature-corrected values.

Interpretation of End Tidal Pco_2

Capnography by infrared analysis or mass spectrometry is a commonly utilized noninvasive monitor (see chap. 15). Exhaled gas measurements will reflect the in vivo (temperature-corrected) Pco_2. With normal alveolar ventilation and a body temperature of 30°C, the end tidal Pco_2 would be 28 mm Hg, while the uncorrected arterial Pco_2 would be 40 mm Hg. The clinician must be aware of this circumstance so that the end tidal Pco_2 will not be inappropriately interpreted.

Oxygenation

Po_2

The balance between oxygen delivery and oxygen demand is well defined for patients at 37°C (see chap. 8). In the absence of data quantifying the changes in the balance between oxygen delivery and demand at temperatures other than 37°C, the clinician is best served by assuming that temperature-induced changes do not significantly alter this balance. Thus, making clinical decisions based upon 37°C requirements (e.g., arterial Po_2 maintained at 60 to 80 mm Hg) are the best guidelines available—even in conditions of significant hyperthermia or hypothermia. Temperature corrected Po_2 values do *not* improve our ability to make clinically relevant interpretations!

Oxygen Content

Oxygen content is most reliably calculated by measuring both the hemoglobin content (gm%) and the percent oxyhemoglobin saturation (So_2) (see chap. 5). Since blood oxygen content in a closed system must remain the same despite temperature changes, variations in So_2 and Po_2 can only occur by transfer of oxygen molecules between the dissolved state and the combined state.

It has been demonstrated that in a closed system So_2 changes by less than 2% over a temperature range of 0°C–42°C.[151, 152] Therefore the So_2 measurement can be considered relatively independent of temperature change in a closed system. When the So_2 is not directly measured but calculated by means of a Po_2-pH nomogram, the in vitro changes in So_2 over the clinically encountered temperature range (18°C to 42°C) are so small that the relationship can be considered temperature-independent.

Since oxygen content can be accurately calculated from 37°C values regardless of patient temperature, there is no need to temperature correct the blood gas values to obtain oxygen-content–based indices such as the arterial-mixed venous oxygen content difference [$C_{(a-v)}O_2$], the intrapulmonary shunt (Qsp/Qt), and the Estimated Shunt (see chap. 9).

Alveolar to Arterial Oxygen Tension Indices

When pulmonary artery blood samples are not available, indices based on alveolar to arterial oxygen tension are often utilized to reflect the pulmonary component of the arterial oxygenation deficit (see chap. 9). The most common indices are the alveolar to arterial tension gradient ($P_{(A-a)}O_2$), the Respiratory Index ($P_{(A-a)}O_2/Pa_{O_2}$), the arterial to alveolar oxygen tension ratio (Pa_{O_2}/PA_{O_2}), and the arterial to inspired oxygen fraction ratio (Pa_{O_2}/FI_{O_2}). The limitations of oxygen tension indices as a reflection of intrapulmonary shunting have been documented[108]; however, when they are utilized, the Pa_{O_2} *should be temperature corrected* to reflect the true difference with the alveolar tension.[153]

CONCLUSION

The popularity of temperature correcting pH, P_{CO_2}, and P_{O_2} values appears to be based on the observation that large differences in the blood gas values are present when the patient's temperature is profoundly hypothermic or hyperthermic. This observation led many to conclude that the 37°C values were "wrong." The real danger in this superficial thought process is the unfounded conclusion that temperature corrected values are "right."

The simple truth is that with significant changes in patient temperature we do not fully understand the complexity of effects on metabolism, vascular function, and respiration. Therefore, both corrected and uncorrected blood gas values are of uncertain usefulness in patients with significant deviations in body temperature. There is not a logical or scientific basis for assuming that temperature corrected values are better than the 37°C values. In fact, the available technical and biologic data pertaining to temperature correction of blood gas values lead to the conclusion that *there is no clinical advantage to using values other than those at 37°C.*

Although temperature correction of blood gases cannot be considered wrong, the process involves several practical disadvantages. First, interpretation of the corrected values demands deviation from the familiar and well-documented guidelines for interpreting the 37°C values. Second, temperature correction assumes the laboratory has received the patient's true temperature at the time of sampling. Our experience reveals that the patient's true temperature is often not reported or erroneously reported. Third, temperature corrected values can be confused with uncorrected values and vice versa. The factor that makes these potential problems significant is that the temperature corrected values are of no clinical advantage over the 37°C values, except when applied to oxygen-tension indices and end tidal CO_2 measurements.

It is ironic that microprocessor availability has made temperature correction effortless and readily available at a time when the biologic and clinical data clearly demonstrate that the process is unnecessary at best and misleading at worst. Available data support the statement that blood gas values should be routinely reported only at 37°C and temperature-corrected values should be calculated only when specifically requested by the physician. In this way, confusion can be avoided and the onus for interpreting the temperature corrected values is placed with the physician who requests the procedure. There is no evidence that patient management is hindered when clinical interpretation of pH, P_{CO_2}, and P_{O_2} is consistently based on 37°C values.

12

Blood Gases and Resuscitation

Carbon dioxide production is normally balanced by CO_2 excretion via the lungs. The efficiency with which alveolar gas exchanges with pulmonary blood flow (alveolar ventilation) determines lung excretion of CO_2 (see chap. 4). Normally the lungs are the limiting factor in CO_2 excretion and the venous to arterial P_{CO_2} gradient $[P_{(v-a)}CO_2]$ is 6 mm Hg or less.

Closed chest cardiac compression in conjunction with positive-pressure ventilation has been the standard cardiopulmonary resuscitative technique for more than a quarter of a century. For almost two decades this method of cardiopulmonary resuscitation (CPR) has been standardized by the American Heart Association. Recent research has documented some fascinating acid-base abnormalities coincident with CPR that call for a reevaluation of the meaning and usefulness of arterial blood gas measurements during the resuscitative effort.

ACID-BASE BALANCE DURING CPR

It appears that in most circumstances cardiac output is so poor with the closed chest compression technique that metabolic acidosis (lactic acidosis) secondary to inadequate tissue perfusion will inevitably occur within 15 to 20 minutes of excellently performed CPR. The severely diminished cardiac output creates significant increases in physiologic deadspace, limiting the efficiency with which the lungs can excrete carbon dioxide despite great increases in minute ventilation and maintenance of acceptable arterial P_{CO_2} values (see chaps. 4 and 10). In other words, *the very low cardiac output becomes the primary factor limiting* CO_2 *excretion!* Since CO_2 production exceeds excretion during CPR, venous CO_2 content increases despite normal lungs and an increased minute ventilation. Although this phenomenon of increased venous P_{CO_2} and decreased venous pH occurs to some degree in most low cardiac output states,[154] it is greatly exaggerated during CPR.[155, 156]

Venous Respiratory Acidosis

An acute increase in venous P_{CO_2} results in a decreased venous pH with little change in plasma bicarbonate concentration (see chap. 3). Systemic capillary blood will be similar to the venous blood, inferring that tissue P_{CO_2} and pH will have similar abnormalities.

During CPR with normal lungs and increased minute ventilation, venous "respiratory acidosis" occurs in conjunction with an arterial "respiratory alkalosis".[155–159] In spontaneously breathing patients with poor cardiac output the $P_{(v-a)}CO_2$ has been observed to increase 50% to 100%; a threefold to tenfold increase has been observed in patients receiving CPR.[155, 156]

Metabolic Acidosis

Inadequate tissue perfusion inevitably leads to anaerobic metabolism and the production of lactic acid. This lactate production has traditionally been considered the primary cause of acidosis during CPR. It is now clear that a significant plasma bicarbonate depletion due to lactic acid accumulation is seldom present early in CPR.[160] The best explanation for this observation is that hepatic function metabolizes lactate to CO_2 as long as liver oxygenation is adequate. As liver oxygenation gradually diminishes, circulating lactic acid gradually accumulates.

The plasma bicarbonate deficit of metabolic acidosis is essentially equal in both the venous and arterial blood. This fact means that the paradoxic venous and arterial pH values seen in early CPR cannot be due to metabolic acidosis. However, early lactate production probably increases CO_2 production by the liver and thereby contributes to the venous respiratory acidosis.

ARTERIAL BLOOD GASES DURING CPR

Arterial P_{O_2}

Arterial oxygen content must be maximal to obtain the best possible oxygenation of heart and brain with the minimal perfusion present during CPR. Therefore, Pa_{O_2} remains an important measurement during CPR.

Arterial P_{CO_2}

The poor cardiac output coincident with CPR greatly increases physiologic deadspace (chaps. 4 and 10). Therefore, a significant increase in total ventilation (minute ventilation) will be required to maintain a "normal" Pa_{CO_2} of 40 mm Hg. In CPR dog models with normal lungs, it is possible to avoid arterial acidemia for up to 18 minutes by providing the required increase in minute ventilation.[160]

Since the $P_{(v-a)}CO_2$ greatly increases during CPR, blood going from the right side of the heart to the left without exchanging with alveolar gas (true shunt mechanisms, zero V/Q—[see chap. 9]) will enter the left side of the heart with a P_{CO_2} significantly greater than the blood that has exchanged with alveolar gas. If the lungs have shunting in excess of 20%, the Pa_{CO_2} may be greatly increased despite adequate minute ventilation.

The arterial P_{CO_2} during CPR cannot be considered to be a reflection of total body CO_2 homeostasis. No particular comfort can be validly derived from a Pa_{CO_2} less than 40 mm Hg, while Pa_{CO_2} values greater than 40 mm Hg reflect either inadequate minute ventilation or intrapulmonary shunting. True shunting in excess of 25% will be associated with hypoxemia despite high FI_{O_2} values.

Arterial pH

Mixed venous pH (pHv̄) is always less than the arterial pH (pHa). During CPR a pHa of less than 7.2 reflects severe tissue acidosis and is a poor prognostic sign.[161] An alkalemic pHa during CPR is almost always due to low Pa_{CO_2} values and does *not* reflect the tissue acid-base state.[162]

The plasma bicarbonate can be calculated from pH and P_{CO_2} (see chap. 3). Bicarbonate deficiency (metabolic acidosis) will not have a significant disparity between the arterial and venous blood. Therefore, the degree of metabolic acidosis in arterial blood is reflective of total body metabolic acidosis.

Summary

Arterial blood gas measurements during CPR are of limited value compared to the information gained in other clinical circumstances. The acid-base status of arterial blood is an unreliable reflection of total body acid-base balance during CPR, especially when there is an alkalemic arterial pH. Arterial plasma bicarbonate levels should be a reasonable reflection of the venous plasma bicarbonate.

A venous hypercarbia must be assumed during CPR; therefore the arterial Pco_2 cannot be assumed to reflect total body CO_2 homeostasis.

Arterial oxygen content greatly determines oxygenation potential to heart and brain during CPR. Arterial Pa_{O_2} values less than 100 mm Hg with FI_{O_2} values greater than 0.60 suggest either inadequate lung ventilation or significant intrapulmonary shunting.

VENOUS BLOOD GASES DURING CPR

Arterial blood gases are sensitive to rapid changes occurring in the pulmonary capillary bed while mixed venous blood gases are sensitive to changes occurring in the systemic capillary bed. With the exception of cardiovascular collapse, arterial blood gases reasonably reflect the total acid-base balance because the respiratory quotient is reasonably consistent and lung function determines total CO_2 excretion. It appears that during CPR the pH$\bar{v}$ (central venous or pulmonary arterial) may be a better clinical guide to tissue acid-base status than pHa.[163, 164]

BICARBONATE ADMINISTRATION

The intravenous administration of sodium bicarbonate solution is the standard therapy for supporting life-threatening metabolic acidemia (see chaps. 3 and 6). With sodium bicarbonate administration, bicarbonate ions are added to the system only after the "CO_2 load" inherent in the sodium bicarbonate solution is eliminated by the lungs. When sodium bicarbonate is administered to a spontaneously breathing patient with acute respiratory acidosis (acute ventilatory failure), the Pa_{CO_2} usually increases and pHa decreases because the "CO_2 load" cannot be eliminated.

It appears that a similar circumstance occurs during CPR since the cardiac output is limiting CO_2 excretion, namely that $P\bar{v}_{CO_2}$ increases and pH$\bar{v}$ decreases with sodium bicarbonate administration. Further, serum osmolality, serum sodium, and excess bicarbonate ion remain after perfusion has been restored.[165] Some have suggested that if a buffer is used in CPR it should be one that does not increase tissue Pco_2, such as TRIS buffer.[166]

13

Metabolic Abnormalities and Blood Gas Interpretation

The primary purpose of this text is to provide a scientifically based rationale for the *clinical* application of blood gas measurements. In this endeavor we have consistently assumed two circumstances to be true: (1) that peripheral carbon dioxide stores are normal and (2) that normal intracellular metabolic pathways are producing a normal respiratory quotient ($RQ = CO_2$ produced/O_2 consumed $= 0.7$ to 1.0). This chapter addresses clinical circumstances in which one of these assumptions is not valid; namely, when peripheral CO_2 stores are altered or when metabolic pathways other than the Kreb cycle are of significance.

CO_2 STORES OF THE BODY

All tissues are exposed to partial pressures of nitrogen (N_2), oxygen (O_2) and carbon dioxide (CO_2). The existence of these tissue partial pressures dictates that some amount of each gas is "stored" in the tissues. Nitrogen stores change when the inspired fraction of N_2 is altered, as with oxygen therapy (see chap. 7). Oxygen stores change at such rapid rates that steady state conditions are almost always present within the confines of biologic viability. On the other hand, CO_2 stores are influenced by several clinically relevant physiologic mechanisms and change at a relatively slow pace. Therefore, it is fair to state that CO_2 stores are continuously readjusting.

Central CO_2 Stores

Each tissue has its own solubility coefficient for CO_2 as well as its own capability to combine CO_2 chemically. These factors determine the degree to which each tissue can potentially "store" CO_2. The most familiar example of CO_2 stores occurs in blood in which CO_2 content comprises carbamino compounds, the carbonic anhydrase-bicarbonate system, and dissolved CO_2. Carbon dioxide transport (chap. 4) is the usual way we refer to changes in these "central CO_2 stores." The regulation of central CO_2 stores is essentially a lung function (alveolar ventilation) as long as cardiac output is adequate to sustain life (see chap. 12).

Prolonged Apnea

Central CO_2 stores must abruptly increase when lung excretion of CO_2 suddenly diminishes. The extreme of this circumstance is prolonged apnea. Available data in anesthetized patients with sudden apnea show a Pa_{CO_2} increase of 4 to 8 mm Hg in the first minute and a 2 to 3 mm Hg rise each minute thereafter.[167, 168] Recent data in awake volunteers suggest the rise in the first minute may be as great as 12 mm Hg.[169] It would appear reasonable to assume that patients with muscular activity or fever would increase central CO_2 stores at an even greater rate.

Peripheral CO_2 Stores

Peripheral CO_2 stores are estimated to be approximately 110 liters in a 70-kg individual. The vast majority (up to 100 liters) is stored in bone and fat that have relatively poor perfusion. Therefore, significant changes in these stores would be expected to take days. Skeletal muscle represents the next largest component (approximately 5 liters) of peripheral CO_2 stores in which significant changes can occur in hours. Visceral tissue stores account for the remainder in which significant changes can occur within minutes.[170]

The Role of Cardiac Output

Venous P_{CO_2} changes will tend to reflect tissue P_{CO_2} changes since carbon dioxide is produced in the cells. For any given tissue, the difference between arterial and venous P_{CO_2} will be a function of both the rate of CO_2 production and the perfusion. When the total body is assessed, the mixed venous to arterial P_{CO_2} difference is not affected to clinically significant degrees by changes in cardiac output until the perfusion is so poor that CPR is required (see chap. 12). Therefore, with

TABLE 13–1.

Theoretical Relationship of P_{CO_2} Changes When Peripheral CO_2 Stores Are Altered*

CO_2 Stores	Tissue P_{CO_2}	$P\bar{v}_{CO_2}$	PA_{CO_2}	Pa_{CO_2}
Normal	50	46	40	40
Decreased	40	36	30	30
Increased	60	56	50	50

*CO_2 production and minute ventilation are assumed normal.

the exception of CPR, the status of peripheral CO_2 stores is not significantly affected by changes in cardiac output.[171]

The Role of Alveolar Ventilation

When the alveolar P_{CO_2} is abruptly changed, the arterial and mixed venous P_{CO_2} values follow with little delay.[172] This represents an abrupt change in central CO_2 stores, with no significant change in peripheral CO_2 stores.[171] Therefore, changes in alveolar ventilation for less than several hours appear to have little effect on the peripheral CO_2 stores. This fact explains why the arterial and mixed venous P_{CO_2} values can rapidly return to baseline following relatively transient changes in alveolar ventilation.

The Role of Minute Ventilation

Assuming a normal CO_2 production, Table 13–1 demonstrates the relationships between CO_2 stores, minute ventilation, and arterial P_{CO_2}. It should be noted that depleted CO_2 stores allow a normal minute ventilation to result in an unexpectedly low Pa_{CO_2}; conversely, increased CO_2 stores allow a normal minute ventilation to result in a greater Pa_{CO_2} than expected.

DEPLETION OF PERIPHERAL CO_2 STORES

Depletion of peripheral stores occurs when CO_2 excretion exceeds CO_2 production for significant periods of time. Skeletal muscle depletion is seen in a few hours[173] and bone depletion within several days.[174] These changes occur slowly enough that blood gas values at any point in time would reflect CO_2 balance as if a stable equilibrium were present.

Alveolar, arterial, and venous P_{CO_2} values are decreased with significant depletion of peripheral CO_2 stores. The diminished alveolar P_{CO_2} is secondary to diminished tissue CO_2 rather than to an increased alveolar ventilation. Therefore, a normal minute ventilation (and normal physiologic deadspace) will be present in conjunction with a diminished alveolar P_{CO_2} (see chap. 10). Such a patient usually presents with a decreased arterial P_{CO_2} in conjunction with a normal or decreased minute ventilation.

This situation emphasizes the necessity for measuring minute ventilation in conjunction with arterial blood gas measurements in critically ill patients. The following case studies are helpful in identifying the patient with depleted peripheral stores.

Case Study 1

A 17-year-old woman who weighed 143 lb (65 kg) was in the front passenger seat of an automobile involved in a head-on accident with a truck. She was wearing a seat belt without shoulder restraints. Her head struck the windshield and she arrived in the emergency room with a depressed skull fracture and subdural hematoma. No other injuries were evident. She was taken to the operating room for evacuation of the hematoma and elevation of the fracture. An intraventricular catheter was placed for intracranial pressure (ICP) monitoring and the patient was taken to the intensive care unit (ICU). She was unresponsive to deep painful stimuli; ICP was 10 mm Hg; FI_{O_2}, 0.35; rectal temperature, 36.5°C; and breathing, spontaneous. The following vital signs and blood gas values were noted:

BP	110/80 mm Hg	pHa	7.52
P	95/min	Pa_{CO_2}	28 mm Hg
RR	22/min	Pa_{O_2}	120 mm Hg
V_T	800 ml	Sa_{O_2}	98%
MV	17.6 L	Hb	12 gm%

Her mental status did not improve over the next two days. She remained stable with ICP values less than 10 mm Hg. Forty-eight hours postoperatively the patient's rectal temperature was 37°C. At FI_{O_2} 0.35, the following were noted:

BP	115/80 mm Hg	pHa	7.51
P	88/min	Pa_{CO_2}	30 mm Hg
RR	17/min	Pa_{O_2}	85 mm Hg
V_T	500 ml	Sa_{O_2}	97%
MV	8.5 L	Hb	11 gm%

The arterial P_{CO_2} remained 28 to 30 mm Hg over 48 hours despite the minute ventilation decreasing by almost 50%. The initial MV of 17.6 L in conjunction with a Pa_{CO_2} of 28 mm Hg is expected (see chap. 6). However, 48 hours later without any apparent change in CO_2 production (body temperature constant, vital signs constant), an 8.5-L MV maintains a Pa_{CO_2} of 30 mm Hg. The best explanation for this circumstance is that the initial hyperventilation excreted more CO_2 than was produced long enough for peripheral CO_2 stores (probably skeletal muscle and bone tissue) to be depleted.

Case Study 2

An 87-year-old woman weighing 110 lb (50 kg) was found comatose on the kitchen floor by her granddaughter who had talked with her 36 hours previously, at which time she seemed normal. There was no evidence found of head injury or myocardial ischemia. Rectal temperature was 36°C. The following values were noted: serum glucose 125 mg%; BUN 12 mg%; Na$^+$ 132 mEq/L; Cl$^-$ 100 mEq/L; K$^+$ 3.2 mEq/L; CO_2 27 mEq/L. With the patient receiving 2 liters by nasal cannula, the following determinations were made:

BP	105/70 mm Hg	pHa	7.53
P	110/min	Pa_{CO_2}	26 mm Hg
RR	15/min	Pa_{O_2}	74 mm Hg
VT	260 ml	Sa_{O_2}	95%
MV	3.9 L	Hb	9.5 gm%

Her MV is probably low normal for her size and age, yet the Pa_{CO_2} is 26 mm Hg. An acute respiratory alkalosis to this extent should be accompanied by a minute volume at least twice normal (see chap. 6). Despite mild hypothermia there is no reason to suspect that metabolic rate is decreased by more than 10%. It is reasonable to assume that this woman was hyperventilating for a number of hours before being found and thus depleted her peripheral CO_2 stores.

Patients such as this tend to replete the peripheral CO_2 stores within several days after regaining consciousness. The reversal process is important because as the stores are repleted either (1) the Pa_{CO_2} must increase and thereby cerebral vasodilation occurs, or (2) the minute ventilation must increase to maintain the lower Pa_{CO_2}. If the cerebrodilation does not create increased ICP the patient will have no problem as Pa_{CO_2} approaches 40 mm Hg. If cerebral vasodilation will create increased ICP and the patient has the ventilatory reserves to increase MV, the Pa_{CO_2} may remain low despite peripheral CO_2 store repletion. If the patient cannot increase ventilatory work readily, significant cardiopulmonary and CNS deterioration may result from repletion of CO_2 stores. Appropriate interpretation of the blood gas values can alert the clinician to these potential dangers.

INCREASED PERIPHERAL CO_2 STORES

Chronic hypercarbia is most commonly seen in patients with chronic obstructive pulmonary disease (COPD). However, it is also seen with chronic restrictive pulmonary disease, morbid obesity (Pickwickian syndrome), and rare CNS disorders.

Chronic CO_2 retention (compensated respiratory acidosis) must involve increased peripheral CO_2 stores. Such patients are able to maintain CO_2 homeostasis (lung excretion equal to cellular production) while maintaining an increased alveolar P_{CO_2}.

Chronic hypercarbia involves intracellular adaptation to increased P_{CO_2}. It appears that such adaptation involves maintenance of mitochondrial function despite intracellular acidosis due to increased intracellular P_{CO_2}. Extracellular acid-base balance is maintained by accumulating an increased bicarbonate ion concentration and a chloride ion deficiency. Available data suggest that water and chloride ion shifts between intracellular and extracellular spaces results in a slightly greater extracellular pH than that in the normal population.[175] Stable chronic hypercarbia is most commonly seen in conjunction with arterial pH values above 7.40 (for further discussion, see chap. 7).

ABERRANT INTRACELLULAR METABOLISM

Increases and decreases in metabolic rate are seen with temperature variation, thyroid dysfunction, and physical activity. These represent quantitative metabolic changes since intracellular pathways remain essentially normal. The general rules applied to interpretation of arterial pH, P_{CO_2}, and P_{O_2} remain valid when only metabolic *rate* is altered since the homeostatic relationship of CO_2 production to O_2 consumption remains constant.

Arterial blood gas interpretation requires additional considerations when intracellular metabolism involves aberrant pathways to a significant extent. Specifically, this becomes clinically relevant with sepsis, lactic acidosis, and parenteral hyperalimentation.

Sepsis

Infection is a common occurrence in critically ill patients and sepsis is a common complication of infection. Sepsis usually involves cellular metabolic dysfunction secondary to systemic circulation of bacterial toxins.

A typical example of hyperdynamic sepsis is a 42-year-old woman with a long history of pelvic inflammatory disease. She is febrile to 40°C and has periodic shaking chills. Arterial blood gas determinations with the patient on room air:

BP	80/30 mm Hg	pHa	7.51
P	120/min	Pa_{CO_2}	29 mm Hg
RR	20/min	Pa_{O_2}	90 mm Hg
VT	600 ml	HCO_3^-	24 mEq/L
MV	12 L	BE	0 mEq/L

Acute alveolar hyperventilation (acute respiratory alkalosis) is most commonly seen with the hyperdynamic phase of septic shock. Blood lactate levels are seldom increased and therefore a significant component of metabolic acidosis is rare.

Hyperdynamic sepsis ("warm shock") involves a decreased oxygen extraction [$C_{(a-v)}O_2$] secondary to decreased oxidative metabolism and systemic arterial to venous shunting.[176] This results in an increased $S\bar{v}_{O_2}$ and thereby an improved arterial oxygenation status (see chap. 8).

The major problem in interpreting blood gases in the patient with hyperdynamic septic shock is that oxygen extraction is decreased independent of the adequacy of cellular oxygenation. The variability of oxygen extraction makes the relationship between arterial PO_2 and tissue oxygenation unpredictable and unreliable.

"Cold septic shock" involves cellular hypoperfusion and manifests blood gases similar to most hypoperfusion states, i.e., increased Pa_{CO_2} and decreased Pa_{O_2}.

Lactic Acidosis

Kreb cycle metabolism requires oxygen utilization and produces CO_2 as the major metabolite. Anaerobic metabolic pathways are less efficient in calorie production but, most importantly, produce hydrogen and lactate ions as metabolites. Thus, inadequate availability of oxygen at the mitochondrial level results in anaerobic metabolism and lactic acid production. The most common cause of anaerobic metabolism is cellular hypoperfusion, clinically referred to as "shock" (hypovolemic, cardiac, septic). Hypoxemia and anemia may potentially produce anaerobic metabolism by themselves, but usually they are combined with a degree of cellular hypoperfusion.

The cellular production of lactic acid is difficult to quantify by laboratory analysis of arterial or central venous blood because organ system perfusion and hepatic function are variable. An adequately oxygenated and perfused liver is dramatically capable of metabolizing lactic acid to carbonic acid. Thus, if some organ systems (e.g., muscle, gastrointestinal tract, skin) produce lactic acid, normal hepatic function may prevent significant accumulation of lactic acid in the core circulation.

The presence of increased blood lactate levels documents the presence of anaerobic metabolism. However, the absence of blood lactate does not infer the absence of anaerobic metabolism. Metabolic acidosis in a patient with severe hypoxemia and/or poor perfusion status must be assumed to be lactic acidotic until proved otherwise. The absence of metabolic acidosis in such a patient should never be interpreted as the absence of anaerobic metabolism!

Severe shivering is a good example of regional lactic acidosis. The extreme increase in skeletal muscle activity rapidly creates anaerobic metabolism and lactic acid production. However, arterial blood will seldom manifest lactic acidosis within the first few minutes. The best explanation is that an adequately perfused liver metabolizes the lactic acid.

The typical arterial blood gases in a shivering patient will manifest hypoxemia due to the increased oxygen consumption unless supplemental inspired oxygen is provided. The transiently increased CO_2 production with shivering is concomitant with the muscle spasms hindering ventilation. This often results in an acute respiratory acidosis.

The presence of metabolic acidemia secondary to lactic acid in a patient with shock, seizures, or shivering is a dire circumstance. The absence of metabolic acidemia infers that vital organs may still be reasonably oxygenated, but by no means is that a certainty.

Parenteral Hyperalimentation

Carbohydrates and proteins have an RQ of 1.0, whereas lipids have an RQ of 0.7. The Kreb cycle in humans averages 0.8 because carbohydrates, proteins, and fats are all normally utilized. Hypertonic glucose solution is usually the principal source of nonprotein calories with total peripheral nutrition (TPN) and leads to an increased level of CO_2 production because the excess glucose must be stored as lipid. Since the metabolic pathway changing carbohydrate to fat has a very high respiratory quotient (approaching 8.0), the overall respiratory quotient significantly increases independent of the relatively stable RQ producing metabolic energy. Patients receiving TPN in which the nonprotein source is glucose will often have an increased CO_2 production. This can be remedied by providing sufficient nonprotein calories as lipid.[177-179]

Patients with increased CO_2 production are required to increase minute ventilation to maintain a normal alveolar P_{CO_2}. In patients receiving TPN, this potentially produces an MV-P_{CO_2} disparity similar to that seen with increased deadspace ventilation (see chap. 10).

14

Common Clinical Causes of Abnormal Blood Gases

Common clinical diseases from the standpoint of blood gas measurement are discussed in this chapter. The diseases are considered in accordance with the following outline (which includes page numbers for future reference):

I. METABOLIC ACID-BASE IMBALANCE

Metabolic acid-base imbalance is common in the critically ill patient. Unfortunately, it is often missed or misjudged clinically until the condition is severe. The clinical availability of blood gas measurements has allowed direct measurement of blood pH and Pco_2. Ready access to this information has allowed the clinician to be alerted to minor changes in pH and blood base. Thus, most of the mystery and complexity that formerly surrounded clinical acid-base imbalance has been removed.

Acidosis and alkalosis are pathophysiologic processes in which the normal quantities of acid and base are skewed (see chap. 3). When metabolic *acidemia* or *alkalemia* is present, it denotes that the metabolic process is *uncompensated*. We have delineated clinically significant *acidemia* as an arterial pH below 7.30 (see chap. 6); it may be life-threatening by itself because: (1) enzyme systems do not function properly; (2) myocardial and central nervous system electrophysiology may be interferred with; (3) electrolyte balance may be acutely upset; (4) acute pulmonary hypertension may be manifested; and (5) autonomic receptors may not react predictably to exogenous drugs. Clinically significant *alkalemia* has been delineated as a pH of more than 7.50 and in and of itself may be threatening to life-supporting systems.

The support and correction of metabolic acidemia and metabolic alkalemia are clinical questions separate from the therapy for the underlying pathophysiologic processes of metabolic acidosis and metabolic alkalosis. At this time, we shall consider the common causes of metabolic acidosis and metabolic alkalosis. Keep in mind that the severity of the accompanying acidemia or alkalemia must be considered as a separate clinical question.

A. Metabolic Acidosis

This is the result of the loss of blood base or the accumulation of excessive nonvolative blood acid, or both. With the exception of lactic acidosis, metabolic acidosis is rarely due to primary pulmonary disease. It usually elicits a compensatory alveolar hyperventilation (decreased Pa_{CO_2}). Hypoxemia is rare as long as the cardiovascular status remains adequate.

Typical Room Air Blood Gases
pH   Below 7.40
P_{CO_2} Below 40 mm Hg
P_{O_2} Above 80 mm Hg
Plasma bicarbonate usually less than normal.
Base excess always negative.
Typical Ventilatory Pattern
V_T Eupnea (normal depth) or hyperpnea (deeper than normal)
RR   Tachypnea (rapid frequency)
MV   Above normal
General Response to Oxygen Therapy
1. Dramatic increase in Pa_{O_2}.
2. Ventilatory state relatively unchanged.
Evaluation of Tissue Oxygenation
1. Oxygen content decreased from normal (shift to the right).
2. Cardiovascular status is the prime determinant of tissue oxygenation.
3. If hypoxemia is present, *hypoxia must be assumed.*

1. Renal Failure (Renal Tubular Acidosis).—The inadequate renal function means that the normal metabolic waste products are not being excreted adequately. Depending on whether the problem is tubular or glomerular, some combination of accumulation of blood acid and decrease of blood base occurs.[180] Primarily there is a disruption of hydrogen ion excretion.

When the diagnosis of renal failure or renal tubular acidosis is made, attention must be paid to the patient's ability to compensate by increasing ventilatory work. A lack of adequate ventilatory reserve or the onset of fatigue could make the acidosis far more life-threatening.

Renal acidosis is generally slow in onset and is seldom accompanied by a significant acidemia.

2. Keto-Acidosis (Diabetic Acidosis or Starvation).—Normal cellular metabolism requires both glucose and oxygen to produce energy. Insulin is essential for the transport of glucose into the cell. When the diabetic patient has a deficit of blood insulin, the glucose cannot adequately enter the cell; therefore, alternative cellular pathways of metabolism are used. The same process occurs when glucose is unavailable due to starvation. The metabolites of the alternative pathways are ketones and the result is a keto-acidosis (see chap. 3).

This patient is usually capable of generating a great deal of ventilatory work, and therefore achieves a state of hyperpnea (deep breaths) and tachypnea (rapid breathing)—referred to as *Kussmaul breathing*. This typical "hyperventilation" of diabetic acidosis is an important diagnostic sign.

3. Lactic Acidosis.—Metabolism continues through metabolic pathways known as *anaerobic pathways* when oxygen is not available to tissues (see chaps. 3 and 12). The metabolic products of these pathways—lactate ion and hydrogen ion—form a nonvolatile acid (lactic acid) in the blood, which has a profound effect on the blood pH.

A severe drop in cardiac output, circulatory shutdown, or severe hypoxemia may result in the accumulation of lactic acid.[181] This is the rule in the patient with profound cardiopulmonary collapse! Lactic acidosis usually dissipates rapidly with the reestablishment of circulation, ventilation, and oxygenation.

B. Metabolic Alkalosis

Metabolic alkalosis is quite common in the critically ill patient. Although not as directly life-threatening as metabolic acidosis, metabolic alkalosis has a dire potential. The immediate compensatory mechanism for metabolic alkalosis is a decrease in ventilatory work (compensatory alveolar hypoventilation); this compensation may be severe enough to cause hypoxemia. It is rare for metabolic alkalosis to cause a "significant" decrease in alveolar ventilation in an alert patient; the tendency is for the alkalemia to remain uncompensated. In the unconscious, semicomatose, or severely debilitated patient, however, metabolic alkalosis may precipitate a marked alveolar hypoventilation.[182]

Typical Room Air Blood Gases
 pH   Above 7.40
 Pco_2 Above 40 mm Hg
 Po_2 60–100 mm Hg
 Plasma bicarbonate usually above normal.
 Base excess always positive.
Typical Ventilatory Pattern
 V_T Usually eupnea or mild hypopnea (shallow breaths)
 RR   Normal or bradypnea (slow frequency)
General Response to Oxygen Therapy
 1. Dramatic increase in Pa_{O_2}.
 2. Ventilatory state relatively unchanged.
Evaluation of Tissue Oxygenation
 1. Oxygen content increased (shift to the left); hemoglobin-oxygen affinity increased.
 2. If significant hypoxemia is present, the tissue oxygenation state depends on the adequacy of the cardiovascular system.

   1. Hypokalemia.—This condition most commonly occurs after several days of intravenous therapy in which potassium replacement has been inadequate. Diuretic therapy and diarrhea are other common causes of hypokalemia.
   Total body potassium depletion results in metabolic alkalosis by two important mechanisms:

   a. The kidneys attempt to conserve potassium, resulting in hydrogen ion excretion and a concomitant increase in blood base.
   b. Potassium (K^+) is the major intracellular cation. Total body depletion induces intracellular potassium to enter the extracellular space in an attempt to maintain near-normal serum levels. As potassium leaves the cell, hydrogen ion must enter. This leads to an increase in blood base.

The measurement of abnormally low potassium ion contents in the serum (hypokalemia) usually reflects a severe depletion of total body potassium. Low normal levels of serum potassium may be maintained in the presence of significant total body potassium depletion. Thus, the metabolic alkalosis (and other manifestations of potassium depletion) may be present while *serum* potassium levels are maintained in the low normal range. As a general rule, abnormally low potassium levels (hypokalemia) reflect a *severe* loss of total body potassium.

Clinically, hypokalemia is manifested as (1) metabolic alkalosis, (2) muscular weakness, and (3) cardiac arrhythmia. *This is a most significant triad in a patient with a borderline ventilatory reserve.* In addition, potassium deficit may precipitate digitalis intoxication.

2. Hypochloremia.—The chloride ion (Cl^-) is the major anion of the body electrolytes; when depleted, the bicarbonate ion must increase in concentration to maintain electric balance with the cations. Thus, decreased blood chloride concentration usually leads to increased blood bicarbonate concentrations.

In addition, the chloride ion is the major exchangeable anion for the renal tubules. If adequate chloride ion is not available, tubular exchange is hindered and usually results in additional potassium loss.[183,184]

3. Gastric Suction or Vomiting.—The primary insult is loss of hydrochloric acid (HCl), but this is soon compounded by potassium loss in the kidney and the gastrointestinal tract.

A common mistake is to attempt to reverse this metabolic alkalosis by the administration of ammonium chloride. This adds to sodium and potassium loss, and the patient deteriorates. Replacement of chloride, water, and potassium will allow the kidneys to reverse the metabolic alkalosis.[183]

4. Massive Administration of Steroids.—This is not unusual therapy in critically ill patients. High doses of sodium-retaining steroids lead to accelerated excretion of hydrogen ion and potassium in the distal tubules of the kidney, and the result is metabolic alkalosis. Steroid preparations such as methylprednisolone sodium succinate (Solumedrol) have little tendency to retain sodium and therefore manifest little, if any, metabolic alkalosis problems in massive doses.

5. Sodium Bicarbonate Administration.—Metabolic alkalosis often occurs after cardiopulmonary resuscitation. Although many factors are involved, one must consider excessive administration of sodium bicarbonate a major factor. However, intact kidneys have a great ability to excrete the excess bicarbonate—as long as there is no potassium depletion.

II. ALVEOLAR HYPERVENTILATION (RESPIRATORY ALKALOSIS)

Alveolar hyperventilation may or may not be secondary to pulmonary disease. Blood gas analysis is most helpful in delineating the cause because there are only *three physiologic causes of alveolar hyperventilation:* (1) chemoreceptor response to arterial hypoxemia, (2) ventilatory response to metabolic acidosis, and (3) central nervous system malfunction.

Alveolar Hyperventilation Due to Hypoxemia.—This is typically a Pa_{CO_2} between 25 and 35 mm Hg, accompanied by a moderate hypoxemia; i.e., the room air Pa_{O_2} is between 40 and 80 mm Hg. To help determine whether the hypoxemia is the cause of the alveolar hyperventilation, one must test the response to oxygen therapy. If the alveolar hyperventilation is secondary to a responsive hypoxemia, oxygen therapy will:

1. Decrease alveolar ventilation; i.e., arterial carbon dioxide tension will increase toward normal and the work of breathing will decrease.
2. Decrease the heart rate if tachycardia is present.
3. Decrease the blood pressure if hypertension is present.

Arterial oxygen tensions will seldom increase above 80 mm Hg with proper oxygen therapy.

Alveolar Hyperventilation Due to Metabolic Acidosis.—This is due to the homeostatic response of attempting to create a respiratory alkalemia to normalize the acid pH. The blood gas findings should immediately reveal the situation: the pH will be less than 7.40, plasma bicarbonate will be less than normal, and the base deficit will be significant. These findings are to be interpreted as *metabolic acidosis*, since that is the primary pathophysiology. The ventilatory response—alveolar hyperventilation—is secondary.

Alveolar Hyperventilation Due to "Central Causes".—This category is reached only after the first two have been ruled out. Such factors as trauma, central nervous system infection, primary brain lesions, systemic sepsis, lung stretch receptor stimulation, and central nervous system depression may lead to central nervous system stimulation of ventilation. As a general rule, these patients do not have pulmonary disease, and in response to oxygen therapy they have dramatic rises in arterial P_{O_2} with little change in ventilatory status.

Immediate clinical assessment of alveolar hyperventilation must center on cardiopulmonary reserve, inasmuch as both the work of breathing and myocardial work are increased. Supportive measures such as oxygen therapy must be instituted while rapid diagnosis of the underlying disease process is being carried out. We will consider the disease entities under three main headings: (1) acute alveolar hyperventilation with hypoxemia, (2) chronic alveolar hyperventilation with hypoxemia, and (3) alveolar hyperventilation without hypoxemia.

A. Acute Alveolar Hyperventilation With Hypoxemia

Typical Room Air Blood Gases
  pH   Above 7.50
  Pco_2 Below 35 mm Hg; below 30 mm Hg when clinically
                significant
  Po_2 40–80 mm Hg
  Plasma bicarbonate within normal range.
  Base excess within normal range.
Typical Ventilatory Pattern
  V_T Hyperpnea (deep)
  RR   Tachypnea (rapid)
  MV   Greater than normal
  Dyspnea frequent.
General Response to Oxygen Therapy
  1. Little rise in Pa_{O_2}.
  2. Decreased ventilatory work (increased Pa_{O_2}).
  3. Decreased myocardial work.
Evaluation of Tissue Oxygenation
  Hypoxia is rare as long as ventilatory and myocardial reserves do
    not fail.

1. Acute Pulmonary Disease.—This category includes pneumonia and atelectasis, adult respiratory distress syndrome (ARDS), and acute asthma.

a. Pneumonia and Atelectasis.—When acute alveolar hyperventilation with hypoxemia is due to an acute pulmonary disease, it is most commonly due to a combination of pneumonia and atelectasis. Almost all acute pulmonary diseases lead to inflammatory changes in the tracheobronchial tree and the alveoli; and this in turn leads to collapse of alveoli, pooling of secretions, and uneven distribution of ventilation. The resulting intrapulmonary shunt causes arterial hypoxemia. The ventilatory system increases its work to compensate for the hypoxemia and in so doing causes a decrease in arterial P_{CO_2}.

The following are groups of patients who commonly manifest pneumonia and atelactasis. These, of course, are in addition to the large number of patients who have primary pulmonary infection.

1.   Patients who have had abdominal or thoracic operations are unable to breathe as deeply or cough as effectively as they were able to do before operation; i.e., vital capacity is greatly decreased.[185] The disability is due primarily to peritoneal irritation, and it results in the pooling of normally produced secretions and the collapse of alveoli at the base of the lung. This combination of microatelectasis and pneumonia is often called *stasis pneumonia*. Acute alveolar hyperventilation with hypoxemia is common in the first several postoperative days.[186] Oxygen therapy may be indicated during this period, as is proper bronchial hygiene therapy.

2. Traumatized patients manifest similar pulmonary problems. If the trauma is causing pain that restricts the ability to cough and to breathe deeply, or if the trauma is to the central nervous system so that the patient has been rendered unconscious, microatelectasis and pneumonia will eventually occur. This may be avoided by *early* application of proper respiratory therapy.

3. Patients with neurologic diseases may have muscular weakness that produces an inability to cough and deep breathe effectively. This leads to atelectasis and pneumonia if aggressive respiratory therapy is not instituted.

4. Patients who aspirate foreign bodies into the tracheobronchial tree have significant atelectasis and, eventually, pneumonia.

5. Segmental or lobar atelectasis is common in many debilitated patients. The sudden onset of fever, dyspnea, and hypoxemia are the usual clinical signs of an acute major atelectasis. The blood gas measurements usually show acute alveolar hyperventilation with hypoxemia.

b. Adult Respiratory Distress Syndrome (ARDS).—This general syndrome is described under many names in the medical literature. Among the best-known descriptive terms are posttraumatic pulmonary insufficiency, shock lung, stiff lung, oxygen toxicity, and ventilator lung. It has been recently described as the severe end of a disease spectrum named Acute Lung Injury.[86, 87] ARDS usually starts as an insidious onset of alveolar hyperventilation and increasing hypoxemia that eventually leads to ventilatory failure.[187]

c. Acute Asthma.—The asthmatic patient in the acute phase has a sudden increase in airway resistance due to bronchospasm and thick, tenacious secretions. Unevenness of distribution of ventilation creates a great deal of venous admixture, which results in a mild arterial hypoxemia. The patient usually is capable of producing enough ventilatory work to provide an increased alveolar ventilation in response to the hypoxemia. *Air trapping* further increases the work of breathing.

The acute asthmatic who is retaining carbon dioxide is undergoing extreme fatigue that threatens his life; in other words, *ventilatory failure in the acute asthmatic is a dire circumstance.*[188] The acute asthmatic attack is typified by acute alveolar hyperventilation with hypoxemia.

2. Acute Myocardial Disease.— In acute myocardial disease, the blood gases usually are close to normal or else show acute alveolar hyperventilation with hypoxemia. The primary cardiopulmonary manifestation of the acute myocardial insult is a decreased cardiac output. Because the metabolic rate stays the same while the capillary blood flow rate deceases, there is a drop in mixed venous oxygen content (see chaps. 5, 7, and 9); therefore, any preexisting intrapulmonary shunt has a far greater hypoxemic effect on the arterial blood. Inasmuch as the cardiovascular system is not capable of readily increasing cardiac output in response to the hypoxemia, the ventilatory system attempts to compensate by increasing the alveolar ventilation. The result is acute alveolar hyperventilation with hypoxemia.

The following is a discussion of the most common cardiopulmonary problems of primary myocardial disease causing acute alveolar hyperventilation with hypoxemia.

a. Acute Myocardial Infarction.—The typical blood gases of a patient with an acute myocardial infarction may be near normal or else show acute alveolar hyperventilation with mild hypoxemia. The hypoxemic patient has a tachypnea and a mild hyperpnea, along with a tachycardia and usually mild hypertension (although hypotension is not uncommon). The ventilatory system is doing much of the compensatory work in response to the hypoxemia, which is secondary to venous admixture plus decreased central venous oxygen content.

These patients benefit greatly from proper oxygen therapy, even when hypoxemia is mild.[189] The benefit is believed to be twofold: a decreased work demand on the injured myocardium and a decreased demand for ventilatory work.

b. Pulmonary Edema.—This entity actually consists of two separate clinical problems.

1. Various diseases can cause an accumulation of fluid in the al-veolar-capillary space—the condition known as *interstitial pulmonary edema*.[190] This can be secondary to either cardiogenic or noncardiogenic pathology.[86] The result is oxygen diffusion impedance and decreased lung compliance. This basic diffusion problem results in a mild arterial hypoxemia, to which the cardiovascular and ventilatory systems respond by increasing work. In many instances, the cardiovascular system is unable to respond to any great degree; therefore, most of the compensatory work is undertaken by the ventilatory system. Obviously, then, alveolar ventilation is greatly increased, and the result is acute alveolar hyperventilation with hypoxemia. The overall response to oxygen therapy is usually dramatic.

2. In *alveolar pulmonary edema*, a transudation of fluid into the al-veolar spaces occurs.[86] The condition may therefore be considered the severe form of interstitial edema. Four basic mechanisms can contribute to this edema: (*a*) increased pulmonary capillary hydrostatic pressure secondary to left ventricular failure or a marked increase in pulmonary artery pressure without arteriolar constriction; (*b*) decreased oncotic pressure in the pulmonary capillary blood, secondary to hypoproteinemia and related diseases; (*c*) decreased alveolar pressures, secondary to upper airway obstruction; and (*d*) destruction of or damage to the alveolar-capillary membrane, secondary to an insult such as inhalation burn.

By far the most common cause of alveolar pulmonary edema is left ventricular failure.[190] The respiratory supportive measures in any pulmonary edema are basically two: proper oxygen therapy and positive-pressure ventilation.

Bubbles forming in the alveoli and the bronchi are the immediate problem in alveolar pulmonary edema. The foaming prevents much of the air that is moving in and out of the lungs from exchanging with the pulmonary blood. In an attempt to overcome the decreased oxygen tension in the "trapped" alveolar air, the pulmonary system attempts to increase air exchange. Thus, alveolar pulmonary edema usually presents as acute alveolar hyperventilation with severe hypoxemia.

In addition to specific corrective measures, there are general respiratory supportive measures that usually help the patient in alveolar pulmonary edema: oxygen therapy, positive-pressure, and alcohol inhalation.

When the insult is beyond the compensating capability of the cardiopulmonary system, acute ventilatory failure ensues—demanding far different therapy.[191] The differentiation of alveolar hyperventilation from acute ventilatory failure in the pulmonary edema patient is by blood gas measurement; clinical examination will not always correlate.

c. Acute Heart Failure.—The basic cardiopulmonary physiologic insult in heart failure is decreased cardiac output in the face of an unchanged metabolic demand. The central venous oxygen content is decreased, and in turn this increases the hypoxemic effect of any preexisting shunt. Because the heart is unable to increase cardiac output in response to the hypoxemic challenge, the ventilatory system responds by increasing alveolar ventilation.

Circumstances differ somewhat, depending on whether the right or the left ventricle has failed:

1. In cases of *right ventricular failure*, the alveolar hyperventilation does *not* mean the patient is in respiratory distress or dyspneic. In fact, this is uncommon in right ventricular failure.

If blood gases are abnormal in right ventricular failure, the abnormality usually is acute alveolar hyperventilation with hypoxemia. If significant venous admixture exists, oxygen therapy may make a dramatic improvement in the arterial Po_2. However, this may make little difference in the state of tissue hypoxia, because tissue hypoxia is primarily dependent on cardiac output and tissue perfusion.

2. In addition to decreased cardiac output, *left ventricular failure* usually includes interstitial or alveolar pulmonary edema. It is the alveolar pulmonary edema that causes respiratory distress and dyspnea in left ventricular failure.

Tissue hypoxia is far more common in left ventricular failure, because poor perfusion of tissues is more common.

d. Effects of Cardiopulmonary Bypass.—Extracorporeal circulation (heart-lung bypass) has many physiologic complications. Generally, the lungs react to this insult by temporarily decreasing the production of surfactant. The decreased compliance, added to the peripheral vascular effects of the bypass, commonly causes a state of alveolar hyperventilation in the early postoperative period. The hyperventilation usually is accompanied by a moderate hypoxemia and a mild acidemia.

It must be remembered that alveolar hyperventilation and hypoxemia are the rule, not the exception, following heart-lung bypass. Because alkalemic pH is not the rule, this entity is not actually an acute alveolar hyperventilation; however, the alveolar hyperventilation and the hypoxemia place it here more appropriately than elsewhere.

B. Chronic Alveolar Hyperventilation With Hypoxemia

Typical Room Air Blood Gases
    pH   7.40–7.50
    P_{CO_2} Below 30 mm Hg
    P_{O_2} Below 70 mm Hg
    Plasma bicarbonate below normal range
    Base excess below normal range
Typical Ventilatory Pattern
    V_T Shallow (hypopnea)
    RR   Tachypnea
General Response to Oxygen Therapy
    1. Ventilatory status may change dramatically.
    2. Cardiovascular status may change dramatically.
    3. Little change in Pa_{O_2}.
Evaluation of Tissue Oxygenation
    Hypoxia is rare as long as perfusion status remains adequate.

Chronic alveolar hyperventilation with hypoxemia is usually due to a primary pulmonary disease that is long-standing. The cardiovascular and hepatorenal systems usually have adequate reserve⁻ to compensate for the pulmonary state.

1. Postoperative Conditions.—It is common to find patients in chronic alveolar hyperventilation with hypoxemia after the second postoperative day. Any degree of pulmonary atelectasis and pneumonia causes an alveolar hyperventilation, for which the renal system will compensate in several days. Such postoperative patients usually require proper oxygen therapy in spite of their apparently excellent clinical cardiopulmonary status. Routine evaluation for respiratory therapy is indicated.

2. Chronic Heart Failure.— This is essentially the same as acute heart failure, except that the renal system has compensated and the alveolar hyperventilation with hypoxemia is now in the presence of a normal or near-normal pH. These patients have little ability to meet physiologic stress, because both the cardiac reserve and the ventilatory reserve are severely limited.

3. Adult Cystic Fibrosis.—This disease is an interesting physiologic study: a severe chronic obstructive pulmonary disease in combination with a very resilient cardiovascular system. Experience with these patients is limited, but they appear to follow a course of chronic alveolar hyperventilation with hypoxemia.[192] The advent of carbon dioxide retention is believed to be primarily due to failure of the myocardial reserve. This occurs when the pulmonary disease is so severe that total cardiopulmonary collapse is at hand. Thus, in these patients, carbon dioxide retention is a dire circumstance, and death usually occurs within one year of onset.

4. Third-Trimester Pregnancy.—The normal respiratory physiology in the third trimester of pregnancy is a restrictive disease;[193] the vital capacity and the total lung capacity have been diminished. With the decrease in residual volume and the functional residual capacity, there is a decrease in physiologic deadspace, and this causes arterial carbon dioxide tensions to fall below normal.[194] (It is also the reason these patients undergo induction of general anesthesia so rapidly.) Various endocrine changes have been postulated to play a role in the decreased arterial carbon dioxide tension.

The mild hypoxemic state is probably secondary to basilar atelectasis and hypoventilation, which result from the restriction of diaphragm movement by the large abdominal mass. The normal blood gas baseline in late pregnancy is chronic alveolar hyperventilation with mild hypoxemia.

5. Noncardiopulmonary Disease.—A number of diseases can prevent normal lungs from functioning properly. Such diseases result in hypoventilation of certain portions of the lung. This hypoventilation creates venous admixture. The resulting hypoxemia is compensated both by increased cardiac output and by increased alveolar ventilation. Such patients usually manifest chronic alveolar hyperventilation with hypoxemia, and all have a decreased ventilatory reserve. We categorize the diseases as follows:

    a. Diseases causing limitation of ventilatory muscular mechanics:
        (1) Neuromuscular disease—e.g., poliomyelitis, peripheral neuritis, myasthenia gravis, porphyria, spinal cord injury.

(2) Skeletal muscle disease—e.g., muscular dystrophy, myotonia.
  b. Disease limiting thoracic expansion—e.g., kyphoscoliosis. Body casts and rib fracture may also have this effect.
  c. Disease limiting descent of the diaphragm—e.g., peritonitis, abdominal tumor, ascites.

C. Alveolar Hyperventilation Without Hypoxemia

Alveolar hyperventilation without hypoxemia is rarely due to primary pulmonary or cardiac disease. In other words, the alveolar hyperventilation is in response to some physiologic stimulus other than hypoxemia. The stimulus may be central nervous system stimulation or insufficient oxygen *supply* to peripheral chemoreceptors—i.e., decreased oxygen-carrying capacity.

Typical Room Air Blood Gases
  pH   Above 7.40
  P_{CO_2} Below 30 mm Hg
  P_{O_2} Above minimal normal
Typical Ventilatory Pattern
  V_T Eupnea or hyperpnea
  RR   Tachypnea
General Response to Oxygen Therapy
  1. Dramatic increase in Pa_{O_2}.
  2. No significant cardiovascular or ventilatory change.
Evaluation of Tissue Oxygenation
  1. Hypoxia may be present.
  2. Oxygen transport *must* be evaluated.

1. Anxiety, Neurosis, Psychosis.—A common cause of alveolar hyperventilation without hypoxemia is *acute anxiety*, which may be aroused by the drawing of the arterial blood, by a fear of doctors or of hospitals, and by other factors. This is always an *acute* alveolar hyperventilation.

True emotional disease may cause hyperventilation; this is more commonly *chronic* alveolar hyperventilation. These patients tend to be on numerous drugs, which often interreact and cause hyperventilation. Cardiopulmonary disease is rare in this kind of patient; therefore, the alveolar hyperventilation is usually without hypoxemia.

2. Pain.—If it does not directly restrict ventilation, pain commonly produces severe anxiety with resultant hyperventilation. There is good evidence to support the belief that afferent pain impulses directly stimulate the respiratory centers. This usually is *acute* alveolar hyperventilation without hypoxemia.

3. Central Nervous System Disease.—Most intracranial disease stimulates ventilation (provided it does not produce coma). The lungs are usually nondiseased and therefore hypoxemia is rare.

4. Anemia.—In addition to acidemia, the peripheral chemoreceptors are usually stimulated by factors that cause a reduction of the *oxygen supply* such as:

    a. Decreased arterial P_{O_2}.
    b. Decreased oxygen content.
    c. Decreased blood flow.

A significantly decreased hemoglobin content places the major burden of tissue oxygenation on cardiac output; i.e., more blood must be circulated per unit of time. The chemoreceptors are more sensitive to lack of oxygen supply than are other tissues, and therefore they will be stimulated prior to other tissues experiencing hypoxia. There is reason to believe that chemoreceptor stimulation plays a major role in stimulating the myocardium to increase cardiac output when the arterial oxygen content is low.

5. Carbon Monoxide Poisoning.—The carbon monoxide molecule has a great affinity for hemoglobin; it preferentially ties up hemoglobin sites and so prevents oxygen from attaching. Thus, carbon monoxide decreases the amount of hemoglobin available for carrying oxygen and, in so doing, decreases the oxygen content. In addition, carbon monoxide in the blood causes the hemoglobin dissociation curve to shift to the left and thus makes the available hemoglobin far less willing to give up oxygen to the tissues.[195]

III. DEADSPACE DISEASES

The deadspace diseases must be discussed separately, because they produce blood gas values that are meaningless if they are not compared with the ventilatory work (see chap. 10).

A. Acute Pulmonary Embolus

This is the classic deadspace-producing disease—the ventilated, unperfused lung. It may be extremely difficult to diagnose clinically. Blood gas measurements are never diagnostic, although they may help rule out acute embolic phenomena or shunt-producing disease (see chap. 10).

Acute pulmonary embolus without cardiopulmonary collapse usually is accompanied by hypoxemia and a pH in the 7.30 to 7.40 range. However, blood gases may be well within acceptable ranges.

There is often a large minute-volume–alveolar-ventilation disparity (see chaps. 6 and 10). Several hours after the embolus, there may no longer be deadspace disease because the unperfused lung often collapses. In fact, the stasis may create collapse of perfused alveoli around the embolic area and true shunting then exists. There are no "typical" blood gases that are reflective of the pulmonary embolic phenomenon!

B. Decreased Cardiac Output

Changes in the distribution of pulmonary blood flow create relatively ventilated, unperfused lung. A minute-volume–alveolar-ventilation disparity usually exists. The hypoxemia is primarily due to decreased mixed venous oxygen content, which accentuates the shunt effect (see chap. 13).

IV. VENTILATORY FAILURE (RESPIRATORY ACIDOSIS)

Ventilatory failure is defined as inadequate alveolar ventilation. This means that the patient is unable to provide enough muscular mechanical work to move a sufficient amount of air into and out of the lungs to meet the carbon dioxide metabolic demands of the body. Ventilatory failure is a severe physiologic state that must be evaluated with great care by the physician and approached with great respect by the respiratory care practitioner.

A. Chronic Ventilatory Failure (Chronic Hypercarbia)

Typical Room Air Blood Gases
   pH   7.40–7.50
   P_{CO_2} Above 50 mm Hg
   P_{O_2} Below 60 mm Hg
   Plasma bicarbonate above normal range.
   Base excess above normal range.

Typical Ventilatory Pattern
VT   Hypopnea (shallow)
RR   Tachypnea (rapid)
General Response to Oxygen Therapy
1. *Decreased alveolar ventilation* (see chap 7).
2. Sensitive to very small increases in inspired oxygen concentrations.
3. Slight improvement in Pa_{O_2}.
Evaluation of Tissue Oxygenation
1. Hypoxia is rare.
2. Adequacy of cardiac output is the prime determinant of tissue oxygenation.
3. Polycythemia is common; increases oxygen content.
4. Hypoxia must be assumed if the patient becomes acidemic.

In clinical medicine, the chronic hypercarbic patient is almost always the severe chronic obstructive pulmonary disease patient—i.e., emphysema and/or chronic bronchitis. Cardiopulmonary reserve is minimal and stress is life-threatening.

This patient presents a particular problem to the clinician who is interpreting blood gases, because the patient is at a different baseline. Alveolar hypoventilation and hypoxemia are "baseline" values and one judges the severity of acute disease on how the blood gases change from the baseline values. In supporting this patient, one cannot demand that he do better than he was doing prior to the acute problem; for example, if his baseline Pa_{O_2} is 50 mm Hg, one cannot try to support him at a Pa_{O_2} of 80 mm Hg, and if his baseline Pa_{CO_2} is 70 mm Hg, one cannot try to support him at a Pa_{CO_2} of 40 mm Hg.

B. Acute Alveolar Hyperventilation Superimposed on Chronic Ventilatory Failure

Typical Room Air Blood Gases
pH   Above 7.50
P_{CO_2} Usually above 40 mm Hg
P_{O_2} Below 60 mm Hg
Plasma bicarbonate usually above normal range.
Base excess usually above normal range.
General Response to Oxygen Therapy
1. Proper concentrations decrease ventilatory work.
2. Too much oxygen causes acute ventilatory failure to be superimposed on the chronic state.

The chronic hypercarbic patient may respond to acute stress by increasing alveolar ventilation. This is difficult to recognize in blood gases unless the age and clinical state of the patient are noted. The initial interpretation should be *uncompensated metabolic alkalosis with hypoxemia!* The condition must be recognized as being acute alveolar hyperventilation superimposed on a chronic ventilatory failure.

C. Acute Ventilatory Failure Superimposed on Chronic Ventilatory Failure

Typical Room Air Blood Gases
    pH   Below 7.30
    P_{CO_2} Above 60 mm Hg
    P_{O_2} Below 50 mm Hg
    Plasma bicarbonate normal or below normal.
    Base excess normal or below normal.
General Response to Oxygen Therapy
    Proper concentration may *improve* ventilatory status.
Evaluation of Tissue Oxygenation
    Hypoxia must be assumed!

It is essential to judge the severity of acute ventilatory failure on the degree of acidemia. These patients have high arterial carbon dioxide tensions with mild degrees of acidemia. This must lead to the conclusion that the patient's "baseline" state is one of high arterial P_{CO_2}.

Oxygen therapy is critical in these patients, because the proper concentrations may improve the ventilatory status and so avoid the need for a ventilator.

Proper oxygen therapy may have little effect on the P_{O_2} but may have a profound effect on tissue oxygenation. These patients are acute medical emergencies; tissue hypoxia must be assumed.

D. Acute Ventilatory Failure

Typical Room Air Blood Gases
    pH   Below 7.30
    P_{CO_2} Above 50 mm Hg
    P_{O_2} Below 60 mm Hg
    Plasma bicarbonate normal.
    Base excess normal.

There is no "typical ventilatory pattern." The patient may be apneic or have severe hyperpnea and tachypnea.

General Response to Oxygen Therapy
   1. Insignificant to mild increase in Pa_{O_2}.
   2. No change in ventilatory status.
Evaluation of Tissue Oxygenation
   Hypoxemia plus acidemia: *hypoxia must be assumed!*

This is a medical emergency! The sudden inability of a patient to move an adequate amount of air into and out of the lungs to meet carbon dioxide demands is a dire condition. This must always be considered an immediate life-threatening situation, because both hypoxemia and acidemia are present. If aggressive supportive and therapeutic measures are not undertaken, the most likely outcome is death.

PART THREE

Bedside Measurement of Blood Gases

15

Capnography

Unlike oxygen and nitrogen, carbon dioxide has a characteristic infrared absorption band allowing for continuous measurement in respiratory gases. In addition to infrared analysis, continuous CO_2 monitoring is also clinically available by mass spectrometry. The technical aspects of CO_2 measurement in respiratory gases are discussed in Chapter 25.

THE NORMAL CAPNOGRAM

The capnogram is a tracing of the inhaled and exhaled CO_2 concentrations with time. The ideal exhalation capnogram was shown previously (see Fig 10–2) in which Phase I represents essentially apparatus and anatomic deadspace gas, Phase II represents increasing CO_2 concentrations resulting from progressive emptying of alveoli, and Phase III (often referred to as the "CO_2 plateau") represents essentially alveolar gas.

An ideal alveolar P_{CO_2} is a mathematical concept based on averaging the continuum of V/Q relationships throughout the lung. Since each alveolus has its own V/Q and compliance/resistance characteristics, alveoli empty in parallel at differing rates and degrees,[196] making it impossible to sample "true" alveolar gas. The arterial P_{CO_2} value is accepted as the physiologic representation of the "true" alveolar P_{CO_2} (see chap. 2 and 4). As illustrated (see the inset of Fig 10–2), CO_2 concentration at the end of exhalation will invariably be less than the arterial P_{CO_2}. A normal capnogram shows a P_{CO_2} within several mm Hg of the arterial P_{CO_2} at the end of the Phase III plateau—the "end tidal CO_2."

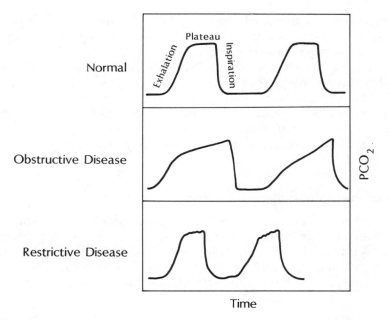

FIG 15–1.
The normal capnograph pattern shows a sharply rising exhalation slope with a clearly identifiable plateau. Inspiration is seen as an abrupt decrease in CO_2 to baseline. Obstructive
disease generally produces a prolonged exhalation slope with a difficult-to-identify plateau.
Restrictive disease generally provides a "choppy" plateau.

THE ABNORMAL CAPNOGRAM

The slope of phase II is influenced by the change in rate and sequence
of alveolar emptying that accompanies lung disease. In general, obstructive disease "flattens" the curve and blurs the distinction between Phases
II and III (Fig 15–1). Restrictive disease may affect Phase II, but more
dependably makes Phase III abnormal. Detailed discussion of capnographic interpretation is beyond the scope of this text and the reader is
referred to other publications for this information.[197] Suffice to say that
an abnormal capnographic analysis is more clinically reliable as an indicator of V/Q inequalities than as a reflector of arterial P_{CO_2}.[198]

END TIDAL CO_2 AND ARTERIAL P_{CO_2}

The most common application of capnography to clinical care is the
use of end tidal CO_2 values as a reflection of the arterial P_{CO_2}. When

the capnogram is abnormal, the end tidal P_{CO_2} must not be considered a reliable reflection of arterial P_{CO_2}. However, as long as the shape of the capnogram remains unchanged, the end tidal P_{CO_2} can be used as a "trending" monitor, providing cardiovascular function is consistent. In other words, the use of end tidal CO_2 as a noninvasive reflection of arterial P_{CO_2} is questionable in the presence of lung disease!

Assuming the capnogram remains normal, end tidal CO_2 measurement can be a reliable reflection of the P_{CO_2} as long as pulmonary perfusion remains consistent and changes in patient temperature are considered.

Alterations in Physiologic Deadspace

Physiologic deadspace is defined as that portion of the ventilation that does not participate in molecular gas exchange with pulmonary blood (see chap. 10). As shown in Figure 15–2, the arterial to end tidal P_{CO_2} difference $[P_{(a-et)}CO_2]$ increases as physiologic deadspace ventilation increases. The most important clinical manifestation of this phe-

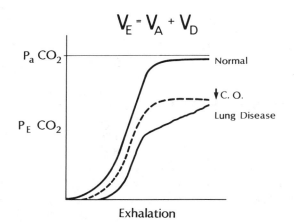

FIG 15–2.
Total ventilation (V_E) is composed of both alveolar ventilation (V_A) and deadspace ventilation (V_D). The $PaCO_2$ is considered the best reflection of alveolar ventilation. The End Tidal P_{CO_2} ($Petco_2$) is the expired P_{CO_2} (P_ECO_2) at the end of the plateau. An increased V_D will be manifest as an increased Pa_{CO_2} − $Petco_2$ gradient.

The two most common causes of increased deadspace ventilation are decreased cardiac output and lung disease. A decreased pulmonary perfusion will result in more alveoli having lower Pco_2; the net result is a decreased expired Pco_2 but no change in lung emptying pattern. This is depicted as the *dashed curve* with a shape similar to normal. Lung disease will involve changing emptying patterns and thus a change in the curve.

nomenon is when cardiac output changes occur. The following case study exemplifies this circumstance.

A 55-year-old man during a posterior spinal fusion of L2-4 experiences a significant blood loss, with mean arterial pressure (MAP) decreasing to 50 mm Hg for approximately 20 minutes while blood and volume replacement were accomplished. Several premature ventricular contractions (PVCs) and ST-segment alterations were noted during the hypotensive episode. After clinical stabilization of cardiovascular function:

MAP	90 mm Hg	pH	7.47		
PR	82/min	P_{CO_2}	38 mm Hg	Pet_{CO_2}	36 mm Hg
MV	7 L	P_{O_2}	256 mm Hg	S_{O_2}	99%
		$F_{I_{O_2}}$	0.5		

End tidal CO_2 was consistent throughout the remainder of the operation. The patient was poorly responsive at the end of the procedure, and it was elected to keep the endotracheal tube in place. In the postanesthesia care unit the vital signs were stable and spontaneous ventilation was deemed adequate with 0.5 $F_{I_{O_2}}$ administered by T-piece. Pulse oximetry revealed S_{O_2} 99% and capnography showed end tidal CO_2 (Pet_{CO_2}) 37 mm Hg. Twenty five minutes later the patient was agitated and diaphoretic:

MAP	130 mm Hg	Pet_{CO_2}	42 mm Hg
PR	125/min	S_{O_2}	99%
RR	35/min		
V_T	300 ml		
MV	10 L		

The assumption that hypercapnea is not responsible for the clinical circumstance is easy to make if one takes the Pet_{CO_2} as a reliable reflection of the arterial P_{CO_2}. In fact, the arterial blood gases were:

pH	7.24
P_{CO_2}	67 mm Hg
P_{O_2}	185 mm Hg

This patient most probably experienced a drop in cardiac output that elicited a sympathetic response resulting in tachycardia and hypertension. The decreased cardiac output increased deadspace ventilation. Both the MV-Pa_{CO_2} disparity (see chap. 10) and the increased $P_{(a-et)}CO_2$ of 25 mm Hg result from the deadspace increase. The assumption that the Pet_{CO_2} reliably reflects Pa_{CO_2} in a situation like this could be disastrous.

Temperature Alteration

Changes in patient temperature alter in vivo blood gas tensions (see chap. 11), e.g., with hypothermia the alveolar and arterial PCO_2 decrease. Since end tidal CO_2 is always a reflection of in vivo alveolar and arterial CO_2 tensions, a misleading $P_{(a-et)}CO_2$ results unless the blood gas is corrected to actual body temperature or the $PetCO_2$ is temperature corrected to 37°C.

CLINICAL MONITORING OF END TIDAL CO_2

Capnography offers two major clinical advantages in that it is noninvasive and provides continuous real-time information about CO_2 elimination. Since capnography requires uncontaminated exhaled gas collection, its application is largely limited to intubated patients.

There are a number of circumstances in which the end tidal CO_2 monitor can be of clinical utility. Emphasis must be placed on the limitations of this monitor in each of the commonly applied clinical circumstances. To date, end tidal CO_2 monitoring has been suggested as a means to: (1) reflect the arterial PCO_2; (2) trend changes in deadspace ventilation; and (3) reflect the adequacy of cardiopulmonary resuscitation (CPR).

Alveolar Ventilation Monitor

In patients with undiseased lungs and stable cardiovascular function, capnography provides a simple noninvasive method to monitor the adequacy of alveolar ventilation rapidly and continuously. These circumstances are most commonly found in patients receiving general anesthesia; patients requiring elective hyperventilation for intracranial disease; neurologically diseased patients requiring ventilatory assistance; and apnea monitoring.

Reliability of this monitor in patients with pulmonary disease or unstable cardiovascular function has not been documented. There are presently no clinical data to justify utilization of $PetCO_2$ as a replacement for Pa_{CO_2} measurement in such patients. A POTENTIALLY MISLEADING MONITOR IS WORSE THAN NO MONITOR!!

Trending Deadspace Ventilation

Changes in the $P_{(a-et)}CO_2$ must be attributed to changes in physiologic deadspace ventilation. The most common causes of alterations in deadspace ventilation are: (1) lung disease; (2) pulmonary embolic phenomena; and (3) changes in cardiac output.

Acute lung pathology alters V/Q and thereby changes the shape of the capnogram. When the $P_{(a-et)}CO_2$ changes in conjunction with the capnographic configuration changing, it is reasonable to assume that deadspace changes are attributable to changes in lung pathology. Since positive end-expiratory pressure (PEEP) therapy is known to decrease deadspace ventilation in adult respiratory distress syndrome (ARDS), $PetCO_2$ in conjunction with continuous transcutaneous PCO_2 monitoring has been suggested as a method for titrating PEEP therapy.[199]

End tidal CO_2 monitors have been utilized in anesthesiology during cranial surgery to detect air emboli.[200] No data are available to evaluate their utility in pulmonary embolic phenomena in intensive care units.

The clinical reality of continuous arterial blood gas monitoring promises the possibility of the $P_{(a-et)}CO_2$ being utilized to trend the adequacy of cardiac output. This is discussed in Chapter 19.

CPR

As discussed in Chapter 12, minimal perfusion of lung during CPR results in minimal CO_2 excretion and development of venous respiratory acidosis.[156] As expected, very low $PetCO_2$ values were observed during CPR, and it was confirmed that reductions in $PetCO_2$ during CPR are associated with comparable reductions in cardiac output. Of more importance was the documentation that increases in $PetCO_2$ during successful resuscitation are associated with corresponding increases in cardiac output.[201-203] Moreover, the extent to which resuscitation maneuvers, especially precordial compression, maintain cardiac output may be more reliably assessed by measurements of $PetCO_2$ than palpation of arterial pressure pulses. Monitoring of $PetCO_2$ to assess the hemodynamic effectiveness of CPR appears to be a practical and noninvasive approach.

16

Pulmonary Artery Oximetry

Oximetry in the right side of the heart was first utilized in the early 1960s in conjunction with diagnostic cardiac catheterization. With the widespread use of flow-directed pulmonary artery (PA) catheters for hemodynamic pressure monitoring in the 1970s and the development of fiberoptic technology in the early 1980s, continuous fiberoptic oximetry of mixed venous blood became a clinical reality. Early oximetric PA catheters were relatively inflexible and difficult to insert, were subject to frequent breakage and malfunction, and required frequent calibration to in vitro $S\bar{v}_{O_2}$ measurements. These problems have been satisfactorily addressed such that the current generation of oximetric PA catheters are readily applied to the management of acutely ill patients.

The technical aspects of fiberoptic oximetry are discussed in Chapter 23. Briefly, the methodology is based on reflectance spectrophotometry where the light wavelength is flashed down the fiberoptic path and the reflected light from the hemoglobin is passed back through the optic fiber and converted into a saturation reading. The catheters are calibrated against an optical standard prior to insertion. Alarm systems have been incorporated as in other monitors that are microprocessor driven and controlled. A 7.5 F, flow-directed thermal dilution PA catheter and a 4 F umbilical artery catheter are commercially available.

CLINICAL ACCURACY

Failure to maintain the catheter tip in the flow of blood can lead to artifactual readings of vessel wall tissue reflectance.[204] As with all spectral analyses of hemoglobin (see chap. 23), the presence of abnormal forms of hemoglobin or other substances with spectral activity in the light wavelength range will result in spurious readings.

There have been relatively few reports assessing the accuracy of the PA fiberoptic oximetric catheter in reflecting $S\bar{v}_{O_2}$. Available data show excellent correlation with in vitro measurements of $S\bar{v}_{O_2}$.[205] An experience with 630 patients showed minimal instrument drift ($<1\%$ in 24 hours) and stable function for up to 102 hours.[204] Clinically acceptable accuracy is apparently unaffected by body temperature, hemoglobin concentration, cardiac index, or method of calibration. The technology appears to be clinically acceptable and reliable when properly functioning and properly applied.

INTERPRETATION OF $S\bar{v}_{O_2}$—PHYSIOLOGIC BASIS

Maintenance of tissue oxygenation in the critically ill requires adequate arterial oxygen content, cardiac output, and tissue perfusion. A hemoglobin of 10 to 12 gm% with a $Pa_{O_2} > 60$ mm Hg or $Sa_{O_2} > 90\%$ is adequate since tissue oxygenation will seldom be significantly enhanced by higher Pa_{O_2} or Sa_{O_2} values (see chap. 5). Chapter 8 discusses evaluation of the cardiovascular and metabolic components of tissue oxygenation via oxygen content measurement of both arterial and pulmonary arterial blood—the $C_{(a-v)}O_2$. Briefly, normal humans have a $P\bar{v}_{O_2}$ of 40 mm Hg, $S\bar{v}_{O_2}$ of 75%, and a $C_{(a-v)}O_2$ of 5 vol%. Table 16–1 lists reference values relating to pulmonary artery oxygenation in the critically ill. These values assume an adequate hemoglobin content and acceptable perfusion status; with anemia, hypoperfusion, acidemia, and sepsis, these guidelines become unreliable.

TABLE 16–1.
Reference Values Relating to Pulmonary Artery Oxygenation in the Critically Ill

CV Status*	$P\bar{v}_{O_2}$	$S\bar{v}_{O_2}$	$C_{(a-v)}O_2$
Healthy resting human volunteer	40 (37–43)	75 (70–76)	5.0 (4.5–6.0)
Critically ill, adequate CV status	37 (35–40)	70 (68–75)	3.5 (2.5–4.5)
Critically ill, borderline CV status	32 (30–35)	60 (56–68)	5.0 (4.5–6.0)
Critically ill, inadequate CV status	< 30	< 56	> 6.0

*CV = cardiovascular.

$S\bar{v}_{O_2}$–$C\bar{v}_{O_2}$ Relationship

The range of clinically encountered $S\bar{v}_{O_2}$ values is 35% to 80%. When hemoglobin concentration is constant, the $S\bar{v}_{O_2}$ closely reflects the $C\bar{v}_{O_2}$ because mixed venous blood always occupies the "steep" portion of the oxyhemoglobin dissociation curve and has a relatively low oxygen partial pressure. For practical purposes a fall of 1 mm Hg in $P\bar{v}_{O_2}$ will result in a fall of 2% in $S\bar{v}_{O_2}$.

$S\bar{v}_{O_2}$ and Hypoxemia

Physiologic stress usually increases cardiac output above increased tissue oxygen requirements, resulting in a decreased $C_{(a-v)}O_2$. This allows maintenance of near normal $S\bar{v}_{O_2}$ despite an increased oxygen consumption, an important mechanism for minimizing the hypoxemic effect of intrapulmonary shunting (see chap 9).

$S\bar{v}_{O_2}$–$C_{(a-v)}O_2$ Relationship

Critically ill patients with adequate cardiovascular reserves are known to maintain $C_{(a-v)}O_2$ values in the range of 2.5 to 4.5 vol% (see chap. 8). Briefly, the $C_{(a-v)}O_2$ is clinically useful as a reflection of oxygen extraction as well as a reflection of the relative adequacy of cardiac output in relation to metabolic demand. Assuming a constant metabolic rate and adequate hemoglobin content, a constant relationship may be expected between $C_{(a-v)}O_2$ and $S\bar{v}_{O_2}$, namely, as $S\bar{v}_{O_2}$ decreases $C_{(a-v)}O_2$ increases. With the availability of pulmonary artery oximetry, this relationship becomes clinically important. For example, if arterial oxygen content remains adequate, deterioration in cardiovascular function may first be manifest in a decreasing $S\bar{v}_{O_2}$.

It has been demonstrated that when the $S\bar{v}_{O_2}$ is greater than 65%, the $C_{(a-v)}O_2$ is most likely less than 4.5 vol%; when $S\bar{v}_{O_2}$ is less than 65%, the $C_{(a-v)}O_2$ is most likely greater than 4.5 vol% as long as the hemoglobin concentration is greater than 10 gm%.[206] In many circumstances, this information obtained by continuous PA oximetry may significantly diminish the need for frequent arterial blood gas measurements and serve to assure the clinician that cardiac output is adequate to meet the oxygen demands of the peripheral tissues.

Conclusions

When arterial blood gas measurements became available in the clinical setting, many expected the Pa_{O_2} measurement to provide an overall reflection of the body's oxygenation status. It quickly became obvious that as helpful as this measurement was, it did not provide all the necessary information; indeed, it was found to be misleading in some circumstances. This led to the general acceptance of the statement that *interpretation* of the Pa_{O_2} value is essential.

The continuous $S\bar{v}_{O_2}$ measurement can contribute greatly to clinical care. However, it is no more of a panacea than was the availability of the Pa_{O_2} measurement 20 years ago. It must be remembered that NO SINGLE OXYGENATION MEASUREMENT HAS ANY SIGNIFICANT ADVANTAGE OVER ANOTHER—THEY ALL DEMAND INTERPRETATION!

INTERPRETATION OF $S\bar{v}_{O_2}$—CLINICAL BASIS

Oxygen delivery $[Ca_{O_2} \times C.O. \times 10]$ represents the milliliters of oxygen delivered to the tissues in one minute. Total body oxygen consumption ($\dot{V}O_2$) represents the milliliters of oxygen extracted by the tissues per minute. The $S\bar{v}_{O_2}$ will be determined by the relationship between oxygen delivery (SUPPLY) and oxygen consumption (DEMAND). Increasing oxygen demand secondary to physiologic stress will normally result in an increase in cardiac output, i.e., an increase in oxygen supply. Since both oxygen supply and demand are increasing, $S\bar{v}_{O_2}$ remains relatively unchanged. In these circumstances the $S\bar{v}_{O_2}$ can be conceptualized as providing a measure of "oxygen reserve" to meet further increases in oxygen demand. An $S\bar{v}_{O_2}$ value greater than 65% represents adequate reserve; 50% to 65% represents limited reserve; 35% to 50% represents inadequate reserve; less than 35% most probably reflects inadequate tissue oxygenation.[207]

$S\bar{v}_{O_2}$ and Cardiac Function

When oxygen delivery is maximal, any increase in $\dot{V}O_2$ will result in a fall in $S\bar{v}_{O_2}$. It has been demonstrated in patients with optimal oxygen content and limited cardiac output that increased ventilatory muscle activity, shivering, convulsions, rewarming after hypothermia, and even movement during routine nursing procedures may result in considerable decreases in $S\bar{v}_{O_2}$.[204]

When arterial oxygenation and oxygen consumption are normal, decreases in cardiac output will be closely paralleled by decreases in $S\bar{v}_{O_2}$.[208] This is especially obvious in low-flow states.

Values of $S\bar{v}_{O_2}$ greater than 60% are seldom associated with cardiovascular instability. Values of $S\bar{v}_{O_2}$ less than 40% usually reflect inadequate cardiac output[209] and may herald the onset of hypotension, vasoconstriction, arrhythmias, respiratory distress, and cardiac arrest.[208, 210] These $S\bar{v}_{O_2}$ changes can occur so rapidly that intermittent sampling would not be effective as a warning prior to clinical extremis, whereas continuous monitoring provides information that may lead to early intervention and prevention of cardiovascular collapse.

$S\bar{v}_{O_2}$ and Sepsis

As discussed in Chapter 13, the combination of a high cardiac output with a small $C_{(a-v)}O_2$ in early sepsis results in a rise in $S\bar{v}_{O_2}$, which has been reported to be an early sign of developing sepsis in critically ill patients.[176, 211]

$S\bar{v}_{O_2}$ and Airway Pressure Therapy

Decreased work of breathing has been reported to result in improvement in $S\bar{v}_{O_2}$. Monitoring $S\bar{v}_{O_2}$ in lieu of measuring cardiac output has been suggested to simplify and speed up the process of titrating positive end-expiratory pressure (PEEP) therapy.[73]

SIMULTANEOUS ARTERIAL–MIXED-VENOUS OXIMETRY

Decreases in arterial oxygen content decrease oxygen delivery and therefore decrease $S\bar{v}_{O_2}$. Since the arterial component of oxygen supply varies enormously in critically ill patients with primary cardiopulmonary disease, any interpretation of $S\bar{v}_{O_2}$ without knowledge of Pa_{O_2} or Sa_{O_2} is open to question. This truism has led to significant interest in combining PA oximetry with pulse oximetry—widely referred to as "dual oximetry."

The theoretic advantage of dual oximetry in monitoring oxygen supply and demand is that changes in the arterial component of oxygen supply are directly monitored rather than inferred, as is the case with PA oximetry alone. Since pulse oximetry is a reliable "trender" of Sa_{O_2} even with significant desaturation, there can be little valid argument with the statement that interpretation of PA oximetry is greatly enhanced by simultaneous monitoring of Sa_{O_2}.

Future Applications of Dual Oximetry

Simultaneous arterial and PA oximetry allow continuous calculation of the oxygen extraction index (O_2EI):

$$O_2EI = \frac{Sa_{O_2} - S\bar{v}_{O_2}}{Sa_{O_2}}$$

It appears that a reasonable correlation exists between total body oxygen utilization and the O_2EI as long as the Sa_{O_2} remains above 89%.[212] The major limitation to dual oximetry rests with the questionable accuracy with which the pulse oximeter quantifies Sa_{O_2} below 90% (see chap. 17).

Another suggested application of dual oximetry is to trend changes in Qsp/Q_T by calculation of the ventilation-perfusion index [VQI = $(1-Sa_{O_2})/(1-S\bar{v}_{O_2})$].[213] More rapid and less costly determination of continuous positive airway pressure levels with this technique has been suggested.[214]

Further study is required to determine the clinical utility of dual oximetry beyond the fact that it greatly enhances proper interpretation of the $S\bar{v}_{O_2}$.

SUMMARY

The major disadvantage of PA oximetry rests in its nonspecificity. The $S\bar{v}_{O_2}$ reflects overall O_2 supply/demand relationships that depend on cardiac output, Sa_{O_2}, $\dot{V}O_2$, and hemoglobin concentrations. Therefore, a decrease in cardiac output can be compensated by a decrease in $\dot{V}O_2$, leaving the $S\bar{v}_{O_2}$ unchanged. Furthermore, patients with good cardiovascular reserves have been shown to be markedly hypoxemic yet show normal $S\bar{v}_{O_2}$ because of reflex cardiovascular compensation.[215]

Pulmonary artery oximetry allows for continuous real-time monitoring of $S\bar{v}_{O_2}$ that can be readily applied in the intensive care unit or the operating room. The patient's risks are essentially those of a PA catheter. Decreases in $S\bar{v}_{O_2}$ can be a reliable predictor of impending low cardiac output states, while improvement in $S\bar{v}_{O_2}$ can be a useful indicator of therapeutic efficacy in patients with decreased cardiac outputs.

When indicated, PA oximetry can be of great benefit to the patient's care. However, it can be potentially misleading if not fully comprehended.

17

Pulse Oximetry

Ear oximetry was the first technique successfully applied to patients for continuous monitoring of arterial oxygen saturation.[216] The need for heating elements to "arterialize" the ear plus the fragility of the equipment prevented this technology from becoming popular for patient monitoring in the perioperative period or during acute critical illness. The advent of pulse oximetry provided a readily applicable clinical tool for noninvasive measurement of arterial oxyhemoglobin.

The technical aspects of pulse oximeters are discussed elsewhere (see chap. 23). Briefly, pulse oximeters are dual wavelength spectrophotometers with plethysmographic capabilities that function by placing a pulsating arterial vascular bed between a 2-wavelength light source and a light detector. The degree of change in transmitted light is proportional to the size of the arterial pulse change, the wavelengths of light used, and the oxyhemoglobin saturations. Assuming that the pulsatile waveform is entirely due to the passage of arterial blood, utilization of the appropriate light wavelengths allows the microprocessor to continuously calculate Sa_{O_2}.

CLINICAL ACCURACY OF PULSE OXIMETERS

Available studies demonstrate that modern pulse oximeters compare well with co-oximetry in the clinical setting. It can be generally stated that Sa_{O_2} values above 80% compare excellently to co-oximetry, while saturations below 80% give reliable trending with clinically acceptable correlations to co-oximetry. Excellent correlations are found in adult volunteers[217, 218] and stable elderly patients,[219] while clinically acceptable correlations are demonstrated in adult and pediatric patients in the intensive care unit.[220-222] When appropriate fetal hemoglobin information is provided to the microprocessor (see chap. 23), clinically acceptable correlations are demonstrated in neonates.[223-225]

Perhaps the most important factor to consider in assessing the accuracy of pulse oximetry is that it offers an excellent continuous real-time trending of Sa_{O_2}. This fact alone gives the technology a significant place in patient monitoring. However, the degree to which it can be used to reliably *quantitate* the actual Sa_{O_2} is open to question. Therefore, we recommend that the clinical use of pulse oximetry should presently be limited to use as a noninvasive reflection of clinically relevant changes in Sa_{O_2}.

CLINICAL LIMITATIONS OF PULSE OXIMETRY

The limitations can be considered with respect to spectrophotometry, pulsatile flow, and the instrument interference.

Spectrophotometric Limitations

The light-emitting diodes utilized for pulse oximetry (see chap. 23) detect reduced (RHb) and oxygenated (O_2Hb) forms of hemoglobin. The presence of hemoglobin moieties such as carboxyhemoglobin (COHb), methemoglobin (METHb), and fetal hemoglobin (FHb) can impair the accuracy of the oxyhemoglobin measurement. Severe anemia (less than 5 gm% Hb) results in unreliable oximeter readings.

Substances with spectral activity in the wavelengths utilized for pulse oximetry would be expected to interfere with the accurate reading of oxyhemoglobin concentration. Dyes such as methylene blue, indocyanine green, and indigo carmine are documented to interfere with oximetry.[226] Intralipid has been reported to have spectral activity in the wavelengths used for in vitro co-oximetry[227] and may interfere with pulse oximetry[217] although this remains to be confirmed. In the pediatric application another source of error is ambient light from infrared heating lamps interfering with oximeter readings.[228] This can be overcome by appropriate shielding of the oximeter probe.

Pulsatile Flow

Pulse oximetry is predicated on the ability to detect arterial blood as separate from venous blood and tissue; the technology depends upon the presence of an adequate pulsatile arterial flow to accomplish this crucial identification (see chap. 23). Conditions such as hypotension, cardiac arrest, cardiopulmonary bypass, and significant hypothermia diminish digital perfusion and alter the pulse oximeters ability to accurately measure Sa_{O_2}.[229, 230]

Conditions that result in significant venous pulsation can render pulse oximetry unreliable. This may be seen with severe right ventricular failure, tricuspid regurgitation, obstruction to venous return, markedly elevated intrathoracic pressure, and the probe on a dependent limb.[230]

Instrument Interference

Motion of the digit on which the unit is placed may be interpreted by the instrument as pulsatile motion and result in artifactual readings.[229] Electrocautery may interfere with the instrument, although this can usually be overcome by use of a separate AC circuit for the electrocautery or the use of rechargeable battery power sources for the oximeter.[229]

CLINICAL ADVANTAGES OF PULSE OXIMETRY

A significant clinical advantage to modern pulse oximeters is that no specialized calibration or sensor site preparation is required. Sensor failure or inappropriate sensor sites are detected by the microprocessor and the clinician is alerted. It appears that the equipment is capable of detecting almost all technical circumstances in which it may be unreliable, and most available products clearly warn the user of such conditions.

Acute deterioration in peripheral circulation is immediately sensed by the pulse oximeter. This is a potential clinical advantage, but again it must be recognized as qualitative rather than quantitative. There are no data to support the contention that the pulse oximeter can be used as a reliable reflection of changes in peripheral perfusion short of acute circulatory collapse.[231] In other words, the pulse oximeter can detect a clinically significant acute deterioration in the peripheral circulatory status, but it does not provide a replacement for either blood pressure monitoring or ECG monitoring. Although research is presently ongoing to develop reliable blood pressure monitoring from pulse oximetry, the present clinically available equipment cannot provide this information.

CLINICAL USES OF PULSE OXIMETRY

The rapid acceptance of this noninvasive technology clearly demonstrates that it is of great advantage to patient care. However, we must constrain enthusiasm with insisting upon documentation of usefulness in each circumstance so that the technology is not misapplied or expected to do more than it is capable of doing.

Operating Room

The pulse oximeter has proved to be a distinct advantage to patient monitoring in the operating room. This makes ultimate sense since the concern is avoidance of arterial desaturation during controlled circumstances of anesthesia and surgery. In less than five years of widespread availability, pulse oximetry has gained status in anesthesiology equal to ECG and blood pressure monitoring. This exuberance and total acceptance of pulse oximetry in the anesthetized patient has "spilled over" to the patient in the intensive care unit with little apparent justification and even less documentation. Recent evidence suggests that these monitors may not detect sudden severe desaturation.[232]

Specific Applications

The easy portability of a pulse oximeter suggests a role in monitoring patients during transport. Diagnostic and therapeutic procedures that potentially threaten adequate oxygenation, such as bronchoscopy and pulmonary lavage, are excellent circumstances for a continuous noninvasive arterial desaturation monitor.

The pulse oximeter can be very useful in the process of decreasing oxygen therapy. We have found that minimization of FI_{O_2} values or discontinuation of oxygen therapy can be accomplished more rapidly in the presence of a reliable desaturation monitor. However, it should not be considered a replacement for arterial blood gas measurement when indicated.

The Critically Ill Patient

Pulse oximetry is not a replacement for blood gas monitoring in the critically ill. Measurement of acid-base and ventilatory status is not provided by pulse oximetry. Although the pulse oximeter may decrease the frequency of blood gas measurement required in some patients, it should not be considered more than a *trend monitor* of Sa_{O_2} in the critically ill.

18

Transcutaneous Gas Monitoring

The technology of transcutaneous gas electrodes is discussed elsewhere (see chap. 24). Briefly, these devices are variants of the blood gas analyzer's Clark and Severinghaus electrodes that measure gas tensions at the skin surface.

PHYSIOLOGY OF SKIN BLOOD FLOW

Human skin is comprised of three layers; the stratum corneum, the epidermis, and the dermis. These three layers form a cohesive covering that ranges in thickness from 0.2 to 2 mm.

Epidermis and Stratum Corneum

The epidermis is a nonvascular layer of living cells that averages 100 μ in thickness, and does not affect the rate of gas diffusion through skin. The epidermal cells consume oxygen and produce carbon dioxide.

The stratum corneum arises from the epidermis and contains no living cells but consists of keratin filaments in a matrix of lipid and nonfibrous protein. The stratum corneum provides the skin's strength and is the rate-limiting factor for gaseous diffusion through the skin.

Dermis

The dermis is a highly vascular layer with papillae projecting into the epidermis. Dermal capillaries in the papillae essentially loop up into the epidermal layer and behave like a countercurrent exchange column.

In other words, lower oxygen concentrations exist at the tips of the papillae as compared to the bases because well-oxygenated blood passing up through the papillae diffuses oxygen to the less well-oxygenated blood in the capillary loop leaving the papillae. A similar process occurs for carbon dioxide, which results in the papillary tip having a higher P_{CO_2} than the base. This countercurrent phenomenon partially explains why the early studies found the transcutaneous P_{O_2} ($P_{tc}O_2$) to be lower than the arterial P_{O_2} and completely explains why the transcutaneous P_{CO_2} ($P_{tc}CO_2$) was found to be higher than the arterial P_{CO_2}.

Heating the Skin Surface

In 1975 it was observed that as the skin surface is heated the regular crystalline structure of the lipids in the statum corneum become disorganized, returning to their normal arrangement on cooling. At 41°C the lipid component "melts" and this transition from a solid to a liquid phase greatly enhances the speed of gas diffusion through the skin.[233] Thus, surface heating to greater than 41°C creates a "diffusion window" in the skin.

Heating the skin surface decreases the countercurrent effect because the increased capillary flow tends to diminish the gas concentration differences between the ascending and descending loops. Although surface heating increases oxygen consumption, the effects of increased blood flow are of much greater magnitude, resulting in papillary tip oxygen concentrations approaching arterial blood concentrations.

Other factors to take into account are that the degree of increased temperature achieved on the skin is related to initial blood flow, body temperature, and electrode temperature. Heating the skin results in decreasing oxygen solubility and a rightward shift of the oxyhemoglobin dissociation curve. The impact of these changes on oxygen tensions depends upon on which part of the curve the arterial values lie.

Despite these complex and conflicting factors, heating the skin surface produces a stable hyperemic flow of arterialized blood in the dermis and reduces the diffusion barrier of the epidermis. The net result is oxygen diffusion through the skin in concentrations resembling the arterial P_{O_2}. If skin circulation falls, the $P_{tc}O_2$ will fall due to both a restoration of the countercurrent exchange mechanism and inadequate oxygen delivery.

The effects of diminished skin circulation on $P_{tc}CO_2$ is insignificant as long as the skin surface is heated. This is most probably due to the fact that restoration of the countercurrent exchange mechanism increases CO_2 concentration in the dermal tips as the blood flow diminishes.

ANIMAL DATA

The relationship between $P_{tc}O_2$ measurements and cardiovascular function has been studied in animal models[234, 235] showing that with inducement and reversal of hypotension the $P_{tc}O_2$ correlates well with cardiac output, mean arterial pressure, and $P\bar{v}_{O_2}$. However, very poor correlation is found between arterial PO_2 and $P_{tc}O_2$ in these studies. Arterial hypoxemia is reliably tracked by $P_{tc}O_2$ as long as cardiac output was maintained. However, hemorrhagic hypotension induced a fall in $P_{tc}O_2$ that paralleled cardiac output, while Pa_{O_2} remained essentially unchanged.[234] A study in dogs rendered hypotensive by sodium nitroprusside infusion while cardiac output was relatively unchanged showed a well-maintained correlation between $P_{tc}O_2$ and Pa_{O_2} at mean arterial pressures below 50 mm Hg.[236] This suggests that $P_{tc}O_2$ values are more sensitive to changes in blood flow than to changes in blood pressure, a conclusion supported by data showing the utility of $P_{tc}O_2$ monitoring in assessing the viability of surgical skin flaps and autografts.[237, 238]

HUMAN DATA

There have been innumerable studies of transcutaneous monitoring in neonates and to a lesser extent in pediatric and adult patients.

Transcutaneous PO_2

Early studies examining the correlation between $P_{tc}O_2$ and Pa_{O_2} in neonates revealed correlation coefficients ranging from 0.92 to 0.99 for patient groups of 11 to 276 newborns.[239] This reliability is found only in conjunction with adequate and stable cardiovascular function. In neonates the $P_{tc}O_2$ tends to overestimate the Pa_{O_2} by 10% to 12%[240]; however, by one year of age the $P_{tc}O_2$ underestimates the Pa_{O_2}[241] and this trend continues in older populations.

The relatively few studies looking at the correlation between $P_{tc}O_2$ and Pa_{O_2} in adults have revealed essentially the same findings as those seen in neonates. Although Pa_{O_2} to $P_{tc}O_2$ correlation coefficients of 0.94 to 0.98 have been reported, the $P_{tc}O_2$ values range from 45% to 108% of the Pa_{O_2}[242]; probably this is due to variations in skin perfusion.

The animal data showing perfusion to be essential to $P_{tc}O_2$ correlating with Pa_{O_2} were supported in human testing[242] where acceptable correlations existed when the Cardiac Index (CI) was greater than 2 L/min/M², while unacceptable correlations existed with CIs below 2 L/min/M².

Interestingly, when $P_{tc}O_2$ remained below 20 mm Hg following successful cardiopulmonary resuscitation, cardiac arrest ensued within 40 to 60 minutes.

Transcutaneous PCO_2

Neonatal and adult studies of $P_{tc}CO_2$ monitoring have shown it to be a reliable trend monitor for Pa_{CO_2} changes in hemodynamically stable patients. In low-flow states the $P_{tc}CO_2$ will rise as flow declines, but generally it remains a reasonable reflector of Pa_{CO_2}.[242]

Transcutaneous PCO_2 Index

Tremper et al.[243] introduced the concept of the $P_{tc}O_2$ Index:

$$\frac{P_{tc}O_2}{Pa_{O_2}}$$

Evaluation of the $P_{tc}O_2$ Index in neonates revealed that the index approached 1 in infants judged to be stable; whereas in infants with pH values less than 7.05, hematocrit readings less than 30%, or mean blood pressure less than 40 mm Hg, the $P_{tc}O_2$ Index ranged from 0.85 to 0.2. This was considered to be a useful monitor of overall hemodynamic function for sick neonates.[244]

An adult study involving 1,073 data sets from 106 critically ill or anesthetized patients showed that a CI of more than 2.2 L/min/M² was associated with a $P_{tc}O_2$ Index of 0.79 +/− 0.12, a CI between 2 and 1.5 L/min/M² was associated with an index of 0.48 +/− 0.07, and a CI of less than 1.5 was associated with an index of 0.12 +/− 0.12.[243] The correlations between $P_{tc}O_2$ and Pa_{O_2} were good for those patients with a CI above 2.2 (R = 0.89) but fell to R = 0.78 when the CI was between 2.2 and 1.5 and to R = 0.06 when the CI was less than 1.5.

CLINICAL APPLICATIONS

Transcutaneous gas monitoring provides a reliable means of trending the values of Pa_{O_2} and Pa_{CO_2} in patients with relatively normal cardiovascular function. Transcutaneous monitoring offers two major advantages over conventional blood gas monitoring in that it provides continuous real-time information and is noninvasive.

Neonatal $P_{tc}O_2$ Monitoring

Routine use of $P_{tc}O_2$ monitoring in neonates revealed that many common diagnostic and therapeutic procedures produced significant hypoxemias that were previously unrecognized. This has resulted in a number of changes in the care of sick neonates.[239] Although pulse oximetry has become the most widely used noninvasive oxygen monitor, the impact and usefulness of transcutaneous Po_2 monitoring in the care of sick neonates must not be forgotten.

Neonatal $P_{tc}CO_2$ Monitoring

Transcutaneous CO_2 monitoring is a reliable means of assessing the adequacy of alveolar ventilation and is more useful than conventional apnea monitors for neonates.[245] Unlike end tidal CO_2 monitoring, the transcutaneous CO_2 electrode is readily applied to unintubated patients. These monitors can be used in a wide range of clinical situations in the intensive care unit and operating room.

Skin Perfusion Monitoring

Simultaneous consideration of $P_{tc}O_2$ and Pa_{O_2} makes it possible to derive the $P_{tc}O_2$ Index ($P_{tc}O_2/Pa_{O_2}$) that has been previously discussed as a direct monitor of the degree of skin perfusion. Since skin receives perfusion far in excess of oxygen demands, the index is reduced early in shock and therefore provides a sensitive early warning sign of decreasing tissue perfusion.

Immediately postresuscitation it has been demonstrated that the $P_{tc}O_2$ Index will be low despite normal blood pressure if the fluid resuscitation has not been sufficient.[246] Persistently low $P_{tc}O_2$ Indices following resuscitation have been reported to precede cardiac arrest by approximately 45 to 60 minutes.[242]

The $P_{tc}O_2$ monitoring can be readily applied to assess the adequacy of vascularization of surgical skin flaps and autografts[237, 238] and they have been used in the assessment of limb perfusion in patients with peripheral vascular disease.[247, 248]

Neonatal Anesthetic Management

The advantages of a noninvasive, continuous monitor that tracks oxygen delivery (Pa_{O_2} and perfusion) offers a tremendous advance in the anesthetic management of neonates and infants. Improved assessment of blood volume replacement, intraoperative hypoxemia, and airway malfunction (kinked endotracheal tube, right main-stem bronchus intubation, accidental extubation), have been demonstrated with transcutaneous monitoring.[242, 249]

Positive End-Expiratory Pressure Therapy

Since transcutaneous oxygen monitoring can be used to evaluate both arterial oxygen tension and perfusion, it is a potential monitor of oxygen delivery. This concept has been demonstrated in an animal model to be as reliable for positive end-expiratory pressure (PEEP) titration as other documented methods.[250] The $P_{tc}CO_2$ has been shown in animal models in conjunction with end tidal CO_2 to evaluate deadspace changes with PEEP therapy.[199]

CLINICAL DISADVANTAGES

The most important disadvantage is blistering or burning of the skin, secondary to the heating element. This can be minimized by changing the site every four hours and avoiding use with hypothermic patients. An equilibration time of 20 to 30 minutes is required each time the site is changed and electrode maintenance is required (see chap. 24).

SUMMARY

Transcutaneous monitoring is relatively simple and potentially useful. Most reports describing unreliable function of transcutaneous gas monitors are due to misapplications of the technology or failure to appreciate the relationships of arterial Po_2 and hemodynamic function. Application of $P_{tc}O_2$ monitors to track arterial gas tensions in hemodynamically unstable patients is inappropriate!

The advent of continuous arterial blood gas monitoring when used in conjunction with transcutaneous gas monitoring will provide the clinician with a means of continual assessment of tissue oxygen delivery unlike any heretofore available (see chap. 19).

19

Continuous Blood Gas Monitoring

A monitor is generally defined as *noninvasive* when application does not require disruption of skin or mucous membrane integrity. Theoretically, a noninvasive monitor should be complication-free when appropriately applied and utilized. An *invasive* monitor is inevitably associated with some risk of complication despite perfect application and maintenance.

A continuous monitor is *proactive*, i.e., it potentially provides information that may lead to therapeutic intervention prior to significant physiologic disruption. Alarm limits may be set to alert the bedside practitioner and thereby improve the ability to detect problems as early as possible. Intermittent monitors are *reactive*, i.e., there must be a reason to initiate the measurement. Of course, intermittent monitors can be automatically cycled very frequently to approach a proactive status.

Table 19–1 classifies clinical monitors in a descending sequence in terms of desirability. Unfortunately, our present techniques for blood gas analysis provide the least desirable form of clinical monitor. It is no wonder that continuous and noninvasive methods of reflecting blood gases have gained such rapid popularity. Indeed, it is fair to state that much of the enthusiasm and acceptance for many technologies resulted more from the undesirability of blood gas analysis than from the accuracy and reliability of the new technologies.

CONTINUOUS BLOOD GAS MEASUREMENT

Fluorescence optode technology holds the greatest promise for achieving continuous blood gas measurements.[251, 252] This technology and an intravascular blood gas system (IBGS)* are discussed elsewhere

TABLE 19–1.

Classification of Clinical Monitors

Classification	Example
Noninvasive, continuous	ECG monitor
Noninvasive, intermittent	Blood pressure cuff
Invasive, continuous	Transduced blood pressure
Invasive, intermittent	Thermal dilution C.O.
Invasive, intermittent, delayed	Arterial blood gases

(see chap. 26). Briefly, three fluorescent optodes specific for pH, P_{CO_2}, and P_{O_2} plus a thermocouple for temperature measurement compose a probe that inserts into a 20-gauge arterial catheter. With the probe in place, a standard continuous flush system is utilized, blood pressure is transduced in the standard manner and blood can be readily withdrawn through the catheter. The microprocessor controls a digital display module that continuously reads pH, P_{CO_2}, and P_{O_2} while up/down arrows signify ongoing changes.

The continuous measurement of pH, P_{CO_2}, and P_{O_2} should have considerable clinical significance because these crucial reflectors of respiratory homeostasis could then be utilized as proactive monitors. A proactive arterial blood gas monitor would allow the clinician to detect significant pH and blood gas changes prior to perturbation of clinical signs, thereby ensuring more timely therapeutic interventions. Additionally, this continuous monitoring capability should enable more rapid and dependable titration of common therapeutic modalities such as oxygen administration, positive-pressure ventilation, positive end-expiratory pressure, and alkali therapy.

A continuous blood gas and pH monitor promises even more if utilized in conjunction with available noninvasive respiratory monitors. As an example, consider the combined continuous monitoring of transcutaneous oxygen tension, capnography, and arterial blood gases. The simultaneous use of these three continuous bedside monitors could theoretically trend cardiac output, categorize the perfusion status, and quantify intrapulmonary shunting without requiring pulmonary artery catheterization.[253]

Continuous Arterial–End Tidal CO_2 Measurement

The $P_{(a-et)}CO_2$ gradient is primarily a manifestation of physiologic

*Cardiovascular Devices, Inc., Irvine, Calf.

deadspace ventilation (see chap. 15). The two major pathologic factors that alter this gradient are lung disease and changes in cardiac output. As illustrated previously (see Fig 15–2), any acute change in the $P_{(a-et)}CO_2$ gradient without simultaneous change in capnographic configuration should indicate a change in cardiac output. This concept offers the possibility of trending cardiac output changes in response to fluid challenge, inotropic therapy, or diuretics, with no more invasion than a 20-gauge arterial catheter.

Continuous Arterial–Transcutaneous P_{O_2} Measurement

The $P_{tc}O_2$ Index $[P_{(a-tc)}O_2/Pa_{O_2}]$ has been discussed previously (see chap. 18). Since the $P_{(a-tc)}O_2$ is a function of skin perfusion, the $P_{tc}O_2$ Index should be a function of the adequacy of skin perfusion. While skin perfusion per se is of limited importance, a diminution in skin blood flow is an early sign of decreasing cardiac output and overall peripheral perfusion in most patients. The $P_{tc}O_2$ Index has been demonstrated to correlate well with cardiac output and perfusion[243] and should provide an early detection of global decreases in the perfusion status.

Continuous Measurement of the Estimated Shunt

Calculation of the intrapulmonary shunt fraction ($\dot{Q}sp/\dot{Q}T$) is generally recognized as the most reliable way to quantitate disruption of pulmonary oxygen transfer and therefore the extent to which pulmonary disease is contributing to arterial hypoxemia (see chap. 9). This calculation requires analysis of pulmonary artery blood. The unavailability of pulmonary artery blood samples in many critically ill patients has led to the description of various indices based on arterial oxygen *tension*-based indices $[P_{(A-a)}O_2,$[96] $Pa_{O_2}/PA_{O_2},$[97] $Pa_{O_2}/FI_{O_2},$[98] $P_{(A-a)}O_2/Pa_{O_2}$[99]$]$ that indirectly reflect Qsp/QT in critically ill patients.[108] An oxygen-*content*-based index, such as the Estimated Shunt (see chap. 9), enables estimation of the intrapulmonary shunt fraction when pulmonary artery blood samples are not available. This Estimated Shunt calculation is based on use of an assumed $C_{(a-v)}O_2$ of 3.5 ml/dl.[95] The Estimated Shunt has been demonstrated to be superior to tension-based indices in reflecting the intrapulmonary shunt fraction.[77, 254] Simultaneous monitoring of the $P_{tc}O_2$ Index and $P_{(a-et)}CO_2$ should allow for verification of the adequacy of cardiac output and peripheral perfusion, thereby confirming the reliability of the Estimated Shunt to quantitate changes in $\dot{Q}sp/\dot{Q}T$.

SUMMARY

Continuous arterial pH, PCO_2, and PO_2 measurement represents a minimally invasive, proactive cardiopulmonary monitoring capability for high-risk surgical and critically ill patients. The simultaneous continuous monitoring of arterial blood gases, $P_{tc}O_2$ and the $P_{et}CO_2$ promises to provide moment-to-moment reflections of cardiac output change, peripheral perfusion status, and oxygen transfer capability of the lungs. These would enable rapid and accurate titration of most therapies used to support cardiopulmonary function in critically ill patients. Additionally, this minimally invasive combination of monitors may provide an objective means of identifying those patients in whom more invasive monitoring, such as pulmonary artery catheterization, is warranted. Further study and development will undoubtedly make all this a clinical reality in the not too distant future.

PART FOUR

Technologic Considerations in Blood Gas Measurement

20

Guidelines for Obtaining Blood Gas Samples

This chapter elucidates the guidelines and techniques used in the critical care areas and central blood gas laboratory of Northwestern Memorial Hospital for almost 20 years. This experience includes nearly 1.5 million blood gas samples from the general hospital patient population; the medical, surgical, and neonatal intensive care areas; the operating rooms; and outpatient services. We believe the criteria are well founded in the medical literature and consistent with the experience of numerous other medical centers. We present the material as *a right way* of obtaining and preparing blood gas samples—by no means do we believe these are the *only* ways!

OBTAINING THE SAMPLE

Blood has been used as a source of laboratory studies for many years because it reflects total body status and is readily available. Since the integrity of a vessel must be violated to obtain a blood sample, it is reasonable to be concerned about the problems that may develop from such an invasion. The three most significant problems are bleeding, obstruction of the vessel, and infection.

Venous puncture would have theoretically fewer problems than arterial puncture because: (1) the pressures are lower and therefore bleeding would be less of a problem, (2) venous collateral vessels are abundant so that obstruction of one peripheral vein is seldom a significant problem, and (3) interruption of venous flow is less significant to tissue viability than interruption of arterial flow. Thus, it is understandable how venous puncture and venous blood samples became the standard for laboratory blood tests.

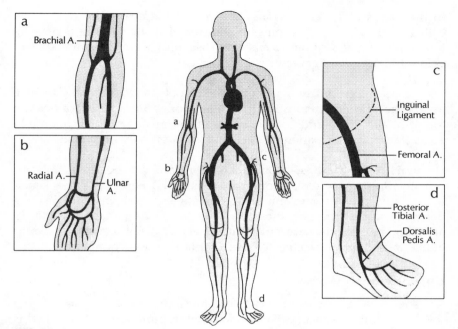

FIG 20–1.
Schematic of collateral circulation. **a,** deep brachial, superior, and inferior ulnar collateral arteries usually provide sufficient flow to the radial and ulnar arteries if the brachial artery is obstructed. **b,** the palmar arches usually provide adequate flow to the hand and fingers when either the ulnar or radial arteries are obstructed. **c,** the deep femoral artery is the only collateral source of flow to the lower extremity—it usually originates well below the level of the inguinal ligament; thus, obstruction to flow in the femoral artery above this point leaves the lower extremity without arterial blood flow. **d,** the arterial arches that provide blood flow to the foot and toes are usually supplied by both the dorsalis pedis and the posterior tibial arteries.

Criteria for Site of Arterial Puncture

The reasons blood gas measurements must be made on arterial blood have been discussed in Section I. It is important to develop a rationale for deciding what criteria should be used to determine the appropriate sampling site and technique.

Collateral Blood Flow.—Arterial puncture may cause vessel spasm, intraluminal clotting, or bleeding with the formation of a periarterial clot (hematoma).[255–257] Any of these factors may result in diminution or total interruption of blood flow to the tissues normally supplied by that vessel. Therefore, an important consideration in choosing arterial puncture sites should be the potential collateral blood flow available in the event the artery becomes obstructed.

Figure 20–1 illustrates the excellent collateral arterial blood supply in the hands and feet. The *brachial artery* at the elbow has reasonable collateral flow when it becomes obstructed. However, there is no adequate collateral flow if the *femoral artery* becomes obstructed immediately below the inguinal ligament.

Vessel Accessibility.—It is easier to palpate, stabilize, and puncture a superficial artery than a relatively deep one. Superficial arteries are found at the distal ends of the extremities—areas that are commonly accessible in the outpatient as well as in the critically ill patient.

Periarterial Tissues.—Muscle, tendon, and fat are reasonably insensitive to pain, whereas bone periosteum and nerves are very sensitive. Thus, arteries surrounded by relatively insensitive tissues are desirable so that the puncture can be as free from pain as possible. In addition, arteries that are not immediately adjacent to veins are preferable to minimize the chance of inadvertent venous puncture.

Upper Extremity Access

The radial artery at the wrist best meets the above criteria as being the safest and most accessible site for arterial puncture.[258] The vessel is located superficially at the wrist and is not adjacent to large veins. The collateral circulation is usually adequate via the ulnar artery. If puncture of the bone periosteum is avoided, the procedure is relatively pain-free.

Puncture of the brachial artery in the antecubital fossa is a logical alternative when the radial arteries are unavailable. It is our opinion that routine arterial punctures by nonphysicians should be limited to the radial artery.

The superficial palmar arch provides the major source of blood flow to the fingers. The arch is derived primarily from the ulnar artery; the radial artery supplies the smaller deep palmar and dorsal arch of the hand. However, 1.6% of patients have incomplete palmar arches so that the hand is perfused primarily by the radial artery.[259] Before invading the radial artery, it is important to determine which of the two arteries is dominant in supplying the palmar arch.

The Modified Allen's Test

Although there are precise methods of assessing collateral circulation,[260, 261] a simple, clinically reliable maneuver for assessing collateral circulation in the hand prior to radial artery puncture is desirable. As originally described in 1929, Allen's test was devised for confirming the presence of radial arterial occlusion.[262] First, the suspected radial artery is occluded at the wrist for 3 minutes and the hand color is compared with that of the other hand. If there is no change in color, the hand has sufficient collateral circulation through the ulnar artery. Second, the ulnar artery is occluded for 3 minutes. Change in the color of the hand leads to a high degree of suspicion of radial artery occlusion. Thus, *a positive Allen's test denotes the presence of radial artery occlusion.*

The test that has been popularized in respiratory care is a *modified* Allen's test (Fig 20–2). The hand is closed tightly to form a fist, thus forcing blood from the hand. Pressure is applied directly at the wrist to compress and obstruct *both* the radial and the ulnar arteries. The hand is then relaxed but not fully extended, revealing a blanched palm and fingers.[263] The obstructing pressure is removed from only the ulnar artery while the palm, fingers, and thumb are observed. They should become flushed within 10 to 15 seconds as blood from the ulnar artery refills the empty capillary beds. The flushing of the entire hand documents that the ulnar artery alone is capable of supplying the entire hand while the radial artery is occluded. Since the purpose of the modified Allen's test is to assess ulnar artery collateral flow to the hand, a positive result confirms the assumption of ulnar artery flow. Therefore, *a positive modified Allen's test denotes the presence of ulnar collateral flow,* suggesting that a radial artery puncture should be safe.

Failure to differentiate clearly the Allen's test from the *modified* Allen's test has resulted in great confusion.[264, 265] A positive Allen's test denotes arterial occlusion and contraindicates radial artery puncture, whereas a positive modified Allen's test denotes intact ulnar collateral flow and suggests that radial arterial puncture will be safe.

We suggest that the modified Allen's test be described only in terms of ulnar collateral flow, since that is its purpose. A positive modified Allen's test denotes adequate ulnar collateral flow, which assumes that transient radial occlusion secondary to arterial puncture will not result in a diminution of the blood supply to the hand. If the ulnar artery does not adequately supply the hand—a negative modified Allen's test—the radial artery should not be used as a routine puncture site for measuring arterial blood gases.[266]

There are limitations to the modified Allen's test: (1) it cannot be performed properly in an unconscious or anesthetized patient; (2) previous radial artery cannulation frequently obliterates the pulse; (3) patients in shock with severe circulatory insufficiency, deeply jaundiced patients, and pallid individuals present a particularly difficult problem in evaluation of the timing of reperfusion; (4) wrist or palm burns make interpretation impossible; and (5) the test is inconclusive if blushing of the palm is delayed 10 to 15 seconds. In these difficult situations the ulnar collateral flow can be evaluated by placing a pulse transducer over the patient's thumb and observing the disappearance of the pulse con-

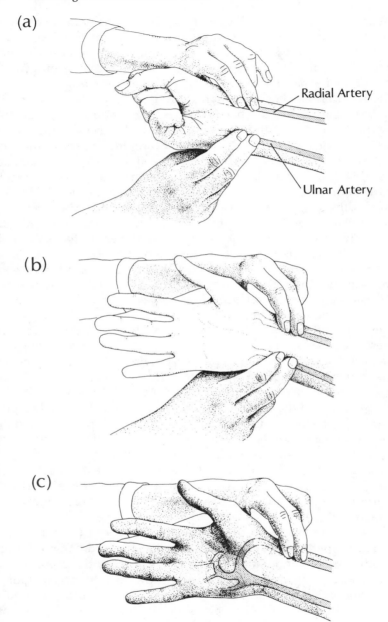

FIG 20–2.
The modified Allen's test. **a,** the hand is clenched into a tight fist and pressure is applied to the radial and ulnar arteries. **b,** the hand is opened (but not fully extended); the palm and fingers are blanched. **c,** removal of the pressure on the ulnar artery should result in flushing of the entire hand.

tour as pressure is placed on the ulnar artery; release of pressure should result in immediate return of the pulse contour.[267]

When the radial artery is the dominant blood supply to the palmar arch, the ulnar artery may be chosen as the puncture site. It is not the wrist vessel of choice because it is harder to stabilize and is more readily subjected to thrombosis because of its smaller diameter.

The brachial artery has been used safely in the intensive care unit[268] and operating room. Catheters placed in larger arteries require close scrutiny for complications and should be removed immediately if signs of hand ischemia appear.

Lower Extremity Access

Percutaneous cannulation of the dorsalis pedis artery is easy to perform, reliable, and relatively safe. The incidence of thrombosis is less than that in radial arteries.[269] The main arterial arch of the foot is supplied by the dorsalis pedis and lateral plantar arteries. To check for collateral flow, occlude the dorsalis pedis artery with external compression and blanch the great toe by compressing the toenail. Release the nail pressure and observe a rapid return of color, which indicates lateral plantar flow is present. Flushing may be difficult to see if the feet are cold[270] or the perfusion status is marginal. A digital pulse transducer over the great toe can be used to detect collateral flow.

The femoral artery has been cannulated for long periods in the intensive care unit without significant problems.[271] Signs of ischemia of the foot are an indication to remove the catheter immediately. We consider this the site of last resort except for patients with aneurysms of the descending aorta.[272]

Technique for Radial Artery Puncture

Most procedures can be accomplished safely and efficiently in many different ways. The following is a protocol we have found very successful in teaching radial artery puncture. We include this stepwise procedure as a prototype, realizing that numerous modifications may be made without affecting the skill or ease with which the procedure can be accomplished.

1. The process is explained to the patient and the radial and ulnar arteries are palpated. A modified Allen's test is performed.
2. The skin at the puncture site is cleansed with an alcohol swab and the area examined for skin rash or other abnormalities that may rule out that site for needle puncture.

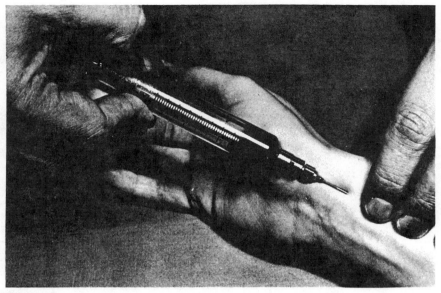

FIG 20–3.
Radial artery puncture technique.

3. A small skin wheal is raised with a local anesthetic through a 25-gauge needle. Experience has shown that the great majority of punctures are accomplished on the first attempt[273]; however, a skin wheal allows another attempt to be made without pain. In addition, most patients appreciate that you are anesthetizing the area prior to needle insertion. There has been no evidence to substantiate the claim that slight breath holding or mild hyperventilation during the puncture significantly affects the blood gas results.

4. We suggest a 20- or 21-gauge needle; however, any gauge in the range of 25 to 19 may be used without affecting the accuracy of the sample.[274] Needle lumens smaller than 22-gauge may require higher arterial pressures to pulsate blood through the needle into the syringe.[275]

5. The angle between the needle and the artery should be as small as possible (Fig 20–3). This makes the hole through the arterial wall oblique so that the circular smooth muscle fibers will seal the hole when the needle is withdrawn. If the needle goes completely through the artery, slowly withdraw the needle until its tip is again within the lumen, as evidenced by free-flowing blood through the needle.

6. After 2–4 ml has been obtained, the needle is withdrawn and pressure is applied to the site for a minimum of 2 minutes. If the needle entry was oblique, the incidence of hematoma (periarterial accumulation of blood) is rare.

ARTERIAL CANNULATION

Our indication for placing an arterial line is when a patient is (or may become) cardiopulmonary unstable—in other words, any patient who needs serial blood gas monitoring and/or continuous arterial pressure monitoring. These general criteria for arterial lines are based on their great contribution to the care of the critically ill patient—especially when compared to their low complication rate.[276]

Complications

Ultrasound flow studies of arteries that have been cannulated have a 7% to 41% incidence of diminished or absent flow for limited times.[277–281] Where adequate collateral circulation is present, these findings do not result in significant complication to the patient.[268, 282] The most severe complications are necrosis and loss of tissue.[283] There have been several case reports of finger and toe loss and numerous cases of lower limb loss or the necessity for femoral endarterectomy. Of more than 20,000 consecutive arterial lines placed by our respiratory care service (none of them femoral), 43 patients (less than 0.1%) have suffered necrosis of fingers or toes. The majority of these patients had either severe four-extremity perfusion deficit or primary vascular disease. None of these patients survived the critical illness.

Infection is a potential problem with all vessel cannulations.[284] Our incidence of systemic sepsis or local infection secondary to arterial cannulation is the same as for venous cannulation.[285] It can be stated that arterial lines properly cared for have no greater complication rate than that of indwelling venous catheters.

Thrombosis is a complication of arterial cannulation. The risk of radial artery thrombosis appears to be diminished if a proper insertion technique is followed[286] or if aspirin is administered beforehand.[287] Additional precautions must be taken when the arterial cannula system incorporates a continuous flush device and/or a pressure monitor. False elevation of pressure readings have been associated with the flush device,[288] and bacteremia has been traced to the pressure transducer.[289]

The extremely low incidence of significant complication compared with the patient care benefits offered by arterial cannulation more than justifies such placement in critically ill patients.

Technique for Indwelling Arterial Cannula

The following technique has proved safe, practical, and dependable in our institution.

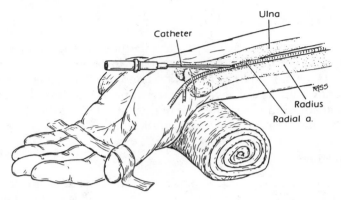

FIG 20–4.
The correct position of the wrist for cannulation, the proper angle for catheter insertion, and the relationship of the radial artery to the bones of the forearm are shown. (From Fragen RJ: Arterial catheterization and maintenance of indwelling arterial lines, in Beal JM (ed): *Critical Care for Surgical Patients.* New York, Macmillan Publishing Co, 1982, p 95.)

I. Equipment
A. Intravenous cannula, consisting of:
    2.5-ml syringe
    Teflon cannula
    Needle stylet
B. 2.5-ml syringe, 25-gauge needle, 1 ampule 1% xylocaine
C. Skin antiseptic swabs
D. Continuous arterial keep-open setup, consisting of:
    1-ml ampule heparin (10 mg/ml)
    500-ml plastic transfer pack
    Intravenous tubing set
    Fenwal pressure bag
    2 fused sterile three-way stopcocks
    Intraflo flushing device (Sorenson)*
    1-ft-high pressure tubing (Cobe)

II. Radial Arterial Cannulation
The supinated arm is placed on an arm board and a folded towel or padding is placed under the wrist to accomplish a 50- to 60-degree angle of extension. The hand including the thumb is taped to a firm surface to help stabilize the artery at the wrist (Fig 20–4). The radial arterial pulse should be palpated at the wrist and the course of the radial artery determined. If the artery is not readily palpable, a small-tipped Doppler flow probe can be placed over the wrist to determine the course of the artery.

The skin is thoroughly cleansed and painted with an iodine solution.

In conscious patients, a skin wheal is raised with local anesthetic at the first skin fold, approximately one inch proximal to the wrist joint. A hole is made in the skin wheal with an 18-gauge needle to facilitate passage of the catheter through the skin. A 20-gauge nontapered, non-radiopaque Teflon catheter, approximately 3 to 3.5 cm in length, is chosen to cannulate the radial artery. This type of catheter is associated with the fewest complications.[290,291] The hub of the catheter should be Luer Lok, and the plug should be removed from the hub before the catheter is inserted into the artery.

The catheter is inserted through the hole in the skin wheal at a 10- to 15-degree angle with the skin, along the course of the artery (see Fig 20–4). As the artery is entered, blood will fill the hub of the needle and spurt out the end; when this occurs, the plastic catheter is carefully advanced up the artery. A pulsatile flow of blood should continue to spurt out the end of the catheter. A halt in the flow of blood indicates that the needle has penetrated the back wall of the artery. To remedy this, only the needle is pulled out and the catheter gradually withdrawn until a spurt of blood appears, signaling that the catheter can again be advanced. A few gauze sponges under the hub of the needle to catch the spurting blood makes this a neater procedure. After flushing, the monitoring assembly is attached to the catheter hub.

The hand and wrist are cleaned and dried, and tincture of benzoin is sprayed over the wrist, the exposed catheter, and a few inches of the connector tubing. A chevron of 0.5-in. tape is placed around the catheter to prevent it from slipping out of place. To prevent disconnection of the connector tubing from the catheter hub, a piece of 1-in. tape, 6 in. long,

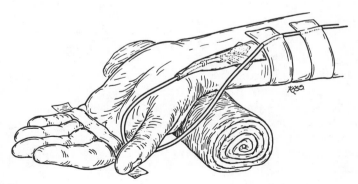

FIG 20–5.
This is the correct method of taping and securing the catheter once it is inserted into the radial artery and attached to the hydraulic system. (From Fragen RJ: Arterial catheterization and maintenance of indwelling arterial lines, in Beal JM (ed): *Critical Care for Surgical Patients.* New York, Macmillan Publishing Co, 1982, p 95.)

is placed along the course of the connector tubing, looped loosely around the thumb, and taped to the wrist and arm with a few strips of 1-in. tape (Fig 20–5). To prevent infection, an antibiotic ointment may be used on the puncture site and covered with a sterile dressing. The fingers should never be included in a dressing over the catheter, because they need to be observed for signs of ischemia. The hand can be released from the arm board or firm surface and the wrist taken out of extension.

III. Continuous Arterial Keep-Open Technique

Note.—Have this prepared before insertion of the cannula.

A. Add 10 mg (1 ml) heparin to 500 ml normal saline.
B. *Important*: Absolutely no air bubbles can be present in the tubing or bag. Eliminate any bubbles by applying firm snapping pressure to the bag or tubing.
C. Insert intravenous tubing into the transfer pack. Make sure that the drip chamber does not completely fill with solution.
D. *Important:* Adhesive tape all junctions of the intravenous tubing so that no medication can be injected into the arterial line.
E. Free the tubing of air; then shut off the tubing control and apply *150 to 300 mm Hg* of pressure from the Fenwal bag to the transfer pack. Maintain at least 50 mm Hg above systolic pressure.
F. Connect Intraflo to the intravenous tubing.
G. Attach three-way stopcocks, with 2.5-ml syringes attached, to the Intraflo. Be sure the stopcocks are "off."
H. Attach the Cobe tubing to the remaining end of the fused stopcocks and connect to the cannula.
I. Rid the entire setup of air and attach it to the arterial cannula (Fig 20–6).

IV. Drawing a Blood Sample

A. A waste syringe is attached to the stopcock farthest from the cannula and solution is withdrawn until undiluted blood enters the syringe. Five to six times the tubing volume is advised.[292]
B. Two milliliters of blood is drawn into the sample syringe through the other stopcock.
C. The plunger is gently pulled on the Intraflo device until the blood is cleared from the tubing.

---

*The Intraflo device flushes approximately 3 ml/hr of the heparinized solution from the transfer pack. This has proved to provide ample flushing to prevent the cannula from clotting. In addition, a tubing that connects to a pressure transducer can be attached directly to the Intraflo device.

CAPILLARY SAMPLES

Improved methods of radial artery cannulation in infants and small children,[293] radial artery puncture,[294] and umbilical artery catheterization[295] have been reported. However, clinical circumstances arise with infants and small children when arterial samples are either not readily available or not indicated. This situation occurs primarily in the well-perfused infant where a Po_2 measurement is desirable but not to the point of warranting arterial sticks or cannulation.

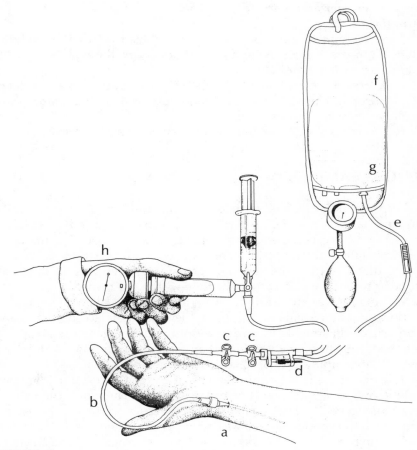

FIG 20–6.
The continuous arterial keep-open technique. **a,** cannula entering radial artery; **b,** Cobe tubing; **c,** fused stopcocks; **d,** Intraflo device; **e,** intravenous tubing; **f,** Fenwal pressure bag; **g,** transfer pack with heparinized solution; **h,** aneroid pressure transducer (electronic transducer may be used).

In a well-perfused infant, arterialized capillary blood will show a consistent correlation with arterial P_{CO_2} and pH and will reflect a *minimal* arterial P_{O_2} value. It must be emphasized that P_{O_2} data from capillary samples are meaningless in a baby whose perfusion status is not perfectly normal.[296–306] When cardiopulmonary instability exists, an arterial cannula is as indicated in the small child and infant as in the adult.[307–311]

Technique for Capillary Samples

1. A highly vascularized capillary bed (earlobe, heel, great toe, or finger) is chosen and warmed for 10 minutes by either heat lamp or warm towels.

2. A *deep* puncture is made with a scalpel blade so that a free flow of blood appears from the wound without squeezing the area. Squeezing will "de-arterialize" the sample.

3. A preheparinized capillary tube (75 to 100 μl) is inserted deep into the drop of blood. The blood should flow easily into the tube. Two capillary tubes provide an ideal sample.

4. The tubes should be immediately sealed and placed in ice.

VENOUS SAMPLES

Appropriately obtained samples of peripheral venous blood in well-perfused patients may be used to grossly reflect the arterial acid-base status.[312, 313] However, peripheral venous blood for assessing the oxygenation state is unacceptable. This is because the distribution of the total cardiac output to the various organ systems depends on the local arteriolar resistance and vasomotor tone within the respective capillary beds. The cardiovascular system always attempts to maintain blood flow to critical organ systems at an optimal level. This is accomplished by appropriate adjustments in cardiac output and changes in regional resistances. Therefore, the various organ systems do not necessarily receive a blood supply proportional to their metabolic demands.

The net effect is differing degrees of oxygen extraction from the blood supplied to the respective organ systems. Therefore, the values of venous oxygen tension would vary depending on the organ system from which the venous sample was taken. These differences exist under basal resting conditions and become even more exaggerated in the critically ill patient. Table 20–1 lists the variations in venous blood gas measurements for blood returning from different organ systems under basal resting conditions.

TABLE 20–1.

Venous Oxygen Tension and Oxygen Contents for Blood Returning From Different Organ Systems*

Organ System	$P\bar{v}_{O_2}$ (mm Hg)	% SAT	$[Ca_{O_2} - Cv_{O_2}]$ (vol%)
Cerebral	37	69	6.3
Coronary	30	56	11.4
Intestinal	45	80	4.1
Renal	74	94	1.3
Skeletal muscle	32	60	8.0
Skin	75	95	1.0

Conditions: Arterial P_{O_2} = 100, Ca_{O_2} = 20.2 vol%, Hb = 15 gm%, cardiac output = 6 L/min, human subject at rest.

PULMONARY ARTERY SAMPLES

When blood samples are aspirated from a PA catheter, the sample must be withdrawn *slowly* since rapid aspiration can result in pulmonary capillary blood being mixed with the pulmonary artery blood.[314] This would cause dramatic increases in oxygen content. Withdrawal rates as high as 30 ml/min may not significantly affect the oxygen saturation,[315] although it still is prudent to withdraw the sample slowly.

PREPARING THE SAMPLE

Blood gas samples are highly susceptible to preanalytic error due to improper methods of obtaining or handling the sample prior to delivery to the laboratory. The following guidelines are the currently accepted practices for eliminating this source of error from blood gas measurement.

Syringes

Earlier studies suggested that plastic substances absorb so much oxygen that their use for blood gas samples would be ill-advised; however, these assumptions have not been substantiated.[316] In essence, pH and P_{CO_2} values have not been greatly affected, whereas P_{O_2} values in excess of 400 mm Hg drop more rapidly in plastic than in glass syringes.[317] Seldom is this circumstance clinically significant.

We *prefer* glass syringes for the following reasons: (1) the barrel has minimal friction with the syringe wall and the pulsating arterial pressure is obvious as the blood fills the syringe; (2) there is seldom a need to "pull back" on the barrel, which can cause air bubbles to enter the sample around the barrel; and (3) small air bubbles adhere tenaciously to the sides of a plastic syringe, making it difficult to expel the air from the sample.[318]

Although glass is preferred, there is no valid objection to the use of appropriate plastic syringes. In fact, we routinely use more than 30,000 plastic syringes per year for sample collection from arterial lines. New designs in expendable plastic syringes have also been marketed that appear to eliminate many of the problems noted above.

Anticoagulants

When blood is removed from a vessel, the clotting mechanisms are immediately activated. This results in a sample of serum plus a blood clot. Blood gas measurements must be accomplished on "whole blood"— i.e., unclotted and unseparated blood. An anticoagulant is used to inactivate the clotting mechanisms so that the sample remains unclotted in the syringe.

Oxylates, ethylenediamine tetra-acetic acid (EDTA), and citrates are commonly used as anticoagulants for blood studies. These are not acceptable for blood gas samples because they significantly alter the blood sample.[319, 320]

Heparin is the anticoagulant of choice; however, too much heparin affects pH, PCO_2, PO_2, as well as the hemoglobin determination.[321–326] The pH of sodium heparin is approximately 7.0; PCO_2 and PO_2 approach room air values. The addition of any diluent potentially alters the hemoglobin concentration measurement.

It can be demonstrated that 0.05 ml sodium heparin (1,000 units/ml or 10 mg/ml) will adequately anticoagulate 1 ml blood; whereas 0.1 ml will not affect pH, PCO_2, or PO_2 values of 1 ml blood.[321] When a 3- to 5-ml syringe with needle is washed with sodium heparin and then ejected, the deadspace of the syringe will contain approximately 0.15 to 0.25 ml sodium heparin. Thus 2 to 4 ml blood will theoretically contain at least 0.05 ml heparin per 1 ml blood but no more than 0.1 ml heparin per 1 ml blood.

Thus, we recommend the syringe be flushed with sodium heparin (10 mg/ml) and then emptied; this will allow adequate anticoagulation of a 2- to 4-ml blood sample with assurance that the results will not be significantly altered by the anticoagulant. Preheparinized blood gas syringes are available with the anticoagulant in either a liquid or a dry state. This potentially eliminates most of the adverse effects of the anticoagulant while still preventing clotting.

Anaerobic Conditions

Room air contains a PCO_2 of essentially 0 and a PO_2 of approximately

150 mm Hg. Air bubbles that mix with a blood sample will result in gas equilibration between the air and the blood. Thus, air bubbles may significantly lower the Pco_2 values of the blood sample with subsequent increase in pH and cause the Po_2 to approach 150 mm Hg. The greater the amount of air mixed with a blood sample, the greater the potential for error. We recommend that any sample obtained with more than minor air bubbles be discarded.

To maintain the anaerobic conditions, the syringe must be immediately sealed with a cap. The sample must be introduced into the electrode chambers without air bubbles.

Delay in Running the Sample

Blood is living tissue in which oxygen continues to be consumed and carbon dioxide continues to be produced, even after the blood is drawn into a syringe. Table 20–2 shows the approximate rate of change of a sample that is held in the syringe at 37°C.[327] If the sample is immediately placed in an ice slush, the temperature rapidly falls to approximately 4°C, and the Pco_2 and pH changes are insignificant over several hours. If the sample is not iced immediately, the changes can be significant.

The white blood cell oxygen consumption is important if the sample is not iced because 0.1 ml oxygen is consumed from 100 ml blood (0.1 vol%) in 10 minutes at body temperature. The effect on oxygen tension depends on the state of hemoglobin saturation.[327] For example, if the Po_2 is 400 mm Hg, it will drop to below 250 mm Hg in 1 hour if the sample is not iced. If the sample is immediately placed in an ice slush, the Po_2 will be more than 350 mm Hg even after 1 hour. If the Po_2 is 50 mm Hg, the loss of 0.1 ml oxygen from 100 ml blood makes a very small change in Po_2, because the primary change is in the hemoglobin saturation.

TABLE 20–2.

In Vitro Blood Gas Changes*

	37°C	4°C
pH	0.01/10 min	0.001/10 min
Pco_2	1 mm Hg/10 min	0.1 mm Hg/10 min
Po_2	0.1 vol%/10 min	0.01 vol%/10 min

*Approximate changes with time and temperature after the sample is drawn into the syringe. Temperature 37°C assumes that the blood remains at body temperature in the syringe. Temperature 4°C assumes that the sample is properly iced immediately after being drawn.

of the blood cells. In fact, immediately placing the sample on ice decreases the metabolic rate to such an extent that the sample may undergo little change over several hours. As a general rule, arterial blood samples should be analyzed within 10 minutes or cooled immediately. Delay of up to one hour for running a cooled sample will have little clinically significant effect on the results. Failure to cool the sample properly is a common source of preanalytic error. Carriers have been developed to assure that the blood gas syringe is properly cooled.

21

Blood Gas Analyzers

The measurement of blood pH, PCO_2 and PO_2 is accomplished by specially designed electrodes, the understanding of which depends on a knowledge of basic electrical physics. In essence, the flow of electrons from one point to another is referred to as an electric *current*. Such an electron flow occurs in response to a *potential difference* between two points in a manner similar to a gas flowing in response to a pressure difference between two points. An electric potential difference *(voltage)* is measured by devices called *voltmeters*. An electric device that can predictably vary potential differences (voltage) is called a *potentiometer*.

pH ELECTRODE

It was discovered more than 70 years ago that if two solutions of different pH values are separated by a particular type of glass membrane, there will be a potential difference across the "pH-sensitive" glass.[328–332] As shown in Figure 21–1,a, if a solution of known pH (6.840) is separated by pH-sensitive glass from a solution of unknown pH, a measurable voltage will be developed across the glass.

Chemical half-cells (Fig 21–1,b) are used to accurately measure the small potential differences accompanying blood pH variations. The *reference electrode* is usually composed of mercury-mercurous chloride (calomel)—a substance that supplies a constant reference voltage as long as the temperature remains stable. The *measuring electrode* is usually composed of a silver-silver chloride substance whose function is to convey the potential difference across the glass membrane to the electronic circuitry.

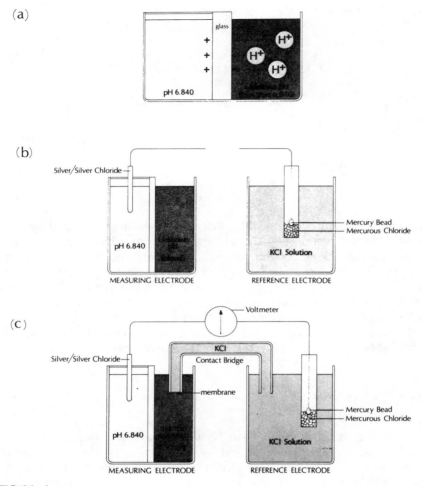

FIG 21–1.
Basic principles of the pH electrode. **a,** voltage developed across pH-sensitive glass when hydrogen ion concentration is unequal in the two solutions. **b,** chemical half-cell is used as the measuring electrode and another half-cell is the reference electrode (see text). **c,** the basic principle of the modern pH electrode (see text).

Modern Electrode

The modern pH electrode (Fig 21–1,c) has the measuring half-cell imbedded within a 6.840 buffer chamber. This half-cell and the adjacent sampling chamber are encased in a constant-temperature environment. The reference half-cell is electronically connected to the measuring half-cell by a *contact bridge*—a potassium chloride (KCl) solution that completes the electronic circuit. The KCl solution is protected from blood contamination either by a membrane or various mechanisms such as pinch valves and/or peristaltic pumps.

Calibration

The relationship between the potential difference ($E_u - E_k$) and the pH values of the known (pH_k) and unknown (pH_u) solutions are defined by the modified Nernst equation:

$$pH_u = pH_k + \left(\frac{E_u - E_k}{2.3026T}\right)\left(\frac{F}{R}\right)$$

where R is the molar gas constant, F is the Faraday constant, and T is the absolute temperature. If the pH of the unknown solution is equal to that of the known solution, the potential difference ($E_u - E_k$) will be zero. A potential of 61.5 millivolts (mV) will be developed for every pH unit difference between the two solutions at 37°C.

Potentiometers adjust the potential differences to the correct pH-scale readout. When a 6.840 buffer solution is in the measuring half-cell, the potential difference is zero and the electronic display is set to 6.840 by a *slope potentiometer*. When the measuring half-cell is filled with a 7.384 buffer solution, the difference between the two half-cells is 0.544 pH units, and a 33.5-mV potential difference can be predicted. Thus, the voltmeter will measure 33.5 mV, and a *balance potentiometer* sets the electronic display at 7.384. Since the potential difference is a linear function of the pH, two-point calibration is usually sufficient for accurate blood pH measurement.

Sanz Electrode

A clinical system for pH measurement must meet three criteria before it can be considered practical and applicable: (1) the blood sample must remain anaerobic; (2) the measuring cycle must require a minimal volume of blood; and (3) a constant temperature must be maintained. Figure 21–2 illustrates the typical design of a modern, ultramicro pH electrode first developed in the mid-1950s and most often referred to as the Sanz electrode.[333] The pH-sensitive glass has been rolled into a fine capillary tube, allowing the necessary blood volume to be as small as 25 μl and remain anaerobic. The entire electrode is small enough to be contained in a thermostatically controlled environment to assure a constant temperature.

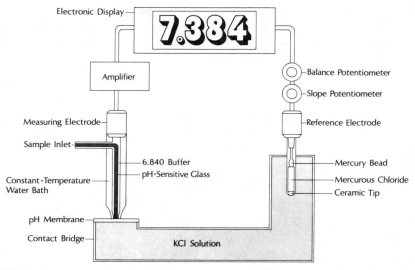

FIG 21–2.
Schematic illustration of the modern, ultramicro pH electrode (see text).

Pco₂ ELECTRODE

Henry's law (see chap. 1) states that the amount of gas diffusing across a permeable membrane is directly proportional to the pressure gradient. As shown in Figure 21–3, if a carbon dioxide partial pressure gradient exists across a permeable membrane with an aqueous bicarbonate solution on the other side, carbon dioxide entering the solution undergoes the following chemical reaction:

$$CO_2 + H_2O \rightarrow H_2CO_3 \rightarrow H^+ + HCO_3^-$$

The hydrogen ion concentration developed is directly proportional to the Pco₂ in contact with the membrane. When the aqueous bicarbonate chamber is used as the measuring half-cell, the pH change can be measured and utilized as an indirect measure of the Pco₂ of the blood.

Modern Electrode

A silicon elastic membrane separates the blood sample from the measuring half-cell (Fig 21–4).[334] The pH-sensitive glass is separated from the membrane by a nylon spacer that allows an aqueous bicarbonate solution (electrolyte) to exist between the glass and the permeable membrane. The measuring half-cell is silver-silver chloride; the reference half-cell is another silver-silver chloride unit rather than calomel.[335, 336]

The entire electrode is in a lucite jacket and is bathed in an electrolyte solution. This electrolyte constantly replenishes the solution at the electrode tip and provides an electric contact bridge between the measuring and reference half-cells.

Calibration

Gases analyzed to precise concentrations are used to calibrate the P_{CO_2} electrode. A gas mixture with a CO_2 concentration of 5% is commonly chosen as the balance point, and a slope point is set with a gas that has approximately 10% CO_2 concentration. The P_{CO_2} will be directly proportional to the hydrogen ion concentration as measured by the pH electrode system.[337]

Severinghaus Electrode

Until the mid-1950s, methods used to measure P_{CO_2} were cumbersome and time-consuming. Some involved the direct measurement of pH and carbon dioxide content; the Henderson-Hasselbalch equation was then used to extrapolate the P_{CO_2}. Another popular method in the

$$\text{GASEOUS } CO_2 \longrightarrow CO_2 + H_2O \rightleftharpoons H_2CO_3 \rightleftharpoons H^+ + HCO_3^-$$

FIG 21–3.
Basic principle of the P_{CO_2} electrode (see text). The *shaded area* represents an aqueous bicarbonate solution.

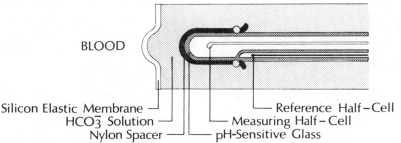

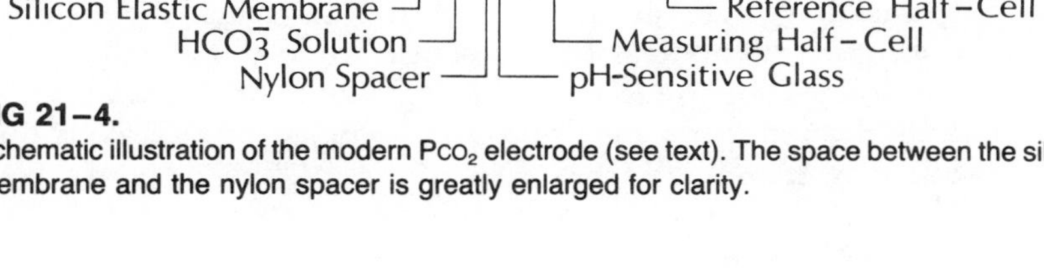

BLOOD

Silicon Elastic Membrane ⎯⎯ ⎯⎯ Reference Half–Cell
HCO_3^- Solution ⎯⎯ ⎯⎯ Measuring Half–Cell
Nylon Spacer ⎯⎯ ⎯⎯ pH-Sensitive Glass

FIG 21–4.
Schematic illustration of the modern P_{CO_2} electrode (see text). The space between the silicon membrane and the nylon spacer is greatly enlarged for clarity.

1940s and 1950s was known as the "CO_2-combining power," which involved the equilibration between blood and a bubble of gas with a known carbon dioxide content. By measuring the carbon dioxide content after equilibration, the P_{CO_2} was extrapolated.[338]

The modern P_{CO_2} electrode was first introduced by Stowe[339] and was further modified by Severinghaus in 1958.[340] This electrode is commonly referred to as the *Severinghaus electrode*.

P_{O_2} Electrode

Gaining electrons in a chemical reaction is known as *reduction* and occurs at a cathode; the loss of electrons in a chemical reaction is known as *oxidation* and occurs at an anode. If oxygen is dissolved in an aqueous medium and exposed to a polarizing voltage at a cathode, the following reaction occurs:

$$O_2 + 2H_2O + 4 \text{ electrons } (e^-) \rightarrow 4OH^-$$

This chemical reduction of oxygen is the principle of the polarographic electrode.

Polarographic Electrode

A silver anode immersed in a potassium chloride electrolyte solution will attract anions (Cl^-) to form silver chloride (Fig 21–5). This oxidation reaction produces a constant flow of electrons (current). An adjacent platinum cathode will react chemically with oxygen to form hydroxyl ions (OH^-)—a reduction reaction that uses electrons. In general, as electrons are consumed at the cathode, the anode reaction is accelerated.

Figure 21–5 illustrates that the amount of oxygen reduced will be directly proportional to the number of electrons used in the cathode reaction. Thus, by measuring the change in current (electron flow) between the anode and the cathode, one can determine the amount of oxygen in the electrode solution.

An external polarizing voltage of approximately -0.6 V is required to minimize the interference of other gases that can also be reduced and to assure rapid oxygen reduction at the cathode. Thus, the common electric concept of an anode as a negative electrode and a cathode as a positive electrode is not applicable. However, the chemical definition of a cathode as the reduction pole and an anode as the oxidation pole remains unchanged.

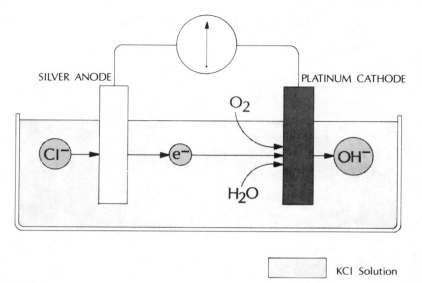

FIG 21–5.
The basic principle of the polarographic electrode. The chloride ion will react with the silver anode to form silver chloride—an oxidation reaction that produces electrons. Oxygen will react with platinum and water, utilizing electrons (a reduction reaction). The flow of electrons can be measured as a current. The greater the concentration of oxygen in solution, the greater the current generated (see text).

Calibration

An analyzed gas mixture with an oxygen concentration of 0% is selected as the slope point; the balance point is set with a gas that has either 12% or 20% oxygen. For convenience and economy, the calibration gases for the PO_2 and PCO_2 electrodes are combined. One gas is usually composed of 5% CO_2 and 12% or 20% O_2, with the remainder composed of nitrogen; the second gas is usually 10% CO_2 and 90% N_2. The influence of the "PO_2" factor (believed due to gas versus liquid measurement) is discussed elsewhere (see chap. 22). Potentiometers are used for display adjustments as described earlier but the electronic circuitry converts this to a current change, therefore the term *amperometric*.

Clark Electrode

The entire electrode system is usually covered by a polypropylene membrane, which allows a slow diffusion of oxygen from the blood into the electrode (Fig 21–6).[341] A slow-diffusing membrane is selected to

P$_{O_2}$ ELECTRODE :

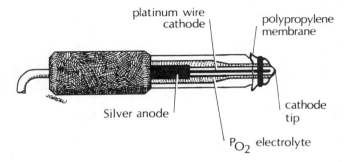

platinum wire cathode

polypropylene membrane

Silver anode

cathode tip

P$_{O_2}$ electrolyte

FIG 21–6.
Schematic illustration of the Clark electrode (see text).

prevent depletion of oxygen while the measurement is taking place.[342, 343] This negates the need for stirring the blood and significantly decreases electrode instability.[344]

Although the first polarographic oxygen electrodes were developed in the late 1930s, the development of the modern electrode in the 1950s for measuring blood and other solutions is attributed to Clark.[345] For this reason the P$_{O_2}$ electrode is commonly referred to as the *Clark electrode*. Conflicting reports of halogenated hydrocarbons affecting the Clark electrode's accuracy and precision raise the possibility that the blood of patients who are anesthetized with these agents may have falsely high P$_{O_2}$ measurements.[346]

THE MODERN BLOOD GAS ANALYZER

The past 20 years have seen a rapid development in blood gas analyzers. Not only does the newest generation of blood gas analyzers accurately and reliably measure pH, P$_{CO_2}$ and P$_{O_2}$ on samples as small as 65 μl, but they are also able to self-calibrate and self-diagnose malfunction and have computer capability for measuring plasma bicarbonate, base excess/deficit, temperature corrections, and other algorithms. Interfacing blood gas analyzers and computer systems allows patient data storage with analysis and "trending" as well as automated blood gas interpretation and billing. Often the capability of manipulating the primary blood gas values of pH, PCO_2 and PO_2 exceeds clinical practicality. The purchase of a blood gas analyzer must depend primarily on the performance of the analyzer in basic blood gas measurements and secondarily on the manipulation of these measurements.

Although there are numerous differences among manufacturers, all modern analyzers contain the following three electrodes:

The Sanz (pH) electrode quantifies the relative acidity and alkalinity of a blood solution by measuring the potential difference across a pH-sensitive glass membrane. Its principle of operation is related to the measurement of voltages, and therefore the electrode is referred to as *potentiometric*.

The Severinghaus (PCO_2) electrode measures carbon dioxide tensions by allowing the carbon dioxide gas to undergo a chemical reaction to produce hydrogen ions. The hydrogen ion concentration is measured by half-cells similar to the Sanz electrode. This system is also *potentiometric*.

The Clark (PO_2) electrode measures oxygen by electron consumption. The electron flow is measured in amperage and is referred to as *amperometric*.

The precision of these measurements is dependent on many things, but the ability to maintain the electrodes at a constant temperature is an important factor. This is accomplished by enclosing the electrodes in a thermostatically controlled water bath, heating blocks, or heated forced-air environments.

22

Quality Assurance in Blood Gas Analysis

The clinician orders blood gas measurements to document, specify, and quantitate abnormalities in cardiopulmonary homeostasis. Significant therapeutic decisions are commonly influenced by these laboratory tests, thus placing overwhelming responsibility on all associated with the laboratory to assure accurate and reliable results. This is best accomplished by dedicated personnel consistently applying meticulous attention to protocol in three areas: (1) preanalytic error, (2) calibration, and (3) quality control. Essential information concerning these three areas will be presented in this chapter. The reader must appreciate that detailed information on laboratory protocol and technique is beyond the intent and scope of this text. However, everyone involved in blood gas analysis should be conversant with these principles; they are the basic and essential steps in quality assurance.

PREANALYTIC ERROR

Preanalytic error is considered to be all factors that cause variance in laboratory results prior to the sample arriving in the laboratory. Few tests are as vulnerable as blood gas analysis to errors introduced by improper sampling, handling, and storage (see chap. 20). Errors such as venous sampling, air bubbles in the syringe, or blood in the "wrong tube" may be obvious to a well-trained, capable, and alert technologist. However, it is a formidable task to discover less obvious factors that significantly affect results.

Our experience allows us to identify four factors associated with significant preanalytic error identifiable by the blood gas technician: (1)

air bubbles in the sample[347, 348]; (2) time delay—specifically, iced samples with more than 60 minutes of delay and uniced samples with more than 15 minutes of delay; (3) blood clots in the sample, reflecting insufficient anticoagulation; and (4) small sample size when excessive anticoagulation is suspect (see chap. 20). Using these narrow criteria, we examined 8,748 consecutive specimens delivered to our Central Blood Gas Laboratory and found that 107 (1.2%) were suspected of preanalytic error.[349] Of the specimens, 6,963 were obtained from indwelling arterial catheters, with a 0.1% incidence of preanalytic error. Of the 173 pulmonary artery samples, 3.5% were suspect. The samples obtained by individual arterial puncture (1,612) had a 5.7% incidence of preanalytic error. Furthermore, samples arriving from intensive care units and operating rooms had an 0.3% incidence (probably due to the prevalence of arterial cannulas), whereas those from the emergency room had a 15.8% incidence.

Although such data are far from conclusive and reflect only one medical center, the basic lesson is obvious—*individual arterial punctures for blood gas analysis are associated with a significant incidence of preanalytic error.*

Since clots are primarily due to inadequate heparin in the syringe and air bubbles often due to improper capping of glass syringes, it is reasonable to expect that preheparinized plastic syringe kits would significantly reduce these problems. However, our study attributed less than 2% of preanalytic error to these factors, emphasizing that technique is still by far the most crucial factor.

CALIBRATION

Calibration is generally defined as the systematic standardization of the graduations of a quantitative measuring instrument. The purpose of calibration is to assure *consistency!* Calibrating standards for blood gas analyzers should simulate the physical properties of blood and meet manufacturers' specifications.

A one-point calibration is an adjustment of the electronic response of an electrode to a single standard. One-point calibration is considered necessary prior to each sample analysis.[350] When two standards are used, the process is referred to as "two-point calibration," which should be done every 8 hours or every 50 blood gas measurements (whichever comes first) as well as after electrode maintenance and repair measures.

Two-point calibration is also indicated when one-point calibration reveals excessive electrode drift, such as: (1) slow electrode response but eventual stabilization at the predicted value; (2) drifting values that do not stabilize; or (3) stable values significantly different from those predicted. Computers now monitor these factors following one-point calibration, but a knowledgeable operator is required to respond intelligently and appropriately to the computer information.

pH Calibration

Several types of buffer solution are acceptable for pH electrode calibration.[351–353] These buffers are excellent standards because of their long shelf life and stability for days after being opened. Since a buffer may be contaminated or mislabeled, a new solution should be introduced immediately following two-point calibration with the old buffer (whose accuracy and consistency have been verified through the laboratory's quality control system). If the pH needs to be adjusted by more than 0.01 unit with the new buffer, it must be seriously questioned since the accuracy of these commercially available buffers is ±0.005 unit of labeled value.

Two-point calibration of the pH electrode is accomplished by setting the slope potentiometer (see chap. 21) to a low pH buffer (e.g., 6.840) and setting the balance potentiometer with a near-normal buffer (e.g., 7.384). One-point calibration is usually done with the near-normal buffer.

P_{CO_2} Calibration

The P_{CO_2} electrode may be calibrated either by introducing a known gas directly or by first equilibrating an aqueous, serum, or blood solution and introducing the liquid. Either method depends on knowing the exact CO_2 content of the gas. Such gas standards are commercially prepared by analytic grade-mixing devices or by gravimetric methods. The contents of the cylinder should be certified by the manufacturer to within ±0.03% and periodically tested by either the Scholander method[354] or mass spectrometry.

Two-point calibration of the P_{CO_2} electrode is commonly accomplished by setting the balance potentiometer (see chap. 20) to a 5% CO_2 standard and the slope potentiometer to a 10% CO_2 standard. A mercury barometer must be in close proximity and checked each time two-point calibration is carried out. The P_{CO_2} is calculated—$(P_B - 47 \text{ mm Hg}) \times \%CO_2$.

P_{O_2} Calibration

Two factors complicate P_{O_2} electrode calibration: (1) the blood gas factor—a gas directly introduced into the electrode results in a higher reading than the same gas first equilibrated with blood and then introduced into the electrode;[355–357] and (2) Po_2 measurement is not linear over the range of 0 to 600 mm Hg.[358]

The *blood gas factor* (Table 22–1) may understate the Po_2 from 2% to 15%[359, 360] but appears to be most apparent in Po_2 values greater than 150 mm Hg.[361] This factor has been implicated to have a substantial effect on the calculation of intrapulmonary shunt.[362] There appears little reason to correct for this factor in the Po_2 range below 100 mm Hg.

Properly calibrated Po_2 electrodes perform within the manufacturer's stated accuracy in Po_2 ranges below 150 mm Hg, but they may vary 20% at 500 mm HG.[363] This has prompted some laboratories to use a higher concentration of oxygen as a balance point;[361–364] one manufacturer published a correction chart for Po_2 values above 150 mm Hg. We have found neither step necessary for accurate calibration or clinical reliability.

The method commonly used for Po_2 electrode calibration is similar to that for the Pco_2 electrode.[353, 359, 365, 366] Most commonly, 0% oxygen is used for the slope point and either 12% or 20% oxygen for the balance point. Some analyzers aspirate room air for the balance point of CO_2 and the balance point of O_2, assuming room air has 0% CO_2 and 20.9% O_2. It is incumbent upon the laboratory to confirm those assumptions regularly.

Electrode Precision

Modern blood gas analyzers carry manufacturer specifications that state electrode reliability assuming the manufacturers' instructions for calibration and sample introduction are followed. Generally, electrode precision is stated as listed in Table 22–2.[367]

Theoretically, proper maintenance and calibration should assure reliability. However, in practice that is not the case and further measures must be taken.

TABLE 22–1.

Blood Gas Factor Calculation for Po_2 Electrode

$$\text{Blood gas factor} = \frac{Po_2 \text{ gas} - Po_2 \text{ blood}}{Po_2 \text{ gas}}$$

Po_2 gas = (Fraction of O_2 in cylinder) (P_B − 47)

Po_2 blood = Recorded result of Po_2 of blood
tonometered with same fraction of O_2

TABLE 22–2.

Electrode Precision

pH	± 0.01 unit
P_{CO_2}	± 2% (approximately ±1 mm Hg at 40 mm Hg)
P_{O_2}	± 3% (approximately ±2.5 mm Hg at 80 mm Hg)
Over 150 mm Hg P_{O_2}, the precision is ±10%.	

QUALITY CONTROL

Quality control refers to a system that documents the accuracy and reliability of the blood gas measurements. The same factors that produce preanalytic error in blood gas analysis have prevented the development of a single standard that has the same properties as blood, is economical and stable, and has pH, P_{CO_2}, and P_{O_2} values that are assayable to the same degree of accuracy as most clinical chemistry controls.[368–370] Therefore, a quality control *system* is essential to assure accuracy in the blood gas laboratory. Following is a review of the basic statistics and methods common to all blood gas quality control systems.

Statistics

A properly functioning electrode that repeatedly analyzes a known value will produce results within a relatively small range. For example, a P_{CO_2} electrode that analyzes a 40.0 mm Hg standard 100 times will produce results in a *frequency distribution* as illustrated in Figure 22–1. More than two thirds of the measurements fall within the 39.0 to 41.0 range and nearly all the values are within the 38.0 to 42.0 range.

The *arithmetic mean* ($\bar{x}$) of the 100 values is calculated as:

$$\bar{x} = \frac{\Sigma x_1}{n} \qquad (1)$$

where Σx_1 is the sum of the values and n is the number of values.[371]

If we wish to choose a single number from our 100 values that best represents the population, we choose the mean value. However, that number does not give information about the distribution pattern; i.e., the mean alone does not give the information that the frequency distribution curve provides. Such information is reasonably accomplished by calculating the *standard deviation from the mean (SD)*:

$$SD = \sqrt{\frac{n\Sigma x_1^2 - (\Sigma x_1)^2}{n(n-1)}} \qquad (2)$$

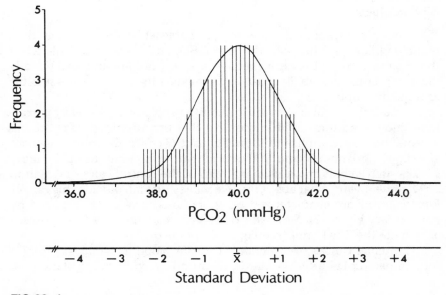

FIG 22–1.
Frequency distribution of Pco_2 measurement, demonstrating bell-shaped distribution and standard deviations.

where Σx_1^2 is the sum of each of the squares.[371]

In our example, the SD is 1.0 mm Hg, which provides some knowledge of the degree to which the values vary from the mean of 40 mm Hg. Assuming a normal distribution of results as in Figure 22–1, 1 SD includes 68% of the values, 2 SD includes 95%, and 3 SD includes 99%. *A value that falls outside of 2 SD of the mean would occur rarely by chance alone.*

Another common statistic in quality control is the *coefficient of variation* (CV), which relates the standard deviation and the mean. This ratio is expressed as a percent (CV%):

$$CV\% = \left(\frac{SD}{\bar{x}}\right)100 \qquad (3)$$

The larger the CV%, the wider the dispersion of the data points around the mean. In our example, the CV% is 2.5%. If any two of the three statistics ($\bar{x}$, SD, or CV%) are known, the third can be calculated.

Methodology

A quality control medium is analyzed at least 20 times on more than one blood gas machine, and the mean, SD, and CV% are calculated. If these values are within the preparer's specifications and additionally meet standards for stability, cost, and other factors, the control is suitable as a quality control.

A quality control *system* must identify problems and specify corrective action in addition to documenting that the machinery is operating acceptably. To accomplish this, quality control charts that plot time (usually days) horizontally and SD vertically are commonly used.[372] Figure 22–2 is such a chart and shows that 95% of the control values fall within 2 SD of the mean. What about the five values that fall outside this range? *Random errors* are characterized by sporadic occurrence as depicted by point A (see Fig 22–2). *Systematic errors* denote a definitive trend toward or outside the 2 SD limit (see Fig 22–2, point B).

The usual causes of systematic error in blood gas analysis are: (1) contaminated pH buffer standards; (2) misanalyzed PCO_2/PO_2 standards;

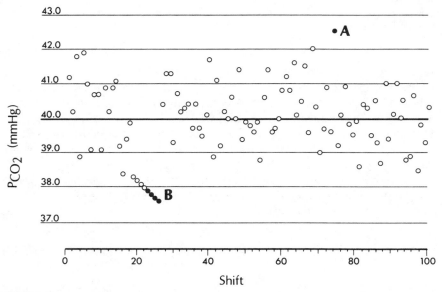

FIG 22–2.
Schematic representation of a quality control chart for PCO_2. Horizontal axis depicts 8-hour shifts. *White circles* represent values within 2 standard deviations of the mean; *black circles* represent values outside 2 standard deviations of the mean. *A* represents a random error; *B* represents systematic errors (see text).

(3) variations in electrode temperatures; (4) inconsistent introduction of the sample into the analyzer; (5) inconsistent calibration technique; (6) change in quality control sample storage or preparation; and (7) functional problems associated with the electrode, such as protein contamination, membrane malfunction, contaminated electrolyte, or electric circuitry problems. All these should be checked on the electrode with the systematic error. Once the problem has been corrected and so indicated on the quality control chart, the control is redone and the results plotted. Troubleshooting must continue until controls are within the 2 SD range.

We recommend that controls be run on at least two levels different from a normal blood gas sample. Control no. 1 could have an acidotic pH, a hypercarbic PCO_2, and a hypoxemic PO_2. Control no. 2 could have an alkalotic pH, a hypocarbic PCO_2, and a hyperoxic PO_2. Some laboratories prefer to add a third level with a normal pH, PCO_2, and PO_2. All levels of quality control should be run more frequently than two-point calibration is performed—i.e., once every 25 blood gas measurements or a minimum of every 4 hours while the machine is operational. The quality control charts should be arranged by type of electrode so that the response to various levels is plotted and observed. Further information on the use and implementation of these systems is readily available.[372–374]

Quality Control Media

Numerous media have been developed as blood gas quality control standards: (1) aqueous buffers,[375–380] (2) glycerin solutions,[353] (3) human/animal serum,[380, 381] (4) human/animal blood,[371, 380, 382–385] and (5) perfluorinated compounds (artificial blood).[386, 387] All these compounds are commercially available or can be prepared in the blood gas laboratory.[383, 387]

External Vs. Internal Systems

Quality control programs are classified as either external or internal, depending on who prepares the control sample. Internal controls are devised within the laboratory, whereas external controls are developed by another laboratory, agency, or commercial firm. *Proficiency testing* describes a mechanism of external quality control in which a laboratory is sent specimens (sometimes without knowledge of their assayed values) and asked to report the results. The agency that receives the results compares them with results from a reference laboratory (typically using the same blood gas equipment) and also from other laboratories that report their results.

An individual quality control system must be developed for each laboratory based on its specific need and capabilities. However, a system must consist of both internal and external controls plus a protocol for making "out of control" decisions.

The "accuracy" of internal quality assurance systems can be monitored by documenting its performance in relation to the external proficiency performance. True machine inconsistency will be reflected in both internal and external quality assurance systems. Inconsistencies shown by the external system not reflected in the internal system demand performance analysis of the internal system.

A supplemental measure to eliminate gross inaccuracies on patient samples is to compare the values from two different technologies. We routinely compare the HbO_2 measurement from spectrophotometry with the PO_2 obtained from the Clark electrode.

23

Oximetric Measurement

In addition to pH, P_{CO_2}, and P_{O_2} measurements, the desirability of also measuring hemoglobin content (Hb) and the percent of oxyhemoglobin saturation (S_{O_2}) in the blood has been discussed (see chaps. 5, 7, and 9). *Oximetry* is a general term pertaining to the various technologies capable of measuring oxyhemoglobin saturation. This chapter discusses three oximetric techniques: (1) spectrophotometry for in vitro analysis of hemoglobin; (2) pulse oximetry for noninvasive measurement of oxyhemoglobin saturation; and (3) fiberoptic oximetry for in vivo measurement of oxyhemoglobin saturation.

SPECTROPHOTOMETRY

All oximetry is based upon *spectrophotometric* principles that measure the portions of light transmitted and/or absorbed by the hemoglobin moiety. Understanding these physical principles requires a basic knowledge of the physics of light.

Basic Physics of Light

Light is an electromagnetic form of energy likened to the waves in a pool of still water following the dropping of a pebble. A wavelength is the distance from one wave peak to another and ranges from about 0.1 nm (10^{-9}) for gamma rays to about 25 cm for radio waves.[388] The continuous waveform from one peak to the next is referred to as a cycle, and the frequency is the number of cycles per second. Thus, the relationship between the two characteristics is fixed and inverse.[389] The energy properties of light are referred to as "packets" or *quanta*. Thus, the *intensity* of a beam of light refers to the number of quanta generated per second.[390]

The atoms in any molecule are constantly vibrating in a pattern not dissimilar to the vibrations generated by light waves. In general, light passing through a substance that has a similar vibrational frequency will tend to be absorbed. The fraction of light absorbed at a specific wavelength is called absorptivity,[388] or extinction coefficient where prescribed conditions are stated for factors such as pH, temperature, specific solvents, etc.[388, 391, 392] The absorptivity characteristics at various wavelengths can be drawn as a spectrum, in essence, a graph of a molecule's absorbance of electromagnetic energies at various wavelengths.

The Spectrophotometer

In the mid-17th century, Isaac Newton observed a "spectrum" of color exiting a prism placed in sunlight. In the 19th century a relationship between light spectra and electricity was noted in that the potential between two electrodes in solution changed when one was illuminated. By the beginning of the 20th century, this observation had been developed into a practical photoelectric cell for the measurement of absorbed light.

Photoelectric principles allow light intensity to be translated to electric current, the basis for modern spectrophotometers. For example, a given light intensity passed through a specific substance would result in some fraction of light transmitted to an oxide-coated metallic surface. The resultant current would be directly proportional to the transmitted light intensity. Embracing these physical principles, solid-state technology of the 1960s made present spectrophotometers possible.

SPECTRAL ANALYSIS

Basic Principles

The transmittance of light through a substance is a logarithmic function of the concentration of that substance, since each molecule absorbs an equal fraction of a particular light wavelength.[393] Since the value of interest is the amount of light absorbed, transmittance (T) can be mathematically converted to absorbance (A):

$$A = 2 - \log\% \, T \tag{1}$$

With absorbance now linearly related to concentration of the substance, Beer's Law can be stated as:

$$A = abc \tag{2}$$

where A is the amount of light absorbed, a is the absorptivity of the substance at a given wavelength, b is the length of the light path in centimeters; and c is the concentration of the substance.[388–391]

For any substance the linear relationship exits only to a certain concentration. Within this limitation a calibration constant can be derived from the concentration and absorbance of a known standard. This constant can then be used to derive the unknown concentration of a substance that has the same absorptivity as the standard.[391] Therefore, Equation (2) can be rewritten:

$$\text{STANDARD} \quad \frac{A}{b\,c} = \frac{A}{b\,c} \quad \text{UNKNOWN} \tag{3}$$

When the light path length (b) is held constant, Equation (3) becomes:

$$\text{STANDARD} \quad \frac{A}{c} = \frac{A}{c} \quad \text{UNKNOWN} \tag{4}$$

Equation (4) can be rewritten:

$$c_u = A_u \frac{c_{st}}{A_{st}} \tag{5}$$

where c_u is the unknown concentration, A_u is the absorbance of the unknown substance and (c_{st}/A_{st}) is the calibration constant.

Spectral Analysis of Hemoglobin

As discussed previously (see chap. 5), the hemoglobin molecule exists in various forms: oxy- (O_2Hb); reduced (RHb); carboxy- (COHb); sulf- (SHb); met- (METHb); and fetal (FHb). Each of these forms has its own light spectrum (Fig 23–1), with SHb being similar to METHb. To minimize spectral shift during analysis, light sources that contain strong emissions of selected wavelengths for the various hemoglobin forms can be utilized. These are referred to as spectral line light sources.[394]

Taking absorbance measurements at two different wavelengths is an appropriate method for determining two of the hemoglobin moieties; three wavelength measurements for three moieties; and four wavelength measurements for four hemoglobin moieties. The specific wavelengths at which measurements are taken are generally chosen so that one wave-

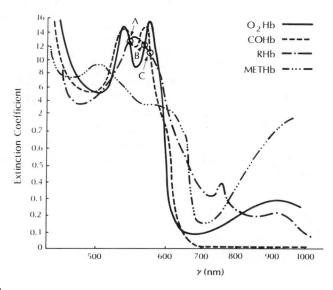

FIG 23–1.
Spectral analysis of hemoglobin. *O₂Hb* is oxyhemoglobin, *COHb* is carboxyhemoglobin, *RHb* is reduced hemoglobin, *METHb* is methemoglobin. Points **A, B,** and **C** identify three wavelengths where different Hb moieties have the same extinction coefficients (isosbestic points): **A,** triple isosbestic point at 548 nm–O2Hb, COHb, and RHb. **B,** double isosbestic point at 568 nm–O2Hb, RHb. **C,** double isosbestic point at 578 nm–COHB, RHb.

length is a maximal difference between the extinction coefficients of the moieties of interest, and the other is an isosbestic point, i.e., the extinction coefficients are the same.[394–398] An assumption is made that the measured absorbance is due to the hemoglobin moieties of interest and no other substances. In practice, however, this is not always true, leading to erroneous determinations.

Incompletely hemolyzed red blood cells can scatter light and produce erroneous measurements. The presence of lipids in the sample also scatters light and distorts the measured absorbances.[227, 393, 395, 399] Intravenous dyes, such as methylene blue and indocyanine green, strongly absorb near-red and infrared light, resulting in lower than actual oxyhemoglobin measured in this region.[400, 401] The presence of COHb will not be detected in a two wavelength method for O₂Hb in the infrared region because the extinction coefficient of COHb is very low in this region, resulting in a higher than actual O₂Hb determination.[398, 402] The presence of METHb in a sample limits the reliability of determinations; even in a four-wavelength method designed for measuring the moiety. When the METHb is greater than 10%, the values are suspect.[398, 399]

All methods are based on adult extinction coefficients. The presence of fetal hemoglobin will have varying effects on the methods in that the spectrum of fetal hemoglobin is different from the adult spectrum. The error effect on results depends on the magnitude of variation between the fetal and adult extinctions at the wavelengths used for absorbance measurements.[399, 403]

THE CO-OXIMETER

Modern co-oximeters are spectrophotometers that simultaneously analyze four hemoglobin moieties—reduced hemoglobin, oxyhemoglobin, carboxyhemoglobin, and methemoglobin. As illustrated in Figure 23–2, a co-oximeter consists of a light source; lenses, and mirrors that focus the beam to the monochromatomator that isolates the four wavelengths of interest using filters or gratings; a beam splitter that divides the beam exiting the monochromatomator so that one is directed to the reference detector and the other is directed through the analytical cuvette to the sample detector; and detectors that are photodiodes that emit electrons in proportion to the amount of light striking their surfaces.

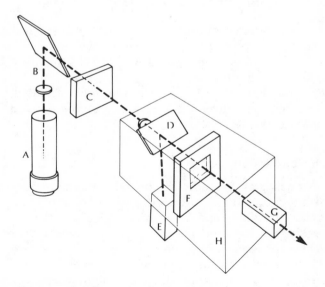

FIG 23–2.
Basic components of co-oximeter. **A,** light source. **B,** lens and mirror. **C,** monochromator. **D,** beam splitter. **E,** reference detector. **F,** cuvette. **G,** sample detector. **H,** temperature regulated block (see text for explanation).

The emitted electrons (current) are fed to a circuit whose output is proportional to the relative absorbance of the sample.

Principles of Operation

Co-oximeters obtain and store absorbance readings on a blank solution at four different wavelengths, λ_1 nm, λ_2 nm, λ_3 nm, and λ_4 nm. The blank absorbances are generally updated every 30 minutes of nonuse or after every sample.

When a diluted, hemolyzed sample is introduced, an absorbance reading is obtained at each wavelength. The corresponding blank absorbances are subtracted from these measurements and the four resulting absorbances are multiplied by the appropriate extinction coefficient to obtain the concentrations (Beer's Law):

$$C_R = K(E_{1R}A_1 + E_{2R}A_2 + E_{3R}A_3 + E_{4R}A_4)$$

$$C_{O_2} = K(E_{1O_2}A_1 + E_{2O_2}A_2 + E_{3O_2}A_3 + E_{4O_2}A_4)$$

$$C_{CO} = K(E_{1CO}A_1 + E_{2CO}A_2 + E_{3CO}A_3 + E_{4CO}A_4)$$

$$C_M = K(E_{1M}A_1 + E_{2M}A_2 + E_{3M}A_3 + E_{4M}A_4)$$

where C = concentration of each Hb moiety; K = a scalar constant set by the Hb calibration procedure; E = each coefficient in the matrix (four Hb moieties at four wavelengths); and A = the absorbance value of the blood at each wavelength.

The total hemoglobin is the sum of the four calculated concentrations. The percentage concentration values are then derived for O_2Hb, COHb, METHb, and RHb.

Co-oximeter Limitations

As previously stated, methylene blue dye has a peak absorbance in the near-red region and will affect measurements in oximetry methods using wavelengths in that and in the infrared region. However, the error is considerably less with co-oximeters utilizing wavelengths in the near-red and visible regions because the near-red is only one of four absorbances used to quantify the hemoglobin moieties.[399, 400]

Any substances in the sample that scatter light will affect co-oximeter measurements since the amount of transmitted light is no longer solely a function of light absorbed by the hemoglobin moieties. Lipids and cell fragments due to incomplete hemolysis are the most common cause of such error.[227, 393, 395, 399]

With adult extinction coefficients, oxygenated fetal hemoglobin will yield a 4% to 7% false carboxyhemoglobin result, while reduced fetal hemoglobin yields a 0.2% to 1.5% false carboxyhemoglobin result.[399] Modern co-oximeters will compensate for the presence of fetal hemoglobin when the operator presses the appropriate keys.

The co-oximeter is the most accurate method available for measuring the four clinically relevant hemoglobin moieties. It is considered the standard against which other methods must be compared.

NONINVASIVE OXIMETRY

In the 1930s, a spectrophotometric instrument transmitting red light measured oxygen saturation on flowing blood in intact vessels.[393] Without compensation for hemoglobin concentration (scattered light from the volume of intact red blood cells) or wavelength drift from the light source, comparisons with van Slyke analyses were excellent. Thus, a potential means for measuring O_2Hb concentrations without obtaining blood samples existed. However, three major obstacles would have to be overcome before such technology would be clinically useful. First, tissue absorbance of light must be separated from blood absorbance. Second, light absorbance due to arterial blood must be separated from capillary and venous blood. Third, the apparatus must be free from environmental influences, reliable, easy to use, and not require frequent calibration.

Ear Oximetry

In 1964, an ear oximeter was introduced that monitored the intensity of incident light by splitting the beam and directing one portion to a detector for continuous measurement. The transmitted light was measured at eight wavelengths between 650 nm and 1050 nm. The ratios of transmitted to incident light and empirically derived constants were used to calculate oxygen saturation. The split-beam concept compensated for pigmentation, other light-absorbing factors, and scattering particles present in the earlobe.[404, 405] It reliably measured oxygen saturations and was the first noninvasive oximeter to be clinically used for cardiopulmonary stress testing, sleep laboratories, and pulmonary rehabilitation programs. However, the device was large, expensive, and the fiberoptic cable connecting the earpiece to the device was delicate. Most importantly, arterial blood was not differentiated from venous blood, rather the site was "arterialized" by a heating mechanism.[404, 405]

Pulse Oximetry

This technology is based on the theory that transilluminated tissue consists of two parts, a venous blood and tissue component (VTC) and an arterial blood component (AC). The attenuation of light by the VTC should remain stable with arterial pulsation, while the AC should fluctuate. Theoretically, the increased light absorbance with arterial pulsation should be due solely to arterial blood flowing into the vascular bed. Thus, the need for "arterializing" the tissue site is eliminated.[406]

In the original method, the AC absorbance was calculated by subtracting the VTC absorbance from the total at each of two wavelengths. One wavelength, at 650 nm, provided a large variation between extinction coefficients for oxyhemoglobin and reduced hemoglobin, while the second at 805 nm provided the isosbestic wavelength. This allowed oxygen saturation to be calculated utilizing a formula requiring extinction coefficients for two moieties and absorbance measurements at two wavelengths.[398, 406] It was assumed the effects of scattered light could be ignored because it was common to both wavelengths and therefore Beer's Law, as related to hemolyzed samples, applied.

This theoretical approach resulted in accuracy when the O_2Hb was greater than 90%. However, at saturations below 90%, there resulted an overestimation by as much as 20% at 50%. Further studies on the effects of scattered light demonstrated this to be a significant source of error that led to modification of the formula, resulting in more reliable values down to saturations of 80%.[407]

Light-Emitting Diode

With the application of the light-emitting diode (LED) in the early 1980s, the mathematical principle of pulse oximetry changed from calculations based on measuring the incident and transmitted light intensities to calculations based only on the intensity of transmitted light striking the detector's surface (signal).[408, 409] The AC signal is identified by the modulating portion and is separated from the VTC signal. Dividing each wavelength's AC by VTC gives corrected AC values that are no longer functions of measured light, but functions of the oxyhemoglobin and reduced extinction coefficients and the path length of the pulsating arterial blood. Thus, a ratio of the corrected AC values is the basis for determining the degree of oxygenation.[408]

With LED technology, an isosbestic wavelength is no longer desirable. To improve accuracy, a second wavelength in the infrared range is chosen where the coefficients vary maximally from those of the wavelength in the red region. Obligingly, the oxyhemoglobin and reduced moieties reverse their positions relative to each other beyond the isosbestic point at 805 nm (see Fig 23–1). The second wavelength used in LED pulse oximetry is 940 nm.

Oxyhemoglobin saturation is calculated by:

$$O_2Hb\% = K_1R^2 + K_2R + K_3$$

where $R = AC_{corr\ 660}/AC_{corr\ 940}$ and K_1, K_2, K_3 are calibration constants.[409]

THE PULSE OXIMETER

The modern pulse oximeter (Fig 23–3) is an enviable technologic triumph made possible only by microprocessor availability. It is the perfect example of modern technology adapted to previously available equipment to accomplish feats unthinkable only 20 years ago.

The LEDs can emit enormous intensities of light that vary almost linearly with drive current. Therefore, they can be modulated to maintain the transmitted light at an optimal intensity for maximum signal-to-noise ratio. A microprocessor continuously monitors the light signals and controls the drive current, overcoming most problems coincident with pigmentation and edema. Since the LED light source is in the probe tip, conventional wires (rather than fiberoptic cable) are used to connect the probe to the oximeter.

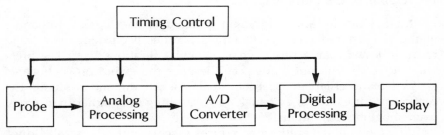

FIG 23–3.
Block diagram of pulse oximeter. Probe consists of 2 LEDs and photodetector. Analog processing amplifies and filters the probe signal. A/D converter converts analog signal to digital. Digital processing performs mathematical computations which is displayed as O2Hb saturation.

The signal detector is a silicon photodiode whose output is linearly proportional to the light striking its surface over a large range of intensities. It has low noise levels, is small and lightweight, and responds to light through the visible region to about 1100 nm. However, it cannot differentiate between the red and infrared light from the LEDs. To solve this problem, the microprocessor alternately turns each LED on, then off, then both off to distinguish the red from the infrared signals. This cycle is repeated hundreds of times per second and additionally solves the problem of ambient light interference since the light measured when both LEDs are off is considered noise and deducted from the light measured when the LEDs are on.

Since the modulating signals of interest are generated by the heart beat, it is reasonable to assume they will not exceed frequencies of 5 cycles/sec (Hz) or 300 beats per minute. Power lines and all electrical equipment in the vicinity generate noise at much higher frequencies that are blocked by an electronic filter that allows only the low-frequency signals to pass. This low pass filter is also used to separate the VTC signal from the modulating signal; a high pass filter separates the AC signal from the modulating signal.

The microprocessor controls all the functions in the oximeter and receives and processes the AC and VTC signals. It can be programmed to interpret the signals and trigger fault messages. If the signals are too high, a "probe off patient" message will display, indicating the absence of tissue between the emitter and detector in the probe. If components are being driven as hard as possible and signals cannot be detected, an "insufficient" message will display. Dark fingernail polish and too much tissue are examples of this condition. The strength of the AC signal is usually displayed with a digital $O_2Hb\%$ that updates every few seconds.

Limitations of the Pulse Oximeter

Methylene blue and indocyanine green dyes have peak absorbances in the red-infrared region. Their presence has been demonstrated to result in lower than actual oxyhemoglobin saturations.[400, 401] The presence of COHb will not be detected because the extinction coefficients for COHb and O_2Hb are isosbestic at almost 660 nm, and at 940 nm the coefficient for COHb is extremely low, resulting in a higher than actual oxyhemoglobin saturation.[402, 410]

Any event that significantly reduces vascular pulsations will reduce the pulse oximeter's ability to calculate saturation. These include hypothermia of a few degrees, hypotension, and infusion of vasoconstrictive drugs.[410]

Clinical applications and limitations of the pulse oximeter have been discussed elsewhere (see chap. 17).

FIBEROPTIC OXIMETRY

The solid state fiberoptic oximeter was developed in the early 1970s. The light source was from LEDs at 685-nm and 920-nm peak emission wavelengths and the detector was a silicon photodiode. The mathematical principles involved with reflectance oximetry[411, 412] were modified for calculating oxygen saturation on nonhemolyzed blood to derive the following formula:

$$O_2Hb\% = A - B (EI/ER)$$

where A is a specific constant supplied with each catheter; B is a constant depending primarily on the light intensity ratio; EI is the reflected light intensity at the infrared wavelength; and ER is the reflected light intensity at the red wavelength.[210, 413, 414] It was found that calibration curves for various catheters were: (1) independent of temperature variations; (2) independent of hematocrit reading variations above 40%; and (3) shifted approximately 1% per 0.1 pH unit change.[413] These predictable and linear factors allow calibration of the instrument to be accomplished by adjusting to a standard sample with a known $O_2Hb\%$ prior to insertion[415] or to an in vitro $O_2Hb\%$ analysis from a blood sample after catheter insertion.[210, 414] Recalibrations, generally required no more than once per day, are accomplished from in vitro analysis.[204]

These solid-state fiberoptic oximeters have been greatly improved and commercially developed as part of a pulmonary artery flotation catheter. Their clinical use is discussed elsewhere (see chap. 16).

TECHNICAL LIMITATIONS OF FIBEROPTIC OXIMETRY

Breakage of Fibers

Breakage is seldom a problem with reasonable handling since plastic has replaced glass as the fiber component. The catheters are reinforced along their length to protect the fibers from inadvertent stress.[204, 210, 414]

Vessel Wall Interference

If the sensor tip contacts the vessel wall, it is unable to analyze the blood accurately spectrophotometrically. Improvements in design of the catheter tip have decreased, but not ablated, the incidence of vessel wall readings. Simple repositioning of the catheter usually corrects the problem.[204, 210, 414, 415]

Clot Formation

Some degree of fibrin formation or clotting occurs on all foreign bodies within the vasculature. Appropriate flushing of the catheter tip during continuous use appears to prevent interference.[204, 210, 414]

COHb

Like all two wavelength oximeters, the fiberoptic oximeter cannot distinguish COHb from the oxyhemoglobin or reduced moiety. By calibrating the fiberoptic instrument to an $O_2Hb\%$ determined by co-oximetry, the fiberoptic saturation will be compensated for the presence of the carboxyhemoglobin moiety as long as the concentration remains reasonably stable.[210]

Hemodilution

With hematocrit readings between 30% and 40%, the variation in Sv_{O_2} is generally < 3%.[210] However, errors > 5% have been reported.[415] Hematocrit readings below 30% cannot be compensated due to the mathematical limitations concerning light scatter in nonhemolyzed blood.

24

Transcutaneous Gas Electrodes

The phenomenon of gas exchange between human skin and the atmosphere was first described in 1851. Adaptations of the Clark and Severinghaus electrodes are capable of measuring the oxygen and carbon dioxide gas tensions diffusing through the skin. Thus, the technical capability for transcutaneous gas measurement became a reality several decades ago and represented the first technology with promise to noninvasively monitor Po_2 and Pco_2. The clinical factors pertaining to this subject are discussed elsewhere (see chap. 18).

Gas diffusion through human skin is greatly enhanced when the skin area is heated to 41° to 45°C.[416-418] Heating the skin area is so crucial to transcutaneous gas tension measurement that the electrodes must include a heating element and a sensitive temperature sensor that varies the current flowing to the heating element to maintain the preset temperature.[419-421] Some commercially available units display the heating element's power consumption so that fluctuations may be used as a reflection of blood flow to the area beneath the electrode surface. This concept depends upon both the ambient temperature and patient temperature remaining constant.

TRANSCUTANEOUS Po_2 ELECTRODE

The $P_{tc}O_2$ electrode (Fig 24–1) is similar to a Clark electrode (see chap. 21) in that it has a silver anode surrounding a platinum or gold cathode and utilizes a polarizing voltage of approximately 600 mV. The electrolyte solution that bathes the surface of the two poles is encased within a polypropylene or polyethylene membrane that allows oxygen

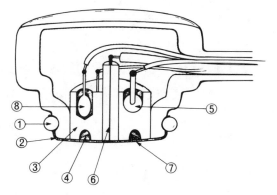

FIG 24–1.
Schematic illustration of the transcutaneous PO$_2$ electrode. **1,** O-ring, securing the membrane. **2,** oxygen-permeable polypropylene membrane. When the electrode is prepared, the membrane covers the electrode surface and the electrolyte and limits the rate of oxygen diffusion. **3,** silver anode, surrounding the cathode. **4,** electrolyte chamber. **5,** heating element. **6,** platinum cathode. **7,** electrolyte, covering the electrode surface. Consists of a solution with an admixture of chloride ions. **8,** NTC resistor, for control of the electrode temperature.

diffusion at a somewhat limited diffusion rate. Thus, oxygen diffuses through the membrane to the cathode where reduction of the oxygen generates a current that is measured and is directly proportional to the concentration of oxygen against the outer membrane surface.

P$_{tc}$O$_2$ Electrode Calibration

The extent of automation varies among transcutaneous monitoring devices, but in all systems the zero point is highly stable. Therefore, a one-point calibration is generally all that is required to assure reliable electrode response.

Ambient air having an oxygen concentration of 20.9% is used for the calibrating gas. In environments where the temperature and relative humidity are a fairly constant 25°C and 50%, respectively, barometric pressure is the only variable and the calibration value can be calculated:

$$P_{tc}O_2 \text{ (calibration)} = P_B (.209)$$

A more precise calibration value can be calculated using the formula:

$$P_{tc}O_2 \text{ (calibration)} = (P_B - P_{H_2O}@^t \times RH) (.209)$$

where $P_{H_2O}^{@t}$ is the saturated water vapor pressure at the temperature of the environment and RH is the relative humidity of the environment. In typical environments the variation between the two formulas is less than 2%.[419-421]

Calibration consists of exposing the electrode to ambient air for several minutes and then comparing the displayed value to the calculated calibration value. A variation of approximately ±2 mm Hg (user-protocol dependent) is generally considered within acceptable drift limits and adjustment to the calibration value is not required; a variation up to ±5 mm Hg is a reasonable drift condition and the display should be adjusted to read the calibration value.

A drift check is recommended every 4 hours during continuous use and after the monitor has been discontinued for any period of time. A one-point calibration is recommended at least once in every 24 hours of continuous use and after changing the membrane and electrolyte solution.

A zero-point check is indicated when a drift condition of >5 mm Hg exists or whenever doubt arises over the clinical reliability of obtained values. The procedure consists of covering a clean membrane surface with a zero oxygen solution (sodium tetraborate, sodium sulphite, and copper [II] sulphate solution), or exposing the electrode to pure nitrogen gas in a closed container.[419-421] Values up to ±5 mm Hg are acceptable. After adjustment to zero, the one-point calibration value is rechecked. Variations greater than ±5 mm Hg indicate problems that must be identified and corrected. Typical problems associated with excessive drift conditions are: inadequately cleaned electrode and membrane surfaces; improperly applied membranes; "exhausted" electrolyte solution; worn-out membranes; and inaccurate calibration values.

TRANSCUTANEOUS P_{CO_2} ELECTRODE

The $P_{tc}CO_2$ electrode (Fig 24-2) structure is that of a miniaturized Severinghaus electrode (see chap. 21). A chlorinated silver wire encased in pH-sensitive glass filled with a buffer solution is the measuring half-cell, and a silver/silver chloride cell is the reference. The electrolyte solution applied to the surface of the two cells is composed of sodium bicarbonate and sodium chloride, and the membrane is permeable to carbon dioxide. Additional components are the same as described for the transcutaneous P_{O_2} electrode, namely a heating element and temperature-sensitive resistor.

The operating principle is the same as the Severinghaus electrode in that the P_{CO_2} present on the outer surface of the membrane diffuses

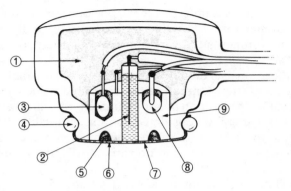

FIG 24–2.
Schematic illustration of the transcutaneous P_{CO_2} electrode. **1,** epoxy resin. **2,** glass electrode with a chlorinated silver wire, a buffer solution (the inner liquid), and a pH sensitive glass membrane. **3,** NTC (negative temperature coefficient) resistor, the temperature sensor. **4,** O-ring, securing the membrane (**7**). **5,** electrolyte chamber. **6,** electrolyte covering the electrode surface (solution of $NaHCO_3^-$ and NaCl). **7,** CO_2 permeable membrane; 12 μ thick PTFE membrane. **8,** heating element (zener diode). **9,** Ag/AgCl reference electrode.

across and reacts with the electrolyte to form hydrogen and bicarbonate ions. The hydrogen ions produced are linearly related to the amount of CO_2 diffusing across the membrane as described in the Henderson-Hasselbalch equation. The hydrogen ions generate a voltage change between the two half-cells that is measured and converted to a $P_{tc}CO_2$ reading in mm Hg.

Transcutaneous P_{CO_2} Electrode Calibration

Physiology dictates that differences between transcutaneous and arterial CO_2 tensions must exist. Although mathematically inaccurate to compensate for the temperature factor in a linear manner, the error is minimal with P_{CO_2} values less than 80 mm Hg.[421] A method[419] for calculating the calibration values is as follows: when the environmental conditions are constant at a temperature of 25°C and a relative humidity of 50%:

$$P_{tc}CO_2 \text{ (calibration)} = P_B (CO_2\%) - X_{@t}{}^{tc}$$

where X is the correction value based on the temperature correction percentages used for Pa_{CO_2}; $_{@t}{}^{tc}$ is the temperature of the electrode. When the environmental conditions are variable:

$$P_{tc}CO_2 \text{ (calibration)} =$$

$$(P_B - P_{H_2O@t})(RH)(CO_2c) - X_{@t}{}^{tc}$$

One-point calibration consists of exposing the electrode surface to a 5% CO_2 gas for several minutes, then comparing the displayed value to the calculated calibration value. A variance of approximately ± 2 mm Hg is within acceptable drift limits and adjusting the display reading to the calculated value is not required; a variance of up to ± 4 mm Hg is a reasonable drift and the display should be adjusted to the calculated value. This one-point calibration should be performed every 4 hours during continuous use and following any discontinuance of use.

A two-point calibration consists of performing the procedure with both 5% and 10% CO_2 gas, with a final check using the 5% gas. A two-point calibration should be performed at least once during a 24-hour period of continuous use, following membrane and electrolyte change, and whenever the clinical reliability of the values is in doubt.

Calibration readings that vary more than 4 mm Hg from the calculated values indicate problems that must be identified and corrected. Typical problems are air bubbles in the electrolyte solution, no gas flow during calibration, the wrong or empty gas cylinders, and the problems discussed for the $P_{tc}O_2$ electrode.

COMBINATION Po_2/Pco_2 TRANSCUTANEOUS ELECTRODE

The components of the combined electrode are the same as the individual electrodes. The calibrating gas is 5% CO_2 and 20.9% O_2 for one-point calibration; 10% CO_2 and 90% N_2 for two-point calibration. The formulas for calculating the calibration values and the procedures are the same as described for the individual electrodes.

TRANSCUTANEOUS ELECTRODE MAINTENANCE

With continuous use, a weekly cleaning of dried electrolyte from the electrode surface and applying a new membrane are recommended. Various cleaning agents are recommended by the manufacturers, but we have found that flushing the surface with distilled water and using cotton swabs to remove any dried particles are usually adequate cleaning methods.

Monitors not in use for more than 24 hours should be turned off to minimize evaporation of the electrolyte by the heating element. If the electrode has a newly applied electrolyte and membrane, it can be stored in this way for up to a week and be returned to service at any time after a one-point calibration for the $P_{tc}O_2$ electrode or a two-point calibration for the $P_{tc}CO_2$ electrode.[419, 420] Electrodes that have not been in service for more than a week require electrode-surface cleaning, membrane change, and one- or two-point calibrations prior to patient application.

PATIENT SAFETY

The skin site for transcutaneous electrodes should be changed at least every four hours to avoid first-degree skin burn. In hypothermic patients this should be accomplished at least every three hours.[419-421]

Any skin with suspect lesions should be avoided as sites for transcutaneous electrode application. An infection-control measure practiced in our neonatal unit is to use a new membrane with each new patient. This was implemented because recommended disinfecting methods varied among manufacturers and the resulting confusion with use of various brands ultimately led to improper disinfection procedures.

25

Exhaled CO$_2$ Measurement

The measurement of CO$_2$ in respiratory gases was first accomplished in 1865 utilizing the principles of infrared absorption.[422] The concept of plotting the CO$_2$ concentration of respiratory gas throughout the ventilatory cycle (capnography) was developed in 1943 and applied in anesthesiology as early as 1950.

INFRARED GAS ANALYSIS

Most gases of interest in respiratory and anesthesia practice have characteristic absorption bands in the infrared region. As illustrated in Figure 25–1, carbon dioxide (CO$_2$) has a strong absorption band at a wavelength of approximately 4200 nm, and nitrous oxide (N$_2$O) has strong absorption bands at wavelengths of approximately 3900 nm and 4500 nm[423, 424]; 3900 nm is generally used for N$_2$O measurements.

Incident light is filtered sequentially, producing beams at the wavelengths specific for peak CO$_2$ and N$_2$O absorption. Each beam alternately traverses a cell chamber containing the gas sample and a reference cell containing room air. The light transmitted through each cell is measured, and the ratio corresponds to the CO$_2$ or N$_2$O content of the sample.[424, 425] Response times are generally fractions of seconds, providing a potential for accurate continuous measurements.[424, 426, 427]

Three problems are inherent with the method of analysis: (1) CO$_2$ sensitivity; (2) water vapor/linearity; and (3) drift.

CO$_2$ Sensitivity

When one gas is capable of absorbing energy from the excited molecules of a second gas, the molecules of the second gas become capable

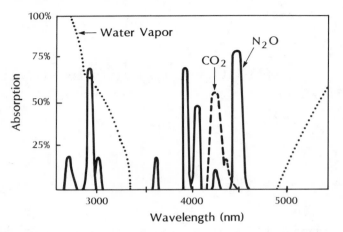

FIG 25-1.
Absorption spectra carbon dioxide, nitrous oxide and water vapor. Water vapor absorbs the largest amounts of infra-red light particularly at wavelengths < 3500 nm and > 5000 nm. The 4000 nm region is not influenced by water vapor and therefore is an ideal range for measuring CO_2 and N_2O absorptions which peak at 4200 nm and 4500 nm, respectively.

of receiving additional photons (absorb more light). This physical property is termed "collision broadening" and is widely utilized to increase sensitivity in light spectral analysis. However, in CO_2 infrared analysis, collision broadening results in CO_2 measurements greater than actual. Seventy percent nitrous oxide (N_2O) produces collision broadening of CO_2 where the CO_2 measurement is increased by a factor of 1.06 the actual value.[427] Correction factors effectively compensate when N_2O is the background gas.[428]

Sampling Linearity

Placing the sampling chamber within the airway would be cumbersome and impractical. This is circumvented by connecting the sampling chamber to the airway via a small bore catheter. The suction used to draw in the sample produces less than atmospheric pressure through the sample chamber and line. Since absorbence is proportional to path length (fixed in a given instrument) and pressure, operating the sample chamber at subatmospheric pressure improves the linearity of the spectrophometric method and reduces water vapor condensation in the sample line and on chamber windows. This has, however, a cost in terms of stability. Water vapor condensation is further minimized by heating the sample chamber.[426]

Electronic Drift

The largest source of drift was found to be due to room temperature changes.[422] Modern instruments incorporate a thermistor in the photometer assembly to monitor thermal drifts.[425] Solid-state components compensate for this problem as well as for N_2O effects and linearity modulations.

INFRARED ANALYZER

Older infrared analyzers have flexible, metal diaphragms separating identical reference and sample detectors filled with pure gas of interest, i.e., CO_2 or N_2O. Light absorbed by the sample under analysis results in less light striking the sample side of the detector relative to the reference side. This results in asymmetrical heating of the detector gas, with a greater pressure exerted on the reference side of the diaphragm moving it toward the sample side. The diaphragm is one plate of a capacitor. Thus, the movement of the diaphragm due to pressure changes results in voltage changes. A chopper disc placed in the path of the incident beam alternately blocks and allows the beam to pass at a frequency between 6 and 60 Hz, producing a modulating beam necessary for the diaphragm-capacitor to function. The output from the detector is rectified (smoothed) and displayed on a meter calibrated in percent concentration.[422, 423, 426]

Modern instruments replaced the diaphragm-detectors with photodetectors whose outputs are proportional to the transmitted light striking their surfaces. Photodetectors eliminate the need for chopper discs and for filling the detector with pure gas of interest, which allows for simultaneous measurement of infrared absorbing gases when the incident light is filtered to produce beams at the peak absorbing wavelengths for those gases. Solid-state components convert the analog outputs from the photodetectors to digital signals that are processed and displayed as percent concentration.[424, 425]

Calibration

Calibration of both older and modern instruments consists of introducing known CO_2 and/or N_2O concentrations into the instruments and adjusting the readouts accordingly. Modern instruments automatically adjust to the values when the operator presses the appropriate keys to initiate a calibration cycle.

Limitations

The modern infrared CO_2 analyzer is a reliable and accurate device in most clinical conditions. The diameter of the sample tubing is approximately 1.5 mm and easily kinked or occluded by mucus. Traps are connected between the sample tubing and analyzer to minimize contamination of the sample chamber by any aspirated substance and to remove water vapor.[424, 426]

Contamination in the sample chamber is evident when room air is sampled as a zero-point check. The contamination blocks light transmission, producing an "absorption" when none should exist. Some instruments are designed so that the sample chamber can be flushed without dismantling the analyzer, thereby minimizing down time.[424, 425]

MASS SPECTROMETRY

All molecules have a distinctive mass. As schematically depicted in Figure 25–2, when molecules are electronically charged and then forced to pass through an electromagnetic field at a constant velocity, the extent to which the direction of the molecular ions deviates will be a function of their mass to charge ratios (m/z).

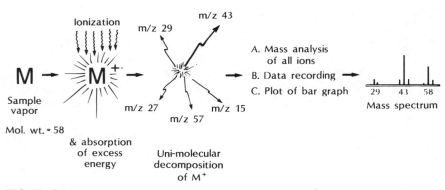

FIG 25–2.
General representation of mass spectrometer analysis. A neutral molecule is bombarded with electrons, giving it sufficient energy to eject one of its own electrons, thereby becoming charged. Excess energy is dissipated by breaking the molecular ion's chemical bonds, producing fragment ions. The production of fragment ions is dependent on the stability of the molecular ion. However, all ions have an electrical charge. Therefore, they can be controlled by various potentials to form a well-collimated beam and be directed into a mass analyzer where they are analyzed according to their abundance along the mass scale.

The Mass Spectrometer

The basic components of a mass spectrometer are schematically depicted in Figure 25–3. The inlet system is either a capillary tube or needle valve assembly that passes a gas sample at atmospheric pressure to an ionization chamber where the pressure is about 10^{-4} mm Hg. The gas molecules are transformed into positively charged ions in the ionization chamber. The ionized gas is extracted from the chamber and accelerated into the quadropole region. The rods are arranged symmetrically with opposite rods connected to direct current and radio frequency voltage regulators. As the voltages are varied from maximum to minimum, only ions of a specific mass to charge ratio traverse the region and strike the detector at the other end. Ions of other masses undergo oscillations as voltages vary, eventually losing their charges as they collide with the rods.

The sensitivity of the detector unit is a few parts per million, and the analog signals generated represent the relative concentrations of dry gases in the sample.[426, 429, 430] The relative fraction of each gas present is determined by summing the signals, then dividing the value for each by the sum total. A typical respiratory mass range is 2 to 100 mass units (u) and can be spanned in approximately 100 milliseconds.[426] Thus, the gas concentration readouts are essentially continuous. Water vapor has a much slower response time than other gases due to its adherence to capillary tube walls, and it cannot be easily measured in a breath by breath analysis. It is generally ignored, but some instruments allow electronic compensation to account for its presence.

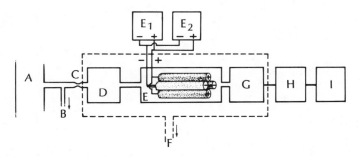

FIG 25–3.
Schematic representation of mass spectrometer. **A,** respiratory gases. **B,** sample pump. **C,** capillary/needle valve inlet leak. **D,** ionization chamber. **E,** quadropole region, E_1 DC generator. E_2 RF generator. **F,** vacuum system. **G,** detector. **H,** signal processing. **I,** display/recorder (see text for explanation).

Applications of Mass Spectrometry

The mass spectrometer was developed over 75 years ago.[431] These instruments were intended for analytical chemistry purposes and spanned a wide range of mass to charge ratios. In 1947, a mass spectrometer was developed to analyze molecules with low mass to charge ratios specifically for the purpose of measuring respiratory gases. This was further improved and described in 1952 as a single-channel commercial mass spectrometer for measurement of respiratory gases.[429] Further improvements in vacuum technology and solid state electronics made the respiratory mass spectrometer a practical addition to most pulmonary function laboratories by the 1960s.

Clinical application of the respiratory mass spectrometer was confined to the pulmonary function laboratories until the 1970s when servo-controlled sampling systems and minicomputers for data accumulation allowed monitoring several patients in intensive care units from one machine. Computerized systems found further application in operating rooms where they monitor anesthetic gases in addition to the respiratory gases.[429,431]

Since less expensive technology is available to monitor both inspired oxygen concentrations and exhaled CO_2 concentrations, the expense of the mass spectrometer limits its clinical justification. Most mass spectrometers are presently devoted to the operating room theater where measurement of gases other than O_2 and CO_2 are required or desirable.

26

Fluorescent Optode Technology

A sensor that operates via electrochemical properties is termed an "electrode"; a sensor that operates via optical detection and quantification of light is termed an "optode." Optodes are commonly classified into three groups: (1) transmission-based optodes; (2) fluorescence-based optodes; and (3) energy-transfer optodes. Each of these may be either reversible (the reagent phase is not consumed) or nonreversible. The utility of a nonreversible sensor is dependent on both the rate of reagent consumption and the ability to replenish the reagent during operation. In vivo sensors should be reversible to allow compactness and longevity.

TRANSMISSION OPTODES

These optodes monitor attenuation in the probe beam at one or more wavelengths. Attenuation may be achieved by absorption, scattering, reflection outside the fiber or reflection at the fiber surface. An absorbence-based, reversible chemical optode has been described for in vivo pH measurement.[432]

FLUORESCENT OPTODES

Luminescence is the emission of light energy resulting from "excited" electrons returning to a basal state. When luminescence is initiated by light (photoluminescence), it is most commonly referred to as fluorescence.

When a fluorescence chemical is exposed to an appropriate light intensity, electrons are activated to an excited state that is essentially maintained while exposed to the light energy source. When the light exposure ends, the electrons return to a basal state and in that process emit a small amount of light energy (luminescence). This emitted light energy is less than the excitation energy and consequently will have a different wavelength.

A fluorescent dye may be conceived as a fluorescent chemical that alters its electron excitation response to a light stimulus as the dye's concentration of a specific substance changes. In other words, the fluorescence is either augmented or quenched as concentration of a specific substance changes within the dye.

A fluorescent optode is composed of a fiberoptic element with a fluorescent dye at the tip. The dye is separated from the environment by a membrane permeable to the specific substance (analyte) to which the dye changes its fluorescence properties. Therefore, the concentration of analyte within the dye is the same as the concentration in the immediate environment. Intermittent flashes of appropriate light intensity are transmitted down the optical fiber to the dye; the resulting photoluminescence intensity will be transmitted back up the optic fiber.

Fluorescent optodes essentially measure the difference between excitation and emission light energy. If the excitation light energy is kept constant, the degree of emission energy that results when a fluorescent indicator is excited by a constant flashing light source is modified only by the concentration of the analyte. Hence, analyte concentration is determined by measurement of the fluorescence change. Examples of fluorescence-based optodes include fiber optic sensors for pH,[432] P_{CO_2},[251] and P_{O_2}.[251, 433]

Flexibility of Fluorescent Optodes

The advantages of fluorescence-based techniques include a high degree of sensitivity, compatibility with laser excitation sources, and a high degree of selectivity. These optodes can be used to measure substances that (1) naturally fluoresce, (2) can be converted to fluorescent compounds (fluorophores), or (3) enhance or quench fluorescence.

Sensors can be constructed that measure a decrease in fluorescence induced by an analyte rather than an increase in fluorescence, a process termed "fluorescence quenching." Although this approach decreases sensitivity, it has the advantage of allowing fiberoptic measurement of substances such as oxygen that will not induce fluorescence.[434, 435]

ENERGY-TRANSFER OPTODES

A limitation of fluorescence-based optodes is the relatively small number of substances that fluoresce. Energy-transfer optodes obviate this problem by combining a colorimetric reagent with a fluorescent indicator. This system combines the advantages of fluorescence measurement with the greater availability of colorimetric chemicals. Optic probes that measure Na^+, K^+, and pH using energy-transfer techniques have been described.[433]

INTRAVASCULAR BLOOD GAS SYSTEM

A recently described intravascular blood gas system (IBGS)* serves as a good example of the application of fluorescent optode technology to the measurement of arterial blood gases.[436] The IBGS probe consists of three optical fibers, each distally tipped with a fluorescence-based sensor affected by either hydrogen ion concentration (pH), carbon dioxide tension (Pco_2), or oxygen tension (Po_2). A silicone matrix is used to house the indicator dye. The fluorescent indicators are enclosed within chambers designed to allow the free passage of excitation light and emitted fluorescence, yet the indicators are isolated from the substance to be measured by a selectively permeable, optically isolated membrane. This arrangement allows for complete isolation of the indicator from all environmental influences except the substance to be measured. The probe also contains a thermocouple for temperature measurement.

The probe has an external diameter of 0.024 (0.62 mm) in. and is configured to allow passage through a 20-gauge vascular catheter without interfering with the fidelity of simultaneously transduced vascular pressures or blood sampling from the catheter. The probe is constructed of nontoxic materials and coated with covalently bonded heparin to diminish potential for thrombus formation.

With in vivo placement, bends in the optical fibers can produce optical misalignment or intensity signal attenuation. The solution to this problem is either (1) the use of fluorescent dyes whose excitation emissions are characterized by 2 different wavelengths of light with ratios proportional to the analyte concentration and independent of system factors, or (2) mixtures of dyes in which one responds to the analyte (active wavelength) and the other is neutral relative to the analyte (reference wavelength).

*Cardiovascular Devices, Inc.

The probe secures to the catheter with a Luer-Lok and a Y extension allows connection to a standard continuous flush line (Fig 26–1). Proximal to the Y fitting, the optic fibers are covered with a protective sheath comprising a flexible cable 6 ft in length that connects to the monitoring instrument.

As schematically illustrated in Figure 26–2, the IBGS is composed of four physically distinct elements: the probe assembly, the patient interface module (PIM), the microprocessor-based analyzer, and the display module. The probe cable plugs into the PIM that provides photo-

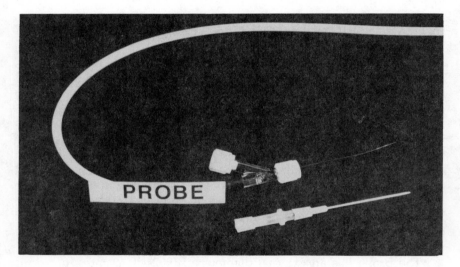

FIG 26–1.
Photograph of probe with Y extension and conventional 20-gauge arterial catheter.

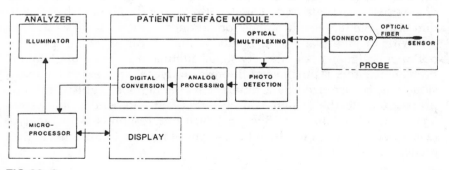

FIG 26–2.
Schematic diagram of major components comprising the IBGS.

detection analog signal processing and analog-to-digital conversion of the returned fluorescence signals. The light source is a stable, high-output, broad-band xenon flash lamp, from which a filter wheel obtains the desired spectrum for each sensor. The resultant excitation light beam passes through a fast-focus condensing lens to direct the maximum emission energy onto the proper optic fiber. To allow for minimal transmission distance of the returning sensor light signals, the PIM is small enough to be conveniently placed close to the patient without impediment to patient access.

All system control functions are performed by a microprocessor in the analyzer. The fluorescence sensor intensity signals are enhanced by digital filtering and stabilized to remove mechanical, electronic, and flash lamp variations by the use of reference signals. Appropriate algorithms are applied to the processed intensity signals to obtain blood gas values.

The display module (Fig 26–3) incorporates the control functions

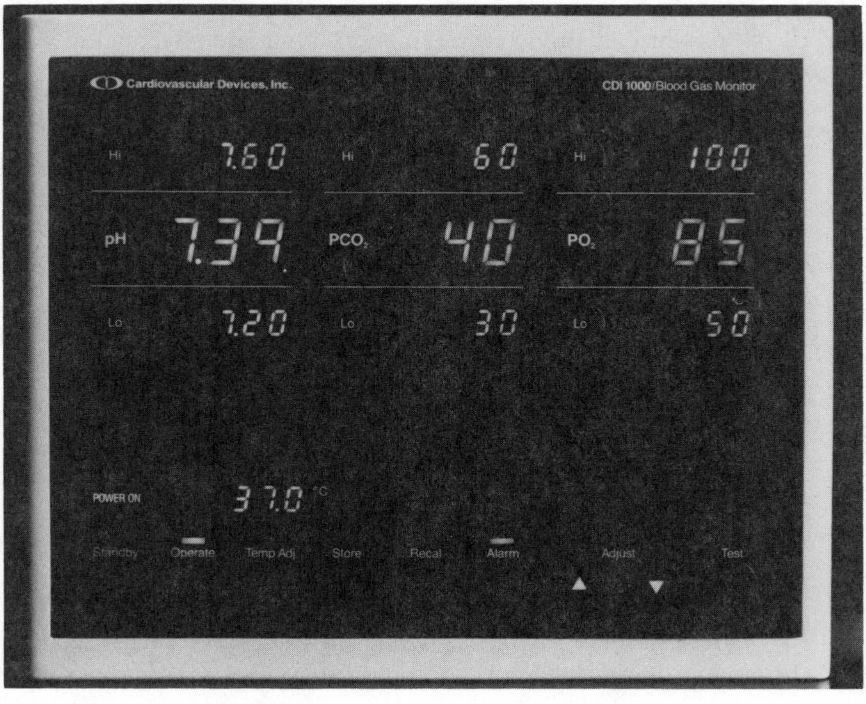

FIG 26–3.
Front panel of display module showing blood gas values, high and low alarm range settings, and temperature and operating controls. The up and down arrows are not shown.

and displays the data; it can readily be mounted on a pole used for intravenous feedings. The pH, PCO_2, and PO_2 are digitally displayed and updated every 6 seconds. High and low alarm limits may be set to give both visual and auditory indications that they have been exceeded. The monitor displays up or down arrows for each value when changes that are not a result of random variation are detected, utilizing algorithms that calculate slope and trends for sensor intensity signals within a sliding time window. The algorithms were optimized for intended function using computer simulations operating on previously recorded data and empirical evaluations.

Two-point calibration of the probe prior to insertion is achieved by tonometry against gases of known O_2, CO_2, and N_2 concentration (Gas 1 has 2.8% CO_2, 5.5% O_2, and 91.7% N_2 and Gas 2 has 8.4% CO_2, 14% O_2, and 77.6% N_2). The automated calibrator system is designed to store the probe and maintain sterility during the calibration routine.

Exhaustive evaluation in a dog model and preliminary evaluation in critically ill patients[436] intimates that this technology is capable of replacing use of the blood gas laboratory in certain patients. Further study and development will surely result in an exciting and challenging vista of continuous blood gas monitoring in the critically ill.

PART FIVE

Case Studies

27

Basic Case Studies in Blood Gas Interpretation

This chapter contains brief presentations of patients treated in the critical care units of Northwestern Memorial Hospital. Each case illustrates a critical point concerning the clinical application of blood gas analysis to supportive care. Reference to portions of the text containing appropriate discussions is made at the end of each case.

This material is intended for self-testing comprehension of the material presented in the text. By no means do these cases represent all possible problems; rather, they represent "typical" or "usual" clinical problems in respiratory care.

CASE 1—METABOLIC KETO-ACIDOSIS

A 17-year-old diabetic entered the emergency room with Kussmaul breathing and irregular pulse.

Room air blood gases:

pH	7.05	HCO_3^-	5 mEq/L
P_{CO_2}	12 mm Hg	BE	−30 mEq/L
P_{O_2}	108 mm Hg		

Interpretation: Severe partly compensated metabolic acidosis without hypoxemia.

Glucose and insulin, intravenously, were immediately started. However, it was believed that the severe acidosis was not being tolerated by the cardiovascular system, and the physician elected to restore the pH to the 7.20 range rapidly.

This was a 106-lb female. Before going on, calculate the amount of sodium bicarbonate you would give.

$$106 \text{ lb} = 48 \text{ kg}$$

$$\frac{1}{4} \times 48 = 12 \text{ L}$$

$$30 \times 12 = 360 \text{ mEq/L total deficit}$$

Because it was considered desirable to partly correct the acidosis, one half was given—i.e., a 180-mEq intravenous push in 15 minutes. Ten minutes later the blood gases were:

pH	7.27	HCO_3^-	11 mEq/L
P_{CO_2}	25 mm Hg	BE	− 14 mEq/L
P_{O_2}	92 mm Hg		

CASE 2—LACTIC ACIDOSIS

A 66-year-old woman with a history of chronic obstructive pulmonary disease entered the emergency room in obvious pulmonary edema.

Room air blood gases:

pH	7.10	HCO_3^-	8 mEq/L	BP	60/?	
P_{CO_2}	25 mm Hg	BE	− 20 mEq/L	P	140/minute, thready	
P_{O_2}	40 mm Hg	S_{O_2}	52%			

Interpretation: Partly compensated metabolic acidosis with severe hypoxemia. (Hypoxia must be assumed when acidemia and hypoxemia coexist.)

In addition to morphine and diuretic therapy, the patient received IPPB with high oxygen concentration and 50% ethyl alcohol in the nebulizer. After 10 minutes:

pH	7.38	HCO_3^-	16 mEq/L	BP	100/40	
P_{CO_2}	28 mm Hg	BE	-7 mEq/L	P	140/minute, strong	
P_{O_2}	110 mm Hg	S_{O_2}	99%			

The lactic acidosis was reversed.

CASE 3—METABOLIC ALKALOSIS

A 17-year-old female with severe kyphoscoliosis entered the hospital with pneumonia.

FI_{O_2} *40%:*

pH	7.37	HCO_3^-	14 mEq/L
P_{CO_2}	25 mm Hg	BE	-7 mEq/L
P_{O_2}	70 mm Hg	S_{O_2}	93%

Interpretation: Chronic alveolar hyperventilation (chronic respiratory alkalosis) with uncorrected hypoxemia.

The patient was given fluids intravenously for 3 days, while the fever and the rales disappeared with antibiotic therapy. However, she began to complain of weakness and difficulty in breathing.

Room air blood gases:

pH	7.53	HCO_3^-	25 mEq/L
P_{CO_2}	31 mm Hg	BE	$+4$ mEq/L
P_{O_2}	62 mm Hg		

Interpretation: In light of this patient's previous gas measurements, this must be interpreted as *uncompensated metabolic alkalosis.*

Serum electrolytes revealed a hypokalemia. After proper KCl replacement, the patient had no complaints.

Room air blood gases:

pH	7.41	HCO_3^-	16 mEq/L

P_{CO_2}	27 mm Hg	BE	-6 mEq/L
P_{O_2}	65 mm Hg		

Interpretation: Her normal state of chronic alveolar hyperventilation with mild hypoxemia.

CASE 4—METABOLIC ALKALOSIS

A 47-year-old man collapsed on the street and was blue with no palpable pulse when the paramedics arrived. The airway was cleared, ventilation was established with 100% oxygen, and closed-chest cardiac massage instituted. Within 20 seconds, there was a palpable pulse and skin color improved. The patient became responsive and uncooperative within 2 minutes.

Twenty minutes following the successful resuscitation, blood gas samples were drawn. The patient had received 100 mEq of sodium bicarbonate and 300 ml of 5% dextrose/water intravenously. What would you expect his blood gases to be on 40% oxygen?

pH	7.51	HCO_3^-	27 mEq/L
P_{CO_2}	35 mm Hg	BE	$+5$ mEq/L
P_{O_2}	62 mm Hg		

Interpretation: Uncompensated metabolic alkalosis with uncorrected hypoxemia. This patient may manifest alveolar hyperventilation without oxygen therapy. The metabolic alkalosis is expected secondary to the sodium bicarbonate administration.

CASE 5—RESPIRATORY ALKALOSIS

A 54-year-old woman with a 10-year history of "heart failure" was taking diuretics regularly. She had a "chest cold" the last week and experienced progressive shortness of breath.

Room air blood gases:

pH	7.54	HCO_3^-	22 mEq/L	V_T	600 ml	BP	160/100
Pco_2	26 mm Hg	BE	+2 mEq/L	RR	25/min	P	110/min
Po_2	48 mm Hg	So_2	89%	MV	15 L	T	100°F

Interpretation: Acute alveolar hyperventilation (acute respiratory alkalosis) with moderate hypoxemia. Hypoxia probably is not present because the cardiovascular system appears intact. This is probably a shunt-producing cardiopulmonary disease because the minute volume is reflected in the alveolar ventilation. The alveolar hyperventilation is most likely due to the hypoxemia. Oxygen therapy is indicated.

FI_{O_2} *40%:*

pH	7.48	HCO_3^-	23 mEq/L	V_T	500 ml	BP	140/90
Pco_2	31 mm Hg	BE	+1 mEq/L	RR	20/min	P	100/min
Po_2	55 mm Hg	So_2	91%	MV	10 L	T	100°F

This patient had a right pleural effusion causing atelectasis and shunting. Three liters of fluid were removed, and the next day:

FI_{O_2} *40%:*

pH	7.42	HCO_3^-	22 mEq/L	V_T	400 ml	BP	120/80
Pco_2	36 mm Hg	BE	−1 mEq/L	RR	12/min	P	90/min
Po_2	90 mm Hg	So_2	97%	MV	4.8 L	T	99°F

Interpretation: Normal ventilatory status with corrected hypoxemia.

CASE 6—PREANALYTIC ERROR

A 47-year-old woman is in the Postanesthesia Care Unit for 3 hours after gallbladder removal. She has been receiving 40% $F_{I_{O_2}}$, and a blood gas sample is drawn to assess the oxygen therapy.

pH	7.44	S_{O_2}	98%	BP	130/90
P_{CO_2}	30 mm Hg	Hb	13.2 gm%	P	95, regular
P_{O_2}	121 mm Hg	BE	-2 mEq/L	RR	20/min
				V_T	350 ml

The physician decides to decrease the $F_{I_{O_2}}$ to 30% and requests a blood gas measurement to be obtained in 30 minutes. One-half hour later, there is no apparent clinical change and the blood gases and vital signs are repeated:

pH	7.41	S_{O_2}	96%	BP	130/90
P_{CO_2}	10 mm Hg	Hb	7.4 gm%	P	95, regular
P_{O_2}	148 mm Hg	BE	-17 mEq/L	RR	22/min
				V_T	350 ml

A technical error is suspected; repeat measurements on 30% $F_{I_{O_2}}$ reveal:

pH	7.45	S_{O_2}	96%
P_{CO_2}	31 mm Hg	Hb	13.1 gm%
P_{O_2}	87 mm Hg	BE	-2 mEq/L

What was the most likely technical error?

A delay in running the sample would decrease the P_{O_2}; exposure to room air would result in an increased pH for the P_{CO_2} drop; too much sodium heparin could explain these erroneous results.

CASE 7—RESPIRATORY ALKALOSIS

A 47-year-old man without previous illness entered the coronary care unit with an ECG diagnosis of "inferior wall infarct" and severe chest pain. He had received morphine in the emergency room. Cardiac monitor showed numerous premature ventricular contractions (PVCs).

Room air blood gases:

pH	7.51	HCO_3^-	23 mEq/L	BP	100/60	
P_{CO_2}	29 mm Hg	BE	0 mEq/L	P	120/min, irregular	
P_{O_2}	64 mm Hg	S_{O_2}	94%	RR	22/min	

Interpretation: Acute alveolar hyperventilation (acute respiratory alkalosis) with mild hypoxemia.

$F_{I_{O_2}}$ *40%:*

pH	7.47	HCO_3^-	24 mEq/L	BP	110/60	
P_{CO_2}	32 mm Hg	BE	0 mEq/L	P	110/min, regular	
P_{O_2}	70 mm Hg	S_{O_2}	96%	RR	18/min	

The oxygen therapy decreased myocardial and ventilatory demand. The arrhythmia disappeared; the chest pain diminished, and the patient felt better.

Note: Oxygen therapy is not the suggested method for treating arrhythmia. However, it is common to have arrhythmia diminish or disappear when oxygen is properly administered.

CASE 8—PREANALYTIC ERROR

A 63-year-old man was admitted for elective knee surgery. Blood gas studies were obtained as part of the preoperative workup. The results obtained with the patient on room air were:

pH	7.36	S_{O_2}	74%	P	80, regular	
P_{CO_2}	46 mm Hg	BE	0 mEq/L	RR	15/min	
P_{O_2}	41 mm Hg	BP	122/84	V_T	450 ml	

Interpretation: Technical error is suspected, since there are no clinical signs of severe hypoxemia. The most likely cause is a venous sample.

CASE 9—ASTHMA

A 9-year-old boy with a history of allergic asthma had been audibly wheezing for 1 week. He had been receiving penicillin, plus oral bronchodilators, for one week. His mother stated he had not slept in two nights. The child was sitting and was using all accessory muscles to breathe. The wheezes could be heard from across the room.

Room air blood gases:

pH	7.41	HCO_3^-	15 mEq/L	VT	500 ml	BP	160/100
PCO_2	25 mm Hg	BE	−7 mEq/L	RR	30/min	P	130/min
PO_2	35 mm Hg	SO_2	62%	MV	15 L	T	101°F

Interpretation: Chronic alveolar hyperventilation (chronic respiratory alkalosis) with severe hypoxemia. Decreased oxygen content and work of breathing make tissue hypoxia a strong possibility. The cardiovascular system is working very hard. Even though this child is not in ventilatory failure, his cardiopulmonary reserve is marginal.

Epinephrine subcutaneously, IPPB with metaproterenol, and intravenous fluids were started.

FI_{O_2} *40%:*

pH	7.44	HCO_3^-	19 mEq/L	VT	400 ml	BP	150/100
PCO_2	29 mm Hg	BE	−4 mEq/L	RR	20/min	P	130/min
PO_2	55 mm Hg	SO_2	90%	MV	8 L		

The rise in pH despite the rise in PCO_2 suggests there had been lactic acidosis present that was corrected by oxygen therapy. Both ventilatory and oxygenation states were markedly improved.

CASE 10—POSTOPERATIVE PATIENT

A 47-year-old woman had her gallbladder removed. On the second postoperative day, she complained of chest pain.

Room air blood gases:

pH	7.45	HCO$_3$$^-$	17 mEq/L	V$_T$	500 ml	BP	130/70
P$_{CO_2}$	25 mm Hg	BE	-5 mEq/L	RR	24/min	P	100/min
P$_{O_2}$	58 mm Hg	S$_{O_2}$	95%	MV	12 L	T	100°F

Interpretation: Chronic alveolar hyperventilation (chronic respiratory alkalosis) with moderate hypoxemia. There is no evidence of deadspace disease. Remember, these are not uncommon blood gas values on the second day after an upper abdominal procedure.

Atelectasis and pneumonia must be ruled out. There is little evidence to support the existence of pulmonary embolus. Oxygen therapy is indicated to reduce ventilatory and myocardial work.

CASE 11—PREGNANCY

A 21-year-old woman in the third trimester of pregnancy fell on the ice and fractured her right forearm.

Room air blood gases:

pH	7.42	HCO$_3$$^-$	19 mEq/L	V$_T$	500 ml
P$_{CO_2}$	29 mm Hg	BE	-4 mEq/L	RR	16/min
P$_{O_2}$	77 mm Hg	S$_{O_2}$	96%	MV	8 L

Interpretation: Chronic alveolar hyperventilation (chronic respiratory alkalosis) with mild hypoxemia. These are normal for the third trimester of pregnancy. Oxygen therapy is *not* indicated.

CASE 12—PAIN AND ANXIETY

A 24-year-old woman entered the emergency room with a broken ankle. She appeared somewhat disoriented and confused.

Room air blood gases:

pH	7.55	HCO_3^-	23 mEq/L
PCO_2	27 mm Hg	BE	0 mEq/L
PO_2	105 mm Hg	SO_2	100%

Interpretation: Acute alveolar hyperventilation (acute respiratory alkalosis) without hypoxemia. Little evidence of tissue hypoxia is present. This is most likely secondary to pain and anxiety.

CASE 13—ANEMIA

A 67-year-old woman was admitted for uncontrolled rectal bleeding of several days' duration.

Room air blood gases:

pH	7.48	HCO_3^-	21 mEq/L	VT	450 ml	BP	160/90
PCO_2	28 mm Hg	BE	−1 mEq/L	RR	20/min	P	120/min
PO_2	95 mm Hg	SO_2	98%	MV	9 L		

Interpretation: Chronic alveolar hyperventilation (chronic respiratory alkalosis) without hypoxemia.

Hemoglobin content was 6 gm%. The chronic hyperventilation was due to the anemia. Control of the bleeding and transfusion resulted in normal blood gas values and vital signs two days later.

CASE 14—SMOKE INHALATION

A 53-year-old fireman was overcome by smoke. In the emergency room with patient receiving 50% oxygen by mask, values were:

pH	7.58	HCO_3^-	21 mEq/L	V_T	760 ml	BP	175/110
P_{CO_2}	23 mm Hg	BE	+1 mEq/L	RR	25/min	P	135/min
P_{O_2}	300 mm Hg	S_{O_2}	61%	MV	19 L		

Interpretation: Acute alveolar hyperventilation (acute respiratory alkalosis) with excessively corrected hypoxemia; in fact, one wonders whether hypoxemia would exist at room air. The cardiopulmonary system is working very hard.

The carboxyhemoglobin level was 40%; that is, 40% of the hemoglobin was saturated with carbon monoxide and unavailable to carry oxygen.

With high oxygen concentrations, the carboxyhemoglobin was reduced by 50% each hour.

CASE 15—PULMONARY EMBOLUS

A 67-year-old woman was convalescing after a leg fracture. Four days after the fracture, she had a sudden onset of severe chest pain and shortness of breath.

Room air blood gases:

pH	7.36	HCO_3^-	18 mEq/L	V_T	720 ml	BP	130/90
P_{CO_2}	33 mm Hg	BE	−5 mEq/L	RR	25/min	P	100/min
P_{O_2}	55 mm Hg	S_{O_2}	88%	MV	18 L	T	99°F

Interpretation: Normal ventilatory status with moderate hypoxemia. The tremendous disparity between minute volume and alveolar ventilation suggests deadspace disease.

Pulmonary angiography revealed massive pulmonary emboli.

CASE 16—MORBID OBESITY

A 450-pound, 42-year-old woman entered the hospital for evaluation of gastrointestinal bypass procedure for obesity.

Baseline blood gases on room air:

pH	7.46	HCO_3^-	50 mEq/L
P_{CO_2}	72 mm Hg	BE	+20 mEq/L
P_{O_2}	45 mm Hg	S_{O_2}	89%

Interpretation: Chronic ventilatory failure (chronic respiratory acidosis) with hypoxemia. This Pickwickian patient has a baseline of severe carbon dioxide retention.

CASE 17—CHRONIC OBSTRUCTIVE PULMONARY DISEASE

A 76-year-old man with a long history of symptomatic chronic obstructive pulmonary disease (COPD) entered the hospital with basilar pneumonia.

Room air blood gases:

pH	7.58	HCO_3^-	40 mEq/L
P_{CO_2}	45 mm Hg	BE	+15 mEq/L
P_{O_2}	38 mm Hg	S_{O_2}	83%

Interpretation: Uncompensated metabolic alkalosis with severe hypoxemia. But this diagnosis must be questioned! The *proper* interpretation is acute alveolar hyperventilation (acute respiratory alkalosis) superimposed on chronic ventilatory failure (chronic respiratory acidosis). Careful oxygen therapy is indicated.

CASE 18—COPD

A 76-year-old man with a long history of symptomatic COPD entered the hospital with basilar pneumonia.

Room air blood gases:

pH	7.25	HCO_3^-	38 mEq/L
P_{CO_2}	90 mm Hg	BE	+5 mEq/L
P_{O_2}	34 mm Hg	S_{O_2}	58%

Interpretation: Acute ventilatory failure (acute respiratory acidosis) superimposed on chronic ventilatory failure (chronic respiratory acidosis). A trial of low-concentration oxygen is indicated.

CASE 19—COPD

A 76-year-old woman with documented CO_2 retention secondary to severe COPD has been in the medical intensive care unit for 3 days with a diagnosis of acute bacterial pneumonitis. She has been stable for 24 hours with the following arterial blood gas values and vital signs on a 28% Venturi mask:

pH	7.44	BP	135/95
P_{CO_2}	63 mm Hg	P	110, regular
P_{O_2}	52 mm Hg	RR	22/min
		V_T	250 ml

She is placed on a nasal cannula at 2 L/minute flow, and the blood gas studies and vital signs are repeated in one hour.

pH	7.36	BP	140/100
P_{CO_2}	75 mm Hg	P	105, regular
P_{O_2}	65 mm Hg	RR	24/min
		V_T	200 ml

CASE 20—PULMONARY ARTERY BLOOD GASES

A 43-year-old man is admitted to the surgical intensive care unit from the operating room. He was in an auto accident 6 hours before and has undergone splenectomy, repair of liver lacerations, and repair of compound femoral fracture. Multiple transfusions were necessary, and his chest is unstable bilaterally due to multiple rib fractures.

The anesthesiologist had difficulty maintaining perfusion during the procedure. Bilateral chest tubes are functioning adequately, and bleeding continues in the chest. Multiple PVCs suggest the possibility of myo-cardial contusion.

Because of cardiovascular instability, a Swan-Ganz catheter is placed. The patient is on 50% $F_{I_{O_2}}$ with controlled volume ventilation and ac-ceptable Pa_{CO_2} and pH. Simultaneous radial artery and pulmonary sam-ples are obtained and show:

	Radial arterial	Pulmonary artery
P_{O_2}	52 mm Hg	31 mm Hg
Hb	14 gm%	14 gm%
HbO_2	83%	50%
CO_2	15.7 vol%	9.5 vol%

What is the man's arterial-venous content difference ($C_{a-v}O_2$) and what is the significance of the finding?

CASE 21—OVERDOSE

A 34-year-old woman entered the emergency room comatose. She was suspected of taking an overdose of an unknown drug.

Room air blood gases:

pH	7.15	HCO_3^-	28 mEq/L
PCO_2	80 mm Hg	BE	0 mEq/L
PO_2	42 mm Hg	SO_2	80%

Interpretation: Acute ventilatory failure (acute respiratory acidosis). Hypoxia must be assumed. Support of ventilation is immediately indicated.

CASE 22—ATELECTASIS

A 53-year-old man with myasthenia gravis was being maintained on a volume ventilator due to a cholinergic crisis, aspiration pneumonia, and withdrawal from all cholinergic medication. For several days, he had been maintained on the same ventilatory parameters and his blood gas values were:

pH	7.43	HCO_3^-	26 mEq/L	VT	800 ml
PCO_2	41 mm Hg	BE	+2 mEq/L	RR	14/min
PO_2	74 mm Hg	SO_2	95%	FI_{O_2}	35%

The next morning his blood gases were:

pH	7.52	HCO_3^-	24 mEq/L	VT	800 ml
PCO_2	30 mm Hg	BE	+2 mEq/L	RR	14/min
PO_2	45 mm Hg	SO_2	86%	FI_{O_2}	35%

Interpretation: Alveolar hyperventilation with respiratory alkalemia and uncorrected hypoxemia. This signals the acute collapse of a lung segment or lobe, producing an acute shunt plus increased air exchange in the ventilated lung.

CASE 23—ADULT RESPIRATORY DISTRESS SYNDROME (ARDS)

A 32-year-old woman had been hospitalized for 18 hours with a diagnosis of pelvic inflammatory disease. She suddenly complained of chills, became very febrile, and was peripherally cold and clammy. She became disoriented and was moved to medical intensive care with a diagnosis of septic shock.

Chest x-ray revealed diffuse infiltrates throughout both lung fields. The patient's breathing was rapid and labored. On 50% oxygen, the arterial blood gases and vital signs were:

pH	7.32	BP	90/?
P_{CO_2}	34 mm Hg	P	140, regular
P_{O_2}	43 mm Hg	RR	36/min
Hb	12.5 gm%	V_T	400 ml

Due to the confusion about the pulmonary vs. cardiovascular components, a Swan-Ganz catheter was placed.

$C_{a-v}O_2$	2.7 vol%
Q_{SP}/Q_T	52%

Was the hypoxemia due to septic shock? Might ARDS be entertained as a possibility?

28

Advanced Case Studies in Blood Gas Interpretation

The purpose of this chapter is to test the readers' comprehension of the more advanced principles of blood gas interpretation. The five case studies in this chapter address critically ill patients with complicated cardiopulmonary and metabolic problems. Appropriate therapy is more likely to be administered to such patients when basic and advanced blood gas interpretation is applied. The suggested answers DO NOT constitute the only solution to the problems; rather, they are based upon logical conclusions extrapolated from the clinical and laboratory findings presented.

ACUTE MYOCARDIAL INFARCTION WITH POOR TISSUE PERFUSION

A 48-year-old white man who weighed 198 lb (90 kg) was admitted to the intensive care unit (ICU) with an acute myocardial infarction. History revealed crushing sternal chest pain, diaphoresis, nausea, and vomiting that started approximately 6 hours prior to admission. The 12-lead ECG on admission showed evidence of ST-segment elevation across the precordial leads, I and AVL. Examination of the chest revealed bilateral moist rales approximately half way up both lung fields. A summation gallop was present without murmurs or evidence of enlargement. The patient's extremities were cold, mottled, and diaphoretic. Urine output was negligible. Chest x-ray film revealed increased lung vascular markings, with diffuse haziness in both lower lung fields.

	Vital signs	*Arterial blood gas (ABG) values*		*Laboratory values*	
BP	150/100	pH	7.31	HCT	38%
P	132/min	P_{CO_2}	29 mm Hg	Hb	13.1 gm%
RR	26/min	P_{O_2}	54 mm Hg	WBC	14,000/mm^3
V_T	500 ml	$F_{I_{O_2}}$	3L nc		
T	101°F	HCO_3^-	14 mEq/L		
		BE	−10 mEq/L		

1. What is the most likely source of the partly compensated metabolic acidosis?

The most likely etiology is lactic acidosis secondary to decreased tissue perfusion.

2. Why is there arterial hypoxemia despite oxygen therapy?

A nasal cannula (nc) is a low-flow system that will deliver minimal oxygen to a patient with an increased minute ventilation of 13 L. A high-flow system would be more appropriate and would allow more reliable interpretation of the arterial P_{O_2} (see chap. 7).

3. To what extent is intrapulmonary shunting responsible for the hypoxemia?

Some increase in physiologic shunting can be assumed secondary to the pulmonary edema. However, the hypoxemic effect of that shunting is most probably accentuated by a decreased mixed venous oxygen content secondary to a decreased cardiac output (see chapters 8 and 9).

Placement of a radial and pulmonary artery (PA) catheter was accomplished and a 50% Venturi mask was applied. The patient received 10 mg morphine sulfate, 80 mg furosemide (Lasix), and a dobutamine drip at 15 μg/kg/min. The following values were obtained:

	Vital signs		*ABG and PA values*		*Hemodynamics*	
BP	138/86	pH	7.24	7.18	PAP	30/20 mm Hg
P	140/min	P_{CO_2}	27	39 mm Hg	MEAN PAP	26 mm Hg
RR	28/min	P_{O_2}	50	28 mm Hg	RA	4 mm Hg
MAP	94	$F_{I_{O_2}}$	0.5		PAOP	22 mm Hg
V_T	400 ml	HCO_3^-	12	11 mEq/L	CO	3.9 L
T	99°R	BE	−15	−14 mEq/L	BSA	2.0 mm^2
		S_{O_2}	79%	37%	Cc_{O_2}	18.5 ml/dl
		C_{O_2}	14.5	6.9 ml/dl		

4. What changes are evident from the arterial blood gas values?

The degree of arterial hypoxemia is more impressive in light of an appropriate delivery of 50% oxygen. Since the base deficit increasing from -10 to -15 mEq/L reflects a more severe metabolic acidemia, the hemoglobin dissociation curve shifts to the right, and a lower saturation is present for the lower PO_2. Unless cardiac output increases, the decreased oxygen delivery further threatens tissue oxygenation (see chap. 5 and chap. 7—refractory hypoxemia).

5. The Cardiac Index (cardiac output [CO]/Body Surface Area [BSA]) is 1.95 L/min/m², which is significantly below the normal range of 2.7 to 4.3. How do the blood gas values reflect the presence of a decreased cardiac output?

The $C_{(a-v)}O_2$ of 7.6 ml/dl is most probably due to a decreased cardiac output since there is no clinical evidence of significantly increased oxygen consumption (see chap. 8). Furthermore, the widened $P_{(v-a)}CO_2$ of 12 mm Hg is most likely secondary to a diminished cardiac output that is beginning to limit the rate of CO_2 excretion in the lungs (see chap. 12).

6. What is the clinical significance of a mixed venous PO_2 of 28 mm Hg?

The mixed venous PO_2 is a reflection of global tissue oxygen extraction, and values less than 30 mm Hg may reflect inadequate tissue oxygenation. The acidemia is responsible for a "shift to the right" and an $S\bar{v}_{O_2}$ of 37% that greatly suggests tissue hypoxia. In this clinical setting of diminished cardiac output, the low $C\bar{v}_{O_2}$ must be highly suspect of reflecting inadequate tissue oxygenation (see chap. 8).

ACUTE PULMONARY EMBOLUS

A 27-year-old, previously healthy female weighing 121 lb (55 kg) is admitted to the ICU with a recent onset of dyspnea, right-sided pleuritic chest pain, and blood-tinged sputum. She claims right leg calf tenderness has been present for two days. She is alert, tachypneic, and diaphoretic, with strong peripheral pulses.

Vital signs		*ABG values*		*Laboratory values*	
BP	134/76	pH	7.47	HCT	36%
P	128/min	PCO_2	33 mm Hg	Hb	12.1 gm%
RR	30/min	PO_2	51 mm Hg	WBC	8,400/mm³
V_T	700 ml	FI_{O_2}	5L nc		

MV	21 L	HCO_3^-	20 mEq/L
T	100.6°F	BE	0 mEq/L
		Sa_{O_2}	86%

When the patient was placed on a 40% venturimask (high-flow system), the Pa_{O_2} increased to 82 mm Hg, with no change in pH or PCO_2.

1. What is the primary V/Q disturbance in pulmonary embolus and how can this be evaluated by blood gas measurement?

Creation of ventilated, unperfused lung regions—physiologic dead-space—is the primary V/Q abnormality. The increased MV to PCO_2 disparity suggests increased deadspace ventilation since metabolic function and cardiac output appear to be appropriate (see chaps. 10 and 13).

2. What is the significance of the response to changes in oxygen therapy?

The low-flow system (nasal cannula) is delivering insufficient augmentation of oxygen when minute ventilation is 3 to 4 times normal (21 L/min). The high-flow system at 40% resulted in significant improvement in Pa_{O_2} without PCO_2 change. This is responsive hypoxemia reflective of shunt-effect mechanism (low V/Q) (see chap. 7).

Although the primary defect in pulmonary embolus is increased physiologic deadspace, the insult classically causes release of vasoactive substances that accentuate low V/Q (shunt effect). Such a shunt effect mechanism creates hypoxemia that is responsive to oxygen therapy (see chaps. 7 and 9).

The patient started to receive heparin therapy and upon returning from a ventilation and perfusion scan, she complained of severe chest pain; this was followed by loss of consciousness and apnea. She was immediately ventilated and intubated, with stabilization of cardiovascular function following intravenous administration of 2 L crystalloid solution. Her sensorium improved and spontaneous ventilation was resumed.

Vital signs		*ABG values*			
BP	88/50	pH	7.42	$PetCO_2$	22 mm Hg
P	134/min	PCO_2	36 mm Hg	$P\bar{E}_{CO_2}$	8
RR	30/min	PO_2	84 mm Hg		
VT	800 ml	FI_{O_2}	0.5		
T	100°F	HCO_3^-	20 mEq/L		
		BE	0 mEq/L		

3. What manifestations of increased physiologic deadspace are now apparent in addition to the MV-P_{CO_2} disparity?

The deadspace to tidal volume ratio (V_D/V_T) can now be calculated: $Pa_{CO_2} - P\bar{E}_{CO_2}/Pa_{CO_2} = 36 - 8/36 = 0.78$. The normal V_D/V_T in a spontaneously breathing patient is 0.2 to 0.4. The $P_{(a-et)}CO_2$ of 14 mm Hg also suggests increased deadspace ventilation (see chaps. 10 and 15).

Although a decreased cardiac output may be contributing to the deadspace ventilation, it is reasonable to assume that pulmonary embolus is responsible for most of the increase in physiologic deadspace.

ACUTE DIABETIC COMA WITH KETOSIS AND SUBSEQUENT CARDIAC ARREST

An 18-year-old female who weighs 110 lb (50 kg) and is a known diabetic is admitted to the Emergency Room. She is obtunded, responding only to deep pain stimuli. Mucous membranes are dry; skin is dry with decreased turgor. Examination of the chest is unremarkable except for tachypnea and tachycardia. Occasional unifocal premature ventricular contractions (PVCs) are noted on the ECG monitor. Administration of normal saline is started intravenously (IV) and 50 cc of 50% dextrose in water is administered without any improvement in mental status. Ten units of regular insulin are given IV.

Vital signs		*Laboratory values*			*ABG values*		*Urine*
BP	102/64	HCT	47%	pH		7.06	4+ sugar
P	126/min	Hb	15.4 gm%	P_{CO_2}		9 mm Hg	4+ ketone
RR	28/min	Na$^+$	132 mEq/L	P_{O_2}		119 mm Hg	
V_T	650 ml	K	5.9 mEq/L	$F_{I_{O_2}}$		0.21	
MV	18.2 L	Cl	92 mEq/L	HCO_3^-		5 mEq/L	
		CO_2	3 mEq/L	BE		−28 mEq/L	
		BUN	32 mg%				
		Glucose	963 mg%				

1. What interpretations can be made from the arterial blood gas values?

Severe acidemia exists despite significant alveolar hyperventilation. Ketosis is the best explanation for the profound acidosis.

No arterial oxygenation deficit exists although this does not guarantee adequate tissue oxygenation. The low Pa_{CO_2} means a similar PA_{CO_2} exists and allows for the alveolar P_{O_2} to be higher than 101 mm

Hg when breathing room air at sea level. Such hyperventilation in healthy lungs results in unusually high room air arterial PO_2 values.

2. What is the "anion gap" and what does it mean?

The routinely measured cations (Na^+ and K^+) account for a greater portion of all cations than the normally measured anions (Cl^- and HCO_3^-) account for all anions. There is normally a 12 to 20 mEq/L difference ("gap") between "measured" cations and anions. The gap increases as "unmeasured" anions (such as ketones or lactate) accumulate. This patient manifests an anion gap of 41 mEq/L.

3. Should this patient receive sodium bicarbonate?

It is generally agreed that a patient with ketoacidosis that is alert and has a stable cardiovascular function should not require sodium bicarbonate therapy unless the arterial pH is less than 7.10. Although this is a complex medical judgment with many factors to be weighed, it can be argued that this patient should receive some bicarbonate therapy solely on the basis of the low pH and very low Pa_{CO_2} (see chap. 14).

As discussed previously (see chap. 6), this 50-kg adult is 80% water, of which one third is extracellular. Therefore, 25% of ideal body weight should be a reasonable estimation of extracellular fluid in liters—12.5 L. There is a 28 mEq/L base deficit, thus 28 × 12.5 (350 mEq/L) should represent the bicarbonate load that returns extracellular fluid to a normal buffer base status. One third to one half of this amount (100 to 150 mEq) should be a reasonable dose since our desire is to achieve a more desirable pH milieu for the heart while treating the ketoacidosis by insulin, fluid, and electrolyte administration.

The managing service decided that bicarbonate therapy was not warranted and instituted therapy to reverse the ketoacidosis. Appropriate IV lines and an arterial line were started and the patient transferred to ICU; an arterial blood gas sample was obtained there and sent to the laboratory. Approximately 10 minutes later the patient had an episode of ventricular tachycardia that degenerated to ventricular fibrillation. As cardiopulmonary resuscitation (CPR) was initiated, the prearrest blood gas results were available. Following are those results and the vital signs at the time the sample was obtained:

Vital signs		*ABG values*	
BP	108/84	pH	6.88
P	142/min	PCO_2	19 mm Hg
RR	32/min	PO_2	89 mm Hg
VT	750 ml	FI_{O_2}	0.30
MV	24 L	HCO_3^-	3 mEq/L
		BE	−30 mEq/L

4. What information do these values offer to explain the patient's deterioration?

The abrupt change in pH is almost entirely due to the increased Pa_{CO_2}. Despite an increased minute ventilation (18.2 to 24 L), the Pa_{CO_2} increased from 9 to 19 mm Hg. This increased physiologic dead-space is best explained by a decreasing cardiac output (see chap. 10).

5. Is bicarbonate therapy now indicated?

The problems of sodium bicarbonate administration during CPR have been discussed (see chap. 12). No bicarbonate therapy was administered.

The patient was ventilated and intubated, and chest compressions were begun. A good femoral pulse was present with CPR and defibrillation returned the heart to a normal sinus rhythm with frequent PVCs. Lidocaine was administered and another blood gas study was obtained.

Vital signs		*ABG values*	
BP	110/90	pH	7.01
MAP	95 mm Hg	P_{CO_2}	14 mm Hg
P	125/min	P_{O_2}	387 mm Hg
RR	28/min (assisted)	$F_{I_{O_2}}$	>0.70
		HCO_3^-	5 mEq/L
		BE	-28 mEq/L

6. Is bicarbonate therapy now indicated?

The same factors now exist that were present before the cardiac deterioration. Since perfusion appears adequate, bicarbonate therapy would now be prudent.

PROLONGED CPR

A 53-year-old previously healthy man experienced a severe myocardial infarction with cardiogenic shock requiring aortic counterpulsation for 27 hours. He remained stable for 18 hours and then manifested electromechanical dissociation (EMD) and was pronounced dead after 40 minutes of CPR.

One hour prior to EMD:

Vital signs

BP	130/70
MAP	90 mm Hg
P	105/min
RR	22/min
V_T	450 ml
MV	9.9 L

ABG values

pH	7.37
P_{CO_2}	42 mm Hg
P_{O_2}	80 mm Hg
$F_{I_{O_2}}$	0.30
HCO_3^-	23 mEq/L
BE	-1 mEq/L
Sa_{O_2}	96%
Ca_{O_2}	17.0 ml/dl

PA values

pH	7.33
P_{CO_2}	50 mm Hg
P_{O_2}	32 mm Hg
HCO_3^-	22 mEq/L
BE	-1 mEq/L
Sv_{O_2}	65%
Cv_{O_2}	11.4 ml/dl

Hemodynamics

PAP	22/12
MEAN PAP	15 mm Hg
RA	9 mm Hg
PAOP	11 mm Hg
CO	4.3 L
BSA	2 m^2
Cc_{O_2}	17.8 ml/dl
Hb	13 gm%

1. What factors delineate borderline cardiopulmonary function?

(a) Cardiac output is low (CI = 2.1 L). This is reflected in the $C_{(a-v)}O_2$ of 5.6 ml/dl as well as the Sv_{O_2} of 65% (see chaps. 8 and 16).

(b) Physiologic deadspace is increased since a minute ventilation of 9.9 L results in an arterial PCO_2 of 42 mm Hg. This is best explained by the decreased cardiac output (see chap. 10).

(c) Qsp/QT is 13%, reflecting a relatively normal lung (see chap. 9). The increased minute ventilation without distress reflects a normal pulmonary system with adequate reserves.

Five minutes after EMD, the trachea is intubated and chest compressions result in palpable femoral pulses and a spike in the arterial line tracing. Arterial and mixed venous blood samples reveal:

ABG values		*PA values*	
pH	7.52	pH	7.31
PCO_2	28 mm Hg	PCO_2	58 mm Hg
PO_2	436 mm Hg	PO_2	25 mm Hg
FI_{O_2}	>0.7	HCO_3^-	22 mEq/L
HCO_3^-	22 mEq/L	BE	-2 mEq/L
BE	-1 mEq/L	Sv_{O_2}	47%
Sa_{O_2}	99%		

2. What clinically important information can be assumed from the arterial blood gas values regarding oxygenation?

Blood going from the right ventricle to the left ventricle is being well oxygenated and ventilated. This reflects a normal lung function but should be little comfort since the venous blood is more reflective of the tissue status.

The absence of metabolic acidosis in the arterial blood can be assumed to reflect the tissue status. This means that either lactate is not being produced in the tissues and thereby tissue oxygenation remains adequate, or a well-oxygenated liver is metabolizing the lactate to CO_2.

Fifteen minutes of appropriate advanced life support has been unsuccessful in restoring cardiac function. Arterial and pulmonary arterial blood samples are obtained.

ABG values		*PA values*	
pH	7.27	pH	7.09

P_{CO_2}	48 mm Hg	P_{CO_2}	84 mm Hg
P_{O_2}	53 mm Hg	P_{O_2}	25 mm Hg
$F_{I_{O_2}}$	>0.7	HCO_3^-	18 mEq/L
HCO_3^-	18 mEq/L	BE	−6 mEq/L
BE	−6 mEq/L	Sv_{O_2}	42%
Sa_{O_2}	85%	Cv_{O_2}	7.4 ml/dl
Ca_{O_2}	15		

3. Why have the arterial values deteriorated?

The profound drop in arterial oxygenation must be assumed due to an increase in the physiologic shunt. This would also explain the increased Pa_{CO_2} since the significantly high Pv_{CO_2} in shunted blood will affect the arterial side.

Examination of the chest reveals decreased breath sounds on the left side. No subcutaneous emphysema or difficulty ventilating is noted. The endotracheal tube is pulled back 1 in., and the breath sounds dramatically improve on the left side. Repeat arterial blood gases:

ABG values

pH	7.39
P_{CO_2}	32 mm Hg
P_{O_2}	345 mm Hg
$F_{I_{O_2}}$	>0.7
HCO_3^-	18 mEq/L
BE	−6 mEq/L
Sa_{O_2}	99%

Thirty-five minutes of resuscitation has not resulted in improved cardiac function. There is now a weak pulse palpable with chest compression.

ABG values		*PA values*	
pH	7.11	pH	6.82
P_{CO_2}	38 mm Hg	P_{CO_2}	96 mm Hg
P_{O_2}	322 mm Hg	P_{O_2}	20 mm Hg
$F_{I_{O_2}}$	>0.7	HCO_3^-	8 mEq/L
HCO_3^-	6 mEq/L	BE	−20 mEq/L
BE	−19 mEq/L	Sv_{O_2}	37%
Sa_{O_2}	99%		

5. What is the significance of the arterial blood gas values?

The severe metabolic acidosis is a reliable reflection of venous and tissue pH. The arterial metabolic acidemia is a dire factor. Successful resuscitation at this point is improbable since significant tissue hypoxia has taken place.

REFERENCES

1. Lavoisier AL: Sur les altérations qui arrivent à l'air dans plusiers circonstances où se trouvent les hommes réunis en société. *Mémories de Médecine en Histoire de la Société de Médecine* 5:569 (1782–1783, read in 1785).
2. Priestley J: *The Discovery of Oxygen, Alembic Club Reprints.* Chicago, University of Chicago Press, 1906.
3. Bert P: *Barometric Pressure: Researches in Experimental Physiology,* Hitchcock MA, Hitchcock FA (trans). Columbus, Ohio, Longs College Book Co, 1943.
4. Cohen P: The metabolic function of oxygen and biochemical lesions of hypoxemia. *Anesthesiology* 1972; 37:148.
5. Warrell DA, et al: Pattern of filling in the pulmonary capillary bed. *J Appl Physiol* 1972; 32:346.
6. Halmaggi DFJ, et al: Pulmonary alveolar-vascular reflex. *J Appl Physiol* 1964; 19:105.
7. Harvey RM, et al: A reconsideration of the origins of pulmonary hypertension. *Chest* 1971; 59:82.
8. Stern LI, et al: Estimation of non-respiratory acid-base abnormalities. *J Appl Physiol* 1969; 27:21.
9. Collier CR, et al: Use of extracellular base excess in diagnosis of acid-base disorders: A conceptual approach. *Chest* 1972; 61:65.
10. Ferguson JKW: Carbamino compounds of CO_2 with haemoglobin and their role in the transport of CO_2. *J Physiol* (Lond.) 1936; 88:40.
11. Ferguson JKW, Roughton FJW: The chemical relationships and physiologic importance of carbamino compounds of CO_2 with haemoglobin. *J Physiol (Lond)* 1934; 83:87.
12. Keilin D, Mann T: Activity of carbonic anhydrase within red blood corpuscles. *Nature* 1941; 148:493.
13. Winters RW: Terminology of acid-base disorders. *Ann Intern Med* 1965; 63:873.
14. Bartels H, et al: Glossary on respiration and gas exchange. *J Appl Physiol* 1973; 34:549.
15. Williams HM: Ventilatory failure. *Medicine* 1966; 45:317.
16. West JB: Causes of carbon dioxide retention in lung disease. *N Engl J Med* 1971; 284:1232.
17. Perutz MF: Structure and function of haemoglobin. Presented at Federation of European Biochemical Societies, First Meeting, London, 1964, pp 143–144.

18. Perutz MF: Stereochemistry of cooperative effects in haemoglobin. *Nature* 1970; 228:726.
19. Rossi L, Roughton FJW: The effect of carbamino-Hb compounds on the buffer power of human blood at 37°C. *J Physiol (Lond)* 1963; 167:15.
20. Chanutin A, Curnish RR: Effect of organic and inorganic phosphates on the oxygen equilibrium of human erythrocytes. *Arch Biochem Biophys* 1967; 121:96.
21. Roughton FJW: The kinetics of haemoglobin: IV. The competition of carbon monoxide and oxygen for haemoglobin. *Proc R Soc Lond [Biol]* 1934; 115:473.
22. Roughton FJW, Darling RC: The effect of carbon monoxide on the oxyhemoglobin dissociation curve. *Am J Physiol* 1944; 141:17.
23. Stewart RD, et al: Experimental human exposure to carbon monoxide. *Arch Environ Health* 1970; 21:154.
24. Darling RC, et al: Some properties of human fetal and maternal blood. *J Clin Invest* 1941; 20:739.
25. Oski FA, et al: The effects of deoxygenation of adult and fetal hemoglobin on the synthesis of red cell 2,3-diphosphoglycerate and its in vivo consequences. *J Clin Invest* 1970; 49:400.
26. Oski FA: Red cell metabolism in the newborn infant: V. Glycolytic intermediates and glycolytic enzymes. *Pediatrics* 1969; 44:84.
27. Vresmold H, et al: Blood oxygen affinity in infancy: The interaction of fetal and adult hemoglobin, oxygen capacity and red cell hydrogen ion and 2,3-diphosphoglycerate concentration. *Respir Physiol* 1973; 18:14.
28. Christiansen, Douglas, Haldane: *J Physiol* (Lond) 1914; 48:244.
29. Bellingham AJ, et al: Regulatory mechanism of haemoglobin oxygen affinity in acidosis and alkalosis. *J Clin Invest* 1971; 50:700.
30. Benesch R, et al: Effect of organic phosphates from the human erythrocyte on the allosteric properties of hemoglobin. *Biochem Biophys Res Commun* 1967; 26:162.
31. Finch C, Lenfant C: Oxygen transport in man. *N Engl J Med* 1972; 286:407.
32. Bryan-Brown CW, et al: Consumable oxygen: Availability of oxygen in relation to oxyhemoglobin dissociation. *Crit Care Med* 1973; 1:17.
33. Severinghaus JW: Blood gas calculator. *J Appl Physiol* 1966: 21:1108.
34. Brewer GJ, Eaton JW: Erythrocyte metabolism: Interaction with oxygen transport. *Science* 1971; 171:1205.
35. Miller D, Lichtman M: Clinical implication of altered affinity of hemoglobin for oxygen, in Weed RI (ed): *Hematology for Internists*. Boston, Little Brown Co., 1971.
36. Torrance J, et al: Intraerythrocytic adaptation to anemia. *N Engl J Med* 1970; 283:165.
37. Laver MB: A fable of our time: Oxygen transport, or does the emperor have new clothes? *Anesthesiology* 1972; 36:105.
38. Comroe JH, et al: The unreliability of cyanosis in the recognition of arterial anoxemia. *Am J Med* 1947; 214:1.

39. Biscoe TJ: Carotid body: Structure and function. *Physiol Rev* 1971; 51:437.
40. Oldham PD: *Measurement in Medicine: The Interpretation of Numerical Data.* London, English Universities Press, 1968.
41. Fleishcer WR, Gambiro SR: *Blood pH, PCO_2, PO_2 and Oxygen Saturation,* ed. 4. Chicago, American Society of Clinical Pathology, Council on Clinical Chemistry, 1972.
42. Severinghaus JW: Measurements of blood gases: PO_2 and PCO_2. *Ann NY Acad Sci* 1968; 148:115.
43. Williams RJ: Standard human beings versus standard values. *Science* 1957; 126:453.
44. Elkinton JR: Acid-base disorders and the clinician. *Ann Intern Med* 1965; 63:893.
45. Asmussen E, Nielsen M: Physiologic deadspace and alveolar gas pressures at rest and during muscular exercise. *Acta Physiol Scand* 1956; 38:1.
46. Jones NL, et al: Physiological deadspace and alveolar-arterial gas pressure differences during exercise. *Clin Sci* 1966; 31:19.
47. Higgs BE, et al: Changes in ventilation, gas exchange and circulation during exercise in normal subjects. *Clin Sci* 1967; 32:329.
48. Bergman NA: Effect of varying respiratory wave forms on distribution of inspired gas during artificial ventilation. *Am Rev Respir Dis* 1969; 100:518.
49. Hedenstierna G, McCarthy G: Mechanics of breathing, gas distribution and functional residual capacity at different frequencies of respiration during spontaneous and artificial ventilation. *Br J Anaesth* 1975; 47:706.
50. Koch G: Alveolar ventilation, diffusing capacity and the A—a PO_2 difference in the newborn infant. *Respir Physiol* 1968; 4:168.
51. Davies CTM: The oxygen-transporting system in relation to age. *Clin Sci* 1972; 42:1.
52. Jarboe TM, et al: Ventilatory failure due to metabolic alkalosis. *Chest* 1972; 61:615.
53. Leigh JM: Variation in performance of oxygen therapy devices. *Ann R Coll Surg Engl* 1973; 52:234.
54. Woolner DF, Larkin J: An analysis of the performance of a variable venturi-type oxygen mask. *Anesth and Intensive Care* 1980; 8:44–51.
55. Wylie WD, Churchill-Davidson GC: *A Practice of Anaesthesia,* ed 3. Chicago, Year Book Medical Publishers Inc, 1978.
56. Scacci R: Air entrainment masks: Jet mixing is how they work; the Bernoulli and Venturi principles is how they don't. *Respir Care* 1979; 24:928–934.
57. Goldstein RS, Young J, Rebuck AS: Effect of breathing pattern on oxygen concentration received from standard face mask. *Lancet* 1982; 2(8309):1188–1190.
58. McPherson SP: Oxygen percentage accuracy of air-entrainment masks. *Respir Care* 1974; 19:658–664.
59. Redding JS, McAfee DD, Parham AM: Oxygen concentration received from commonly used delivery systems. *South Med J* 1978; 71:169–172.

60. Cohen JI, Demers RR, Saklad M: Air-entrainment oxygen masks: A performance evaluation. *Respir Care* 1977; 22:277–282.
61. Gibson RI, Comer RB, Beckham RW, et al: Actual tracheal oxygen concentration with commonly used oxygen equipment. *Anesthesiology* 1976; 44:71–73.
62. Schachter EN, Littner MR, Luddy P, et al: Monitoring of oxygen delivery systems in clinical practice. *Crit Care Med* 1980; 8:405–409.
63. Davidson FF, et al: The components of the alveolar-arterial oxygen tension difference in normal subjects and in patients with pneumonia and obstructive lung disease. *Am J Med* 1972; 52:754.
64. Dines DE, Titus JL, Sessler D: Aspiration pneumonitis. *Mayo Clin Proc* 1970; 45:347–360.
65. Lewinski A: Evaluation of methods employed in the treatment of the chemical pneumonitis of aspiration. *Anesthesiology* 1965; 26:37–44.
66. Glasser SA, Domino KB, Lindgren L, et al: Pulmonary blood pressure and flow during atelectasis in the dog. *Anesthesiology* 1983; 58:225–231.
67. Bishop MJ, Cheney FW: Effects of pulmonary blood flow and mixed venous O_2 tension in gas exchange in dogs. *Anesthesiology* 1983; 58:130–135.
68. Domino KB, Wetstein L, Glasser SA, et al: Influence of mixed venous oxygen tension (PvO_2) on blood flow to atelectatic lung. *Anesthesiology* 1983; 59:428–434.
69. Carlon GC, Howland WS, Turnbull AD, et al: Pulmonary venous admixture during mechanical ventilation with varying FIO_2 and PEEP. *Crit Care Med* 1980; 8:616–619.
70. Douglas ME, Downs JB, Dannemiller FJ, et al: Changes in pulmonary venous admixture with varying inspired oxygen. *Anesth Analg* 1976; 55:688–693.
71. McAslan TC, Matjasko-Chiu J, Turney SZ, et al: Influence of inhalation of 100% oxygen in intrapulmonary shunt in severely traumatized patients. *J Trauma* 1973; 13:811–821.
72. Shapiro BA, Cane RD, Harrison RA, et al: Changes in intrapulmonary shunting with the administration of 100% oxygen. *Chest* 1980; 77:138–141.
73. Suter PM, Fairley HB, Isenberg MD: Optimum end-expiratory pressure in patients with acute pulmonary failure. *N Engl J Med* 1975: 292:284–289.
74. Suter PM, Fairley HB, Scholobohm RM: Shunt, lung volume and perfusion during short periods of ventilation with oxygen. *Anesthesiology* 1975; 43:617–627.
75. Markello P, Winter P, Olszowka A: Assessment of ventilation-perfusion inequalities by arterial-venous nitrogen differences in intensive care patients. *Anesthesiology* 1972; 37:4–15.
76. Smith JL: The influence of pathological conditions on active absorption of oxygen by the lungs. *J Physiol* 1897; 22:307.

77. Smith JL: The pathological effects due to increase of oxygen tension in the air breathed. *J Physiol* 1899; 24:19.
78. Winter P, et al: The toxicity of oxygen. *Anesthesiology* 1972; 37:210.
79. Crapo J, Tierney D: Superoxide dismutase and pulmonary oxygen toxicity. *Am J Physiol* 1974; 226:1401–1407.
80. Stevens JB, Autor AP: Oxygen induced synthesis of ethylene oxide. *Anesthesiology* 1969; 30:349.
81. Freeman B, Crapo J: Hyperoxia increases O_2 radical production in rat lungs and lung mitochondria. *J Biol Chem* 1981; 256:10986–10988.
82. Cross C: The granular type II pneumocyte and lung antioxident defense. *Ann Intern Med* 1974; 80:409.
83. Kistler GS, Caldwell PRB, Weibel ER: Development of fine structural damage to alveolar and capillary lining cells in oxygen-poisoned rat lungs. *J Cell Biol* 1967; 32:605.
84. Mason FJ: Phospholipid synthesis in primary cultures of type II alveolar cells (abstr). *Am Rev Respir Dis* 1977; 115 (part 2):352.
85. Steinberg H, Greenwald RA, Moak SA, et al: The effect of oxygen adaptation on oxyradical injury to pulmonary epithelium. *Am Rev Respir Dis* 1983; 128:94–97.
86. Shapiro BA, Cane RD: Metabolic malfunction of the lung noncardiogenic edema and adult respiratory distress syndrome. *Surg Annu* 1981; 13:271–298.
87. Shapiro BA, Cane RD, Harrison RA: Positive end-expiratory pressure therapy in adults with special reference to acute lung injury: A review of the literature and suggested clinical correlations. *Crit Care Med* 1984; 12:127–141.
88. Weil JV, Zwillich CW: Assessment of ventilatory response to hypoxia: Methods and interpretation. *Chest* 1976; 70:124.
89. King T, Briscoe W: Abnormalities of blood gas exchange in COPD. *Postgrad Med* 1973; 54:101.
90. Robin ED: Abnormalities of acid-base regulation in chronic pulmonary disease with special reference to hypercapnia and extracellular alkalosis. *N Engl J Med* 1963; 268:917.
91. Forster RE: Exchange of gases between alveolar air and pulmonary capillary blood: Pulmonary diffusing capacity. *Physiol Rev* 1959; 37:391.
92. Berggren SM: The oxygen deficit of arterial blood caused by nonventilation to parts of the lung. *Acta Physiol Scand* [suppl 11] 1942; 4:9.
93. Cane RD, Shapiro BA, Harrison RA, et al: Minimizing errors in intrapulmonary shunt calculations. *Crit Care Med* 1980; 8:294–297.
94. Cournand A, et al: Measurements of cardiac output in men using the technique of catheterization of the right auricle or ventricle. *J Clin Invest* 1945; 24:106.
95. Harrison RA, Davison R, Shapiro BA, et al: Reassessment of the assumed A-V oxygen content difference in the shunt calculation. *Anesth Analg* 1975; 54:198–202.

96. Liliental JL, Riley RL, Proemmel DD, et al: An experimental analysis in man of the oxygen pressure gradient from alveolar air to arterial blood. *Am J Physiol* 1946; 147:199–216.

97. Peris LV, Boix JH, Salom JV, et al: Clinical use of the arterial/alveolar oxygen tension ratio. *Crit Care Med* 1983; 11:888–891.

98. Lecky JH, Ominsky AJ: Postoperative Respiratory Management. *Chest* 1972; 62:505.

99. Seigel JH, Farrell EJ, Miller M, et al: Cardio-respiratory interactions as determinants of survival and the need for respiratory support in human shock states. *J Trauma* 1973; 13:602.

100. Kanber GJ, King FW, Eshchar YR, et al: The alveolar-arterial oxygen gradient in young and elderly men during air and oxygen breathing. *Am Rev Respir Dis* 1968; 97:376–381.

101. Lawrence M: Abbreviating the alveolar gas equation: An argument for simplicity. *Respir Care* 1985; 30:964–968.

102. Hess, D, Maxwell C: Which is the best index of oxygenation: $P(A-a)O_2$, PaO_2/PAO_2 or PaO_2/FIO_2? *Respir Care* 1985; 30:961–963.

103. Pepe PE, Hudson LD, Carrico CJ: Early application of positive end-expiratory pressure in patients at risk for the adult respiratory-distress syndrome. *N Engl J Med* 1984; 311:281–286.

104. Cohen A, Taeusch HW Jr, Stanton C: Usefulness of the arterial/alveolar oxygen tension ratio in the care of infants with respiratory distress syndrome. *Respir Care* 1983: 28:169–173.

105. Maxwell C, Hess D, Shefet D: Use of the arterial/alveolar oxygen tension ratio to predict the inspired oxygen concentration needed for a desired arterial oxygen tension. *Respir Care* 1984; 29:1135–1139.

106. Covelli HD, Nessan VJ, Tuttle WK: Oxygen derived variables in acute respiratory failure. *Crit Care Med* 1983; 11:646–649.

107. Dean JM, Wetzel R, Gioria FR, et al: Use of oxygen-derived variables for estimation of pulmonary shunt in critically ill children (abstract). *Crit Care Med* 1984; 12:280.

108. Cane RD, Shapiro BA, Templin R, et al: The unreliability of oxygen tension based indices in reflecting intrapulmonary shunting in the critically ill. *Crit Care Med* 1988; in press.

109. Gilbert R, Keighley JF: The arterial/alveolar oxygen tension ratio: An index of gas exchange applicable to varying inspired oxygen concentrations. *Am Rev Respir Dis* 1974; 109:142–145.

110. Gilbert R, Auchincloss JH, Juppinger M, et al: Stability of the arterial/alveolar oxygen partial pressure ratio: Effects of low ventilation/perfusion regions. *Crit Care Med* 1979; 7:267–272.

111. Horovitz JH, Carrico CJ, Shires T: Pulmonary response to major injury. *Arch Surg* 1974; 108:349–355.

112. Lecky JH, Ominsky AJ: Postoperative respiratory management. *Chest* 1972; 62:505–575.

113. Covelli HD, Nessan VJ, Tuttle WK: Oxygen derived variables in acute respiratory failure. *Crit Care Med* 1983; 11:646–649.

114. Robinson NB, Weaver LJ, Carrico CJ, et al: Evaluation of pulmonary dysfunction in the critically ill (abstract). *Am Rev Respir Dis* 1981; 123:92.

115. Martyn JAJ, Aikawa N, Wilson RS, et al: Extrapulmonary factors influencing the ratio of arterial oxygen tension to inspired oxygen concentration in burn patients. *Crit Care Med* 1979; 7:492–496.

116. Wallfisch HK, Tonnesen AS, Huber P: Respiratory indices compared to venous admixture (abstract). *Crit Care Med* 1981: 9:147.

117. Sjanga G, Seigal JH, Coleman W, et al: Physiologic meaning of the respiratory index in various types of critical illness. *Circ Shock* 1985; 17:179–193.

118. Fisher SR, et al: Comparative changes in ventilatory deadspace following micro and massive pulmonary emboli. *J Surg* 1976; 29:195.

119. Duranceau A, et al: Ventilatory deadspace in diagnosis of acute pulmonary embolism. *Surg Forum* 1974; 25:229.

120. Deal CW, et al: Veno-arterial shunting in experimental pulmonary embolism. *J Surg Res* 1970; 10:579.

121. Wilson JE, et al: Hypoxemia in pulmonary embolism: A clinical study. *J Clin Invest* 1971; 50:481.

122. Johansson H, Lofstrom JB: Effects on breathing mechanics and gas exchange of different inspiratory gas flow patterns during anesthesia. *Acta Anaesthesiol Scand* 1975; 19:8.

123. Bergman NA: Effect of varying respiratory waveforms on distribution of inspired gas during artificial ventilation. *Am Rev Respir Dis* 1969; 100:518.

124. Otis AB, et al: Mechanical factors in distribution of pulmonary ventilation. *J Appl Physiol* 1956; 8:427.

125. Daly BDT, Edmonds CH, Norman JC: In vivo alveolar morphometrics with positive end expiratory pressure. *Surg Forum* 1973; 24:217–219.

126. Dueck R, Wagner PD, West JB: Effects of positive end expiratory pressure on gas exchange in dogs with normal and edematous lungs. *Anesthesiology* 1977; 47:359–366.

127. Hammon JW, Wolfe WG, Moran JF, et al: The effect of positive end expiratory pressure on regulated ventilation and perfusion in the normal and injured primate lung. *J Thorac Cardiovasc Surg* 1976; 72:683–689.

128. Ashwood ER, Kost G, Kenny M: Temperature correction of blood gas and pH measurement. *Clin Chem* 1983; 29:1977–1985.

129. Andritsch RF, Muravchick S, Gold MI: Temperature correction of arterial blood-gas parameters: A comparative review of methodology. *Anesthesiology* 1985; 55:311–315.

130. Mustafa MKY, Khogali M, Elkhatib G, et al: Sequential pathophysiological changes during heat stress and cooling in sheep, in Hales JRS (ed): *Thermal Physiology.* New York, Raven Press, 1984, pp 515–518.

131 Hart GR, Anderson RJ, Crumpler CP, et al: Epidemic classical heat stroke: Clinical characteristics and course of 28 patients. *Medicine* 1982; 61:189–197.

132. McNicol MW, Smith R: Accidental hypothermia. *Br Med J* 1964; 1:19–21.

133. Rahn H, Reeves RB, Howell BJ: Hydrogen ion regulation, temperature and evaluation. *Am Rev Respir. Dis* 1975; 112:165–172.

134. Majewska AA, Morris LE, Lee DC, et al: Blood gas determination in hypothermic mammals. *Acta Anaesthesiol Scand* [Suppl] 1966; 23:688–695.

135. Moore B: The cause of the exquisite sensitivity of living cells to changes in hydrogen and hydroxyl in concentration. *J Physiol (Lond)* 1919; 53:LVII–LVIII.

136. Austin JH, Sunderman FW, Camack JG: Studies in serum electrolytes: Serum electrolyte composition and the pH of a poikilothermous animal at different temperatures. *J Biol Chem* 1927; 72:677–685.

137. Reeves RB: The interaction of body temperature and acid-base balance in ectothermic vertebrates. *Annu Rev Physiol* 1977; 39:559–586.

138. Malan A: Acid-base regulation during hibernation, in Rahn H, Prakash O (eds): *Acid-Base Regulation and Body Temperature.* Dordrecht, Martinus Nijhoff, 1985, pp 33–54.

139. Reeves RB: Temperature-induced changes in blood acid-base status = pH and pCO_2 in a binary buffer. *J Appl Physiol* 1976; 40:752–761.

140. Ream AR, Reitz BA, Silverberg G: Temperature correction of pCO_2 and pH in estimating acid-base status. *Anesthesiology* 1982; 56:41–44.

141. Williams JJ, Marshall BE: A fresh look at an old question. *Anesthesiology* 1982; 56:1–2.

142. Carson SAA, Morris LE: Controlled acid-base status with cardiopulmonary bypass and hypothermia. *Anesthesiology* 1962; 23:618–626.

143. Nisbet HIA: Acid-base disturbance in hypothermia. *Int Anesthesiol Clin* 1964; 2:829–855.

144. Becker H, Vinten-Johansen J, Buckley GD, et al: Myocardial damage caused by keeping pH 7.40 during system deep hypothermia. *J Thorac Cardiovasc Surg* 1981; 82:810–820.

145. Becker H, Vinten-Johansen J, Maloney JV, et al: Effect of pH adjustment in deep hypothermia and circulatory arrest. *Chir Forum Exp Klin Torsch* 1980; 80:291–294.

146. McConnel D, White F, Nelson RL, et al: Importance of alkalosis in maintenance of "ideal" blood pH during hypothermia. *Surg Forum* 1975; 26:263–265.

147. Ohmura A, Wong KC, Westenskow DR, et al: Effect of hypocarbia and normocarbia on cardiovascular dynamics and regional circulation in the hypothermic dog. *Anesthesiology* 1979; 50:293–298.

148. Matthews AJ, Stead AL, Abbott TR: Acid-base control during hypothermia. *Anaesthesia* 1984; 39:649–654.

149. Ohmura A, Wong KC, Lu TS, et al: The effect of deep hypothermia and circulatory arrest on CSF-Na, K, pH, bicarbonate and pCO_2 in newborn lambs. *Cryobiology* 1984; 15:192–198.

150. Hornbein TF, Fortner RWF, Casselle DC: The effect of ventilation on cerebral oxygenation during hypothermia. *Anesthesiology* 1969; 30:342.

151. Roughton FJW, Severinghaus JW: Accurate determination of an O_2 solubility in unmodified human blood form 0 to 37°C. *J Appl Physiol* 1973; 35:861–869.

152. Van Steckelenburg GJ: The influence of temperature changes on the pO_2 of normal anaerobic blood samples. *Resp Physiol* 1970; 8:245–259.

153. Severinghaus JW: Respiration and hypothermia. *Ann NY Acad Sci* 1959; 80:384–394.

154. Benjamin E, Paluch TA, Berger SR, et al: Venous hypercarbia in canine hemorrhagic shock. *Crit Care Med* 1987; 15:516–518.

155. Nowak RM, Martin GB, Carden DL, et al: Selective venous hypercarbia during human CPR: Implications regarding blood flow. *Ann Emerg Med* 1987; 16:527–530.

156. Weill MH, Rackow EC, Trevino R, et al: Difference in acid-base state between venous and arterial blood during cardiopulmonary resuscitation. *N Engl J Med* 1986; 315:153–156.

157. Grundler W, Weill MH, Rackow EC, et al: Selective acidosis in venous blood during human cardiopulmonary resuscitation: A preliminary report. *Crit Care Med* 1985; 13:886–887.

158. Beyar R, Kishon Y, Kimmel E, et al: Blood gas and acid-base balance during cardiopulmonary resuscitation by intrathoracic and abdominal pressure variations. *Basic Res Cardiol* 1986; 81:326–333.

159. Grundler W, Weill MH, Rackow EC: Arteriovenous carbon dioxide and pH gradients during cardiac arrest. *Circulation* 1986; 74:1071–1074.

160. Sanders AB, Ewy GA, Taft TV: Resuscitation and arterial blood gas abnormalities during prolonged cardiopulmonary resuscitation. *Ann Emerg Med* 1984; 13:676–679.

161. Suljaga-Pechtel K, Goldberg E, Strickon P, et al: Cardiopulmonary resuscitation in a hospitalized population: Prospective study of factors associated with outcome. *Resuscitation* 1984; 12:77–95.

162. Ornato JP, Gonzalez ER, Coyne MR, et al: Arterial pH in out of hospital cardiac arrest: Response time as a determinant of acidosis. *Am J Emerg Med* 1985; 3:498–502.

163. Ralston SH, Voorhees WD, Showen L, et al: Venous and arterial blood gases during and after cardiopulmonary resuscitation in dogs. *Am J Emerg. Med* 1985; 3:132–136.

164. Martin GB, Carden DL, Nowak RM, et al: Comparison of central venous and arterial pH and PCO_2 during open chest CPR in the canine model. *Ann Emerg Med* 1985; 14:529–533.

165. Weill MH, Ruiz CE, Michaels S, et al: Acid-base determinants of survival after cardiopulmonary resuscitation. *Crit Care Med* 1985; 13:888–892.

166. Wiklund L, Soderberg D, Henneberg S, et al: Kinetics of carbon dioxide during cardiopulmonary resuscitation. *Crit Care Med* 1986; 14:1015–1022.

167. Holmdahl MH: Pulmonary uptake of oxygen, acid-base metabolism and circulation during prolonged apnea. *Acta Chir Scand* 1956; 212:108.

168. Henneberg S, Soderberg D, Groth T, et al: Carbon dioxide production during mechanical ventilation. *Crit Care Med* 1987; 15:8–13.

169. Stock MC, McDonald JS, Silver MJ, et al: How fast does CO_2 really rise during apnea? *Anesth Analg* 1986; 65:S153.

170. Farhi LE, Rahn H: Dynamics of changes in carbon dioxide stores. *Anesthesiology* 1960; 21:604.

171. Farhi LE, Rahn H: Gas stores of body and unsteady states. *J Appl Physiol* 1955; 7:472.
172. Farhi LE: Gas stores of the body, in Fenn WO, Rahn H (eds): *Handbook of Physiology: Respiration.* Baltimore, Williams & Wilkins Co., 1965, Vol 1, pp 873–885.
173. Ward SA, Whipp BJ, Koyal S, et al: Influence of body CO_2 stores on ventilatory dynamics during exercise. *J Appl Physiol* 1983; 55:742–749.
174. Bolot JR, Berstein S, Guerin MA, et al: Iliac crest bone CO_2 and CO_2/Ca ratio in man during respiratory failure. *Bull Eur Physiopathol Respir* 1976; 12:39–47.
175. Robin ED: Abnormalities of acid-base regulation in chronic pulmonary disease, with special reference to hypercapnia and extracellular alkalosis. *N Engl J Med* 1963; 268:917.
176. Nishijima H, Weil MH, Shubin H, et al: Hemodynamic and metabolic studies on shock associated with gram negative bacteremia. *Medicine* 1973; 52:287–294.
177. Askanazi J, Nordstrom J, Rosenbaum SH, et al: Nutrition for the patient with respiratory failure: Glucose vs. fat. *Anesthesiology* 1981; 54:373.
178. Baker JP, Detsky AS, Stewart S, et al: Randomized trial of total parenteral nutrition in critically ill patients: Metabolic effects of varying glucose-lipid ratios as energy source. *Gastroenterology* 1984; 87:53.
179. Askanazi J, Elwyn DH, Silverberg PA, et al: Respiratory distress secondary to the high carbohydrate load of TPN: A case report. *Surgery* 1980; 87:596.
180. Morris RC: Renal tubular acidosis. *N Engl J Med* 1969; 281:1405.
181. Weil MH, et al: Experimental and clinical studies on lactate and pyruvate as indications of the severity of acute circulatory failure (shock). *Circulation* 1970; 41:989.
182. Jarboe TM, et al: Ventilatory failure due to metabolic alkalosis. *Chest* 1972; 61:615.
183. Kassirer JP, et al: The critical role of chloride in the correction of hypokalemic alkalosis in man. *Am J Med* 1965; 38:172.
184. Schwartz WB, et al: Role of anions in metabolic alkalosis and potassium deficiency. *N Engl J Med* 1968; 279:630.
185. Hamilton WK: Atelectasis, pneumothorax and aspiration as postoperative complications, review. *Anesthesiology* 1961; 22:708.
186. Sellery CR: A review of the causes of postoperative hypoxia. *Can Anaesth Soc J* 1968; 15:142.
187. Petty T, et al: The adult respiratory distress syndrome. *Chest* 1971; 60:233.
188. McFadden ER Jr, et al: Arterial blood gas tension in asthma. *N Engl J Med* 1968; 278:1027.
189. Loeb HS, et al: Effects of low-flow oxygen on the hemodynamics and left ventricular function in patients with uncomplicated acute myocardial infarction. *Chest* 1971; 60:352.
190. Robin ED, et al: Pulmonary edema. *N Engl J Med* 1973; 288:239.

191. Miller, A, et al: Acute reversible respiratory acidosis in cardiogenic pulmonary edema. *JAMA* 1971; 216:1315.

192. Addington WW, et al: Cystic fibrosis of the pancreas: A comparison of the pulmonary manifestations in children and young adults. *Chest* 1971; 59:306.

193. Gaensler EA, et al: Pulmonary function in pregnancy. *Am Rev Tuberc* 1953; 67:779.

194. Lucius H, et al: Respiratory functions, buffer system and electrolyte concentrations of blood during human pregnancy. *Respir Physiol* 1970; 9:311.

195. Boutros A, et al: Management of carbon monoxide poisoning in the absence of hyperbaric oxygenation chamber. *Crit Care Med* 1976; 4:144.

196. Nunn JF: Respiratory deadspace and distribution of the inspired gas, in Nunn JF (ed): *Applied Respiratory Physiology,* ed. 2. London, Butterworths, 1977.

197. Smallhout B, Kalenda Z: *An Atlas of Capnography.* vol 1, Zeist, the Netherlands, Kerckebosch, 1975.

198. West JB: *Ventilation/Blood Flow and Gas Exchange,* ed 2. Oxford, England Blackwell Scientific Publications, 1970.

199. Murray IP, Modell JH, Gallagher JJ, et al: Titration of PEEP by the arterial minus end-tidal carbon dioxide gradient. *Chest* 1984; 85:100–104.

200. Brechner VL, Bethune RW: Recent advances in monitoring pulmonary air embolism. *Anesth Analg* 1971; 50:255–261.

201. Trevino RP, Bisera J, Weil MH, et al: End-tidal CO_2 as a guide to successful cardiopulmonary resuscitation: A preliminary report. *Crit Care Med* 1985; 13:910.

202. Sanders AB, Ewy GA, Bragg S, et al: Expired PCO_2 as a prognostic indicator of successful resuscitation from cardiac arrest. *Ann Emerg Med* 1985; 14:948.

203. Garnett AR, Ornato JP, Gonzalez ER, et al: End-tidal carbon dioxide monitoring during cardiopulmonary resuscitation. *JAMA* 1986; 257:512.

204. Divertie MB, McMichan JC: Continuous monitoring of mixed venous oxygen saturation. *Chest* 1984; 85:423–428.

205. Baele PL, McMichan JC, Marsh HM, et al: Continuous monitoring of mixed venous oxygen saturation in critically ill patients. *Anesth Analg* 1982; 61:513–517.

206. Stock MC, Shapiro BA, Cane RD: Reliability of SvO_2 in predicting A-VDO2 and the effect of anemia, abstract. *Crit Care Med* 1986; 14:402.

207. Schmidt CR, Frank LP, Forsythe SB, et al: Continuous SVO_2 measurement and oxygen transport patterns in cardiac surgical patients. *Crit Care Med* 1984; 12:523–527.

208. Krauss XH, Verdouw PD, Hugenholtz PG, et al: On-line monitoring of mixed venous oxygen saturation after cardiothoracic surgery. *Thorax* 1975; 30:636–643.

209. Lee J, Wright F, Barber R, et al: Central venous oxygen saturation in shock: A study in man. *Anesthesiology* 1972; 36:472–478.

210. Martin WE, Cheung PW, Johnson CC, et al: Continuous monitoring of mixed venous oxygen saturation in man. *Anesth Analg* 1973; 52:784–793.

211. Nishijima H, Weil MH, Shubin H, et al: Hemodynamic and metabolic studies on shock associated with gram negative bacteremia. *Medicine* 1973; 52:287–294.

212. Rasanen J, Downs JB, Seidman P, et al: Estimation of oxygen utilization by dual oximetry, abstract. *Crit Care Med* 1987; 15:404.

213. Rasanen J, Downs JB, Malec DJ, et al: Oxygen tensions and oxyhemoglobin saturations in the assessment of pulmonary gas exchange. *Crit Care Med* 1987; 15:1058–1061.

214. Rasanen J, Downs JB, Dehaven B: Titration of continuous positive airway pressure by real time dual oximetry, abstract. *Crit Care Med* 1987; 15:395.

215. Cohen E, Eisenkraft JB, Thys DM, et al: Continuous monitoring of mixed venous oxygen saturation during one lung anesthesia: Effects of CPAP and PEEP. *Anesthesiology* 1984; 61:A512.

216. Chapman KR, Rebuck AS: Oximetry, in Nochomowitz ML, Cherniack NS (eds): *Non-invasive Respiratory Monitoring.* New York, Churchill Livingstone, Inc., 1986, pp 203–221.

217. Hess D, Kochansky M, Hassett L, et al: An evaluation of the Nellcor N-10 portable pulse oximeter. *Respir Care* 1986; 31:796–802.

218. Yelderman M, New W: Evaluation of pulse oximetry. *Anesthesiology* 1983; 59:349–352.

219. Mihm FG, Halperin BD: Non-invasive detection of profound arterial desaturations using a pulse oximetry device. *Anesthesiology* 1985; 62:85–87.

220. Fait CD, Wetzel RC, Dean JM, et al: Pulse oximetry in critically ill children. *J Clin Monit* 1985; 1:232–235.

221. Taylor MB, Whitwam JG: The current status of pulse oximetry. *Anaesthesia* 1986; 41:943–949.

222. Fanconi S, Doherty P, Edmonds JF, et al: Pulse oximetry in pediatric intensive care: Comparison with measured saturations and transcutaneous oxygen tension. *J Pediatr* 1985; 107:362–366.

223. Ramanathan R, Durand M. Larrazabal C: Pulse oximetry in very low birth weight infants with acute and chronic lung disease. *Pediatrics* 1987; 79:612–617.

224. Jenni MS, Peabody JL: Pulse oximetry: An alternative method for the assessment of oxygenation in newborn infants. *Pediatrics* 1987; 79:524–528.

225. Durand M, Ramanathan R: Pulse oximetry for continuous oxygen monitoring in sick newborn infants. *J Pediatr* 1986; 109:1052–1056.

226. Scheller MS, Unger RJ, Kelner MJ: Effects of intravenously administered dyes on pulse oximetry readings. *Anesthesiology* 1986; 65:550–552.

227. Cane RD, Harrison RA, Shapiro BA, et al: The spectrophotometric absorbance of Intralipid. *Anesthesiology* 1980; 53:53–55.

228. Brooks TD, Paulus DA, Winkle WE: Infrared heat lamps interfere with pulse oximeters. *Anesthesiology* 1984; 61:630.

229. New W: Pulse oximetry. *J Clin Monit* 1985; 1:126–129.

230. Kim J-M, Arakawa, K, Benson KT, et al: Pulse oximetry and circulatory kinetics associated with pulse volume amplitude measured by photoelectric plethysmography. *Anesth Analg* 1986; 65:1333–1339.

231. Lawon D, Norley, I, Korbon G, et al: Blood flow limits and pulse oximeter signal detection. *Anesthesiology* 1967; 67:599–603.

232. Severinghaus JW, Naireh KH: Accuracy of response of several pulse oximeters to profound hypoxia. *Anesthesiology* 1987; 67:551–558.

233. Van Duzee BF: Thermal analysis of human stratum corneum. *J Invest Dermatol* 1975; 65:404.

234. Tremper KK, Waxman KS, Shoemaker WC: Effects of hypoxia and shock on transcutaneous PO_2 values in dogs. *Crit Care Med* 1979; 7:526.

235. Rowe MI, Weinberg G: Transcutaneous oxygen monitoring in shock and resuscitation. *J Pediatr Surg* 1979; 14:773.

236. Tremper KK, Waxman KS, Konchigeri J: Effects of sodium nitroprusside on the relationship between transcutaneous and arterial PO_2: Experimental and clinical studies. *Anesthesiology* 1983; 59:A158.

237. Keller HP, Klaye P, Hockerts T: Transcutaneous PO_2 measurement on skin transplants. *Birth Defects* 1979; XV: 511.

238. Achauer BM, Black KS, Beran AV: Transcutaneous PO_2 monitoring of flap circulation following surgery. *Birth Defects* 1979; XV:517.

239. Lucey JF: Clinical uses of transcutaneous oxygen monitoring. *Adv Pediatr* 1981; 28:27–56.

240. Huch R, Lubbers DW, Hutch A: Reliability of transcutaneous monitoring of arterial PO_2 in newborn infants. *Arch Dis Child* 1974; 49:213.

241. Monaco F, Nickerson BG, McQuitty JC: Continuous transcutaneous oxygen and carbon dioxide monitoring in the pediatric ICU. *Crit Care Med* 1982; 10:765.

242. Tremper KK, Waxman KS, Bowman R: Continuous transcutaneous oxygen monitoring during respiratory failure, cardiac decompensation, cardiac arrest and CPR. *Crit Care Med* 1980; 8:377.

243. Tremper KK, Shoemaker WC: Transcutaneous oxygen monitoring of critically ill adults, with and without low flow shock. *Crit Care Med* 1981; 9:706.

244. Versmold HT, Linderkamp O, Holzman M: Transcutaneous monitoring of PO_2 in newborn infants: Where are the limits? Influences of blood pressure, blood volume, blood flow, viscosity and acid base state. *Birth Defects* 1979; 15(4):285–294.

245. Peabody JL, Gregory GA, Willis MM: Failure of conventional monitoring to detect apnea resulting in hypoxemia. *Birth Defects* 1979; XV:275.

246. Waxman KS, Sadler R, Eisner ME: Transcutaneous oxygen monitoring of emergency department patients. *Am J Surg* 1983; 146:35.

247. Burgess EM, Matsen FA, Wyss CR, et al: Segmental transcutaneous measurements of PO_2 in patients requiring below knee amputation for peripheral vascular insufficiency. *J Bone Joint Surg* 1982; 64A:373–382.

248. White RA, Nolan L, Harley D, et al: Noninvasive evaluation of peripheral vascular disease using transcutaneous oxygen tension. *Am J Surg* 1982; 144:68–75.

249. Marshall TA, Kattwinkel J, Bevry FA, et al: Transcutaneous oxygen monitoring of neonates during surgery. *J Pediatr Surg* 1980; 15:797.
250. Halden L: Monitoring of optimal oxygen transport by the transcutaneous oxygen tension method in the pig. *Acta Anaesthesiol Scand* 1982; 26:209.
251. Gehrich JL, Lubbers DW, Opitz N, et al: Optical fluorescence and its application to an intravascular blood gas monitoring system. *IEEE Trans Biomed Eng* 1986; 33:117–132.
252. Shapiro BA, Cane RD, Chomka CM, et al: Evaluation of a new intra-arterial blood gas system in dogs, abstract. *Crit Care Med* 1987; 15:361.
253. Shapiro BA, Cane RD: Personal communication.
254. Hess D, Maxwell C, Shefet D: Determination of intrapulmonary shunt: Comparison of an estimated shunt equation and a modified shunt equation with the classic equation. *Respir Care* 1987; 32:268.
255. Eriksen HC, Sorenson HR: Arterial injuries: Iatrogenic and noniatrogenic. *Acta Chir Scand* 1969; 135:133.
256. Mortensen JD: Clinical sequelae from arterial needle puncture cannulation and incision. *Circulation* 1967; 35:1118.
257. Mathieu A, et al: Expanding aneurysm of the radial artery after frequent puncture. *Anesthesiology* 1973; 38:401.
258. Sackner MA, Avery WG, Sokolowski J: Arterial puncture by nurses. *Chest* 1971; 59:97.
259. Baker RJ, Chunpraph B, Nyhus LN: Severe ischemia of the hand following radial artery catheterization. *Surgery* 1976; 80:449–457.
260. Barnes RW, et al: Noninvasive assessment of altered limb hemodynamics and complications of arterial catheterization. *Radiology* 1973; 107:505.
261. Kazamias TM, et al: Blood pressure measurement with Doppler ultrasonic flowmeter. *J Appl Physiol* 1971; 30:585.
262. Allen EV: Thromboangiitis obliterans: Methods of diagnosis of chronic occlusive arterial lesions distal to the wrist with illustrative cases. *Am J Med Sci* 1929; 178:237.
263. Greenhow DE: Incorrect performance of Allen's test—ulnar artery flow erroneously presumed inadequate. *Anesthesiology* 1974; 37:356.
264. Peters KR, Chapin JW: Allen's test—positive or negative? *Anesthesiology* 1980; 53:85.
265. Messick JM: Allen's test—neither positive nor negative. *Anesthesiology* 1981; 54:523.
266. Ryan JF, et al: Arterial dynamics of radial artery cannulation. *Anesth Analg* 1973; 52:1017.
267. Brodsky JB: A simple method to determine patency of the ulnar artery intraoperatively prior to radial-artery cannulation. *Anesthesia* 1975; 42:626–627.
268. Barnes RW, et al: Safety of brachial arterial catheters as monitors in the intensive care unit—prospective evaluation with the Doppler ultrasonic velocity detector. *Anesthesiology* 1976; 44:260.
269. Youngberg JA, Miller ED: Evaluation of percutaneous cannulations of the dorsalis pedia artery. *Anesthesia* 1976; 44:80–83.

270. Johnstone RE, Greenhow DE: Catheterization of the dorsalis pedis artery. *Anesthesia* 1973; 39:654–655.

271. Ersoz CJ, Hedden M, Lain L: Prolonged femoral arterial catheterization for intensive care. *Anesth Analg* 1970; 49:160–164.

272. Kopman EA, Ferguson TB: Intraoperative monitoring of femoral artery pressure during replacement of aneurysm of descending thoracic aorta. *Anesth Analg* 1977; 56:603–605.

273. Petty TL, Bigelow B, Levine BE: The simplicity and safety of arterial puncture. *JAMA* 1966; 195:181.

274. Bageant RA: Variations in arterial blood gas measurements due to sampling techniques. *Respir Care* 1975; 20:565.

275. Ansel G, Douce FH: Quantitative study on the effects that syringe material and needle size exert on minimum filling pressure of arterial blood gas syringes, abstracted. *Respir Care* 1980; 25:1234.

276. Miller MG, Hedley-Whyte J: Intra-arterial monitoring: A routine and safe procedure, in Eckenhoff JE (ed): *Controversy in Anesthesiology*. Philadelphia, WB Saunders Co, 1979, pp 257–265.

277. Barnes RW, et al: Complications of brachial artery catheterization: Prospective evaluation with the Doppler ultrasonic velocity detector. *Chest* 1974; 66:363.

278. Bedford RF: Long-term radial artery cannulation: Effects on subsequent vessel function. *Crit Care Med* 1978; 6:64.

279. Bedford RF: Radial artery function following percutaneous cannulation with 18- and 20-gauge catheters. *Anesthesiology* 1977; 47:37.

280. Bedford RF: Wrist circumference predicts the risk of radial-arterial occlusion after cannulation. *Anesthesiology* 1978; 48:377.

281. Comstock MK, Ellis T, Carter JG, et al: Safety of brachial vs. arterial catheters, abstracted. *Anesthesiology* 1979; 51:S158.

282. Downs JB, Chapman RL, Hawkins IF: Prolonged radial-artery catheterization. *Arch Surg* 1974; 108:671.

283. Katz AM, et al: Gangrene of the hand and forearm: A complication of radial artery cannulation. *Crit Care Med* 1974; 2:270.

284. Stamm WE, et al: Indwelling arterial catheters as a source of nosocomial bacteremia: An outbreak caused by flavobacterium species. *N Engl J Med* 1975; 292:1099.

285. Gardner RM, et al: Percutaneous indwelling radial-artery catheters for monitoring cardiovascular function: Prospective study of the risk of thrombosis and infection. *N Engl J Med* 1974; 290:1227.

286. Jones RM, Hill AB, Nahrwold ML, et al: The effect of method of radial artery cannulation on postcannulation blood flow and thrombus formation. *Anesthesiology* 1981; 55:76.

287. Bedford RF, Ashford TP: Aspirin pretreatment prevents postcannulation radial artery thrombosis. *Anesthesiology* 1979; 51:176.

288. Schwartz AJ, Stoner BB, Jobes DR: A hazard of the Intraflo continuous flush system. *Crit Care Med* 1977; 5:115.

289. Waton JR, Shapiro BA, Harrison RA, et al: Serratia bacteremia from mean arterial pressure monitors. *Anesthesiology* 1975; 43:113.
290. Kim MJ, Arakawa K, Bliss J: Arterial cannulation factors in the development of occlusion. *Anesth Analg* 1975; 54:836–841.
291. Bedford RF: Radial arterial function following percutaneous cannulation with 18-20 gauge catheters. *Anesthesiology* 1977; 47:37.
292. Bourke DL: Errors in hematocrit determination. *Anesthesiology* 1976; 45:357.
293. Chinyanga HM, Smith JM: A modified Doppler flow detector probe: An aid to percutaneous arterial cannulation in infants and small children. *Anesthesiology* 1979; 50:256.
294. Kisling JA, Schreiner RL: Techniques of obtaining arterial blood from newborn infants. *Respir Care* 1977; 22:513.
295. Cole AFD, Rolbin SH: A technique for rapid catheterization of the umbilical artery. *Anesthesiology* 1980; 53:254.
296. Banister A: Comparison of arterial and arterialized capillary blood in infants with respiratory disease. *Arch Dis Child* 1969; 44:726.
297. Dell RB, Winters RW: Capillary blood sampling for acid-base determinations: Technique and validity. Copenhagen, Radiometer, No. A48, 1970.
298. Docrat K, Kenny S: The accuracy of capillary sampling for acid-base estimations. *Br J Anaesth* 1965; 37:840.
299. Gandy G, et al: The validity of pH and PCO_2 measurements in capillary samples in sick and healthy newborn infants. *Pediatrics* 1964; 34:192.
300. Glasgow JFT, Flynn DM, Swyer RR: A comparison of descending aortic and "arterialized" capillary blood in the sick newborn. *Can Med Assoc J* 1972; 106:660.
301. Jung RC, Balchum OJ, Massey FJ: The accuracy of venous and capillary blood for the prediction of arterial pH, PCO_2 and PO_2 measurements. *Am J Clin Pathol* 1966; 45:129.
302. Koch G: The validity of PO_2 measurement in capillary blood as a substitute for arterial PO_2. *Scand J Clin Lab Invest* 1968; 21:10.
303. Koch G, Wendel H: Comparison of pH, carbon dioxide tension, standard bicarbonate and oxygen tension in capillary blood and in arterial blood during the neonatal period. *Acta Paediatr Scand* 1967; 56:10.
304. Laughlin DE, McDonald JS, Bedell GN: A microtechnique for measurement of PO_2 in "arterialized" earlobe blood. *J Lab Clin Med* 1964; 64:330.
305. Mountain KR, Campbell DG: Reliability of oxygen tension measurements on arterialized capillary blood in the newborn. *Arch Dis Child* 1970; 45:134.
306. Siggard-Andersen O: Acid-base and blood gas parameters: arterial or capillary blood? *Scand J Clin Lab Invest* 1968; 21:289.
307. Galvis AG, Donahoo JS, White JJ: An improved technique for prolonged arterial catheterization in infants and children. *Crit Care Med* 1976; 4:166.
308. Neal WA, et al: Umbilical artery catheterization: Demonstration of arterial thrombosis by aortography. *Pediatrics* 1972; 50:6.

309. Tooley WH: What is the risk of an umbilical artery catheter? *Pediatrics* 1972; 50:1.
310. Gupta JM, Robertson NRC, Wigglesworth JS: Umbilical artery catheterization in the newborn. *Arch Dis Child* 1968; 43:382.
311. Cochran WD, Davis HT, Smith CA: Advantages and complications of umbilical artery catheterization in the newborn. *Pediatrics* 1968; 42:769.
312. Gambino SR, Thiede WH: Comparisons of pH in human arterial, venous and capillary blood. *Am J Clin Pathol* 1959; 32:298.
313. Phillips B, Peretz DI: A comparison of central venous and arterial blood gas values in the critically ill. *Ann Intern Med* 1969; 70:745.
314. Shapiro HM, et al: Errors in sampling pulmonary artery blood with a Swan-Ganz catheter. *Anesthesiology* 1974; 40:291.
315. Mihm F, Feeley TW, Rosenthal M, et al: The lack of effect of variable blood withdrawal rates on the measurement of mixed venous oxygen saturation. *Chest* 1980; 78:452.
316. Evers W, Racz GB, Levy AA: A comparative study of plastic (polypropylene) and glass syringes in blood gas analysis. *Anesth Analg* 1972; 50:92.
317. Scott PV, Horton JN, Mapleson WW: Leakage of oxygen from blood and water samples stored in plastic and glass syringes. *Br Med J* 1971; 3:512.
318. Winkler JB, et al: Influence of syringe material on arterial blood gas determinations. *Chest* 1974; 66:518.
319. Gambino SR: Heparinized vacuum tubes for determination of plasma pH, plasma CO_2 content, and blood oxygen saturation. *Am J Clin Pathol* 1959; 32:285.
320. Ad Hoc Committee on Acid-base Terminology of the New York Academy of Sciences: Current concept of acid-base measurement. *Ann NY Acad Sci* 1966; 133:251.
321. Yoshimura H: Effects of anticoagulants on the pH of the blood. *J Biochem (Tokyo)* 1935; 22:297.
322. Hamilton RD, Crocket AJ, Alpers J: Arterial blood gas analysis: Potential errors due to the addition of heparin. *Anaesth Intensive Care* 1978; 6:251.
323. Cole JK: The effect of heparin on blood gas analysis. *Med J Aust* March 24, 1979, p 221.
324. Gast LR, Scacci R, Miller WF: The effect of heparin dilution on hemoglobin measurement from arterial blood samples. *Respir Care* 1978; 23:149.
325. Bradley JG: Errors in the measurement of blood PCO_2 due to dilution of the sample with heparin solution. *Br J Anaesth* 1972; 44:231.
326. Hansen JE, Simmons DH: A systematic error in determination of blood PCO_2. *Am Rev Respir Dis* 1977; 115:1061.
327. Kelman GR, Nunn JF: Nomograms for correction of blood PO_2, PCO_2, pH and base excess for time and temperature. *J Appl Physiol* 1966; 21:1484.
328. Cremer M: *Z Biol* 1906; 47:562.
329. Haber F, Klemensiewicz Z: *Z. Physik Chem* 1909; 67:385.
330. Borelius G: *Ann Physik* 1914; 45:929.

331. Gold V: *pH Measurements: Their Theory and Practice.* London, Methuen, 1958.
332. Bates RG: *Electrometric pH Determinations.* New York, John Wiley & sons, 1954.
333. Sanc MC: Ultramicro methods and standardization of equipment. *Clin Chem* 1957; 3:406.
334. Adams AP, Morga-Hughes JO, Sykes MK: pH and blood gas analysis. *Anaesthesia* 1968; 23:47.
335. Severinghaus JW, Stupfel M, Bradley AF: Accuracy of blood pH and PCO_2 determinations. *J Appl Physiol* 1956; 9:189.
336. Severinghaus JW: Measurements of blood gases: PO_2 and PCO_2. *Ann NY Acad Sci* 1968; 148:115.
337. Linden RJ, Ledsome JR, Norman J: Simple methods for the determination of the concentrations of carbon dioxide and oxygen in blood. *Br J Anaesth* 1965; 37:77.
338. Riley RI, Proemmel DD, Franke RE: A direct method of determination of oxygen and carbon dioxide in blood. *J Biol Chem* 1945; 161:621.
339. Stow RW, Baer RF, Randall BF: Rapid measurement of the tension of carbon dioxide in blood. *Arch Phys Med Rehabil* October 1957, p 646.
340. Severinghaus JW, Bradley AF: Electrodes for blood PO_2 and PCO_2 determinations. *J Appl Physiol* 1958; 13:515.
341. Kreuzer F, Watson TR Jr, Ball JM: Comparative measurements with a new procedure for measuring the blood oxygen tension in vitro. *J Appl Physiol* 1958; 12:65.
342. Heitmann H, Buckles RG, Laver MB: Blood PO_2 measurements: Performance of microelectrodes. *Respir Physiol* 1967; 3:380.
343. Polgar G, Forster RE: Measurement of oxygen tension in unstirred blood with a platinum electrode. *J Appl Physiol* 1960; 15:706.
344. Sproule BJ, et al: An improved polarographic method for measuring oxygen tension in vitro, *J Appl Physiol* 1957; 11:365.
345. Clark LC Jr: Monitor and control of blood and tissue oxygen tensions. *Trans Am Soc Artif Intern Organs* 1956; 2:41.
346. Hood LC, Noble WE, Smith E: Negligible halothane carryover in the IL-813 blood gas analyzer. *Clin Chem* 1980; 26:675.
347. Ishikawa S, et al: The effects of air bubbles and time delay on blood gas analysis. *Ann Allergy* 1974; 33:72.
348. Mueller RG, Lang GE, Beam JM: Bubbles in samples for blood gas determinations. *Am J Clin Pathol* 1976; 65:242.
349. Walton JR, Shapiro BA, Wine C: Pre-analytic error in arterial blood gas measurement, abstracted. *Respir Care* 1981; 26:1136.
350. Moran RG: External factors influencing blood gas analysis: Quality control revisited. *Am J Med Tech* 1979; 45:1009–1011.
351. Drinker PA, et al: Use of a sodium chloride-phosphate buffer for pH standardization in a new blood gas analyzer with an isotonic sodium chloride bridge. *Clin Chem* 1973; 19:1243.
352. Durst RA, Staples BR: Tris/Tris HCl: A standard buffer for use in the physiologic pH range. *Clin Chem* 1972; 18:206–208.

353. Veefkind AH, Van den Camp RAM, Maas AHJ: Use of carbon dioxide and oxygen-tonometered phosphate-bicarbonate-chloride-glycerol-water mixtures for calibration and control of pH, PCO_2 and PO_2 electrode systems. *Clin Chem* 1975; 21:685–692.

354. Scholander PF: Analyzer for accurate estimation of respiratory gases in one half cubic centimeter samples. *J Biol Chem* 1947; 167:235.

355. Adams AP, Morgan-Hughes J: Determination of the blood-gas factor of the oxygen electrode using a new tonometer. *Br J Anaesth* 1967; 39:107–113.

356. Bird BD, Williams J, Whitwam JG: The blood gas factor: A comparison of three different oxygen electrodes. *Br J Anaesth* 1974; 46:249–252.

357. Rhodes PG, Moser KM: Sources of error in oxygen tension measurements. *J Appl Physiol* 1966; 21:729–734.

358. Severinghaus JW, Bradley AF: *Blood Gas Electrodes or What the Instructions Didn't Say.* Copenhagen, Radiometer, 1971, pp 12–31.

359. Herring K, et al: Response of the oxygen electrode to various calibration materials, abstracted. *Respir Care* 1979; 24:59–60.

360. Leary ET, Delaney CJ, Kenny MA: Use of equilibrated blood for internal blood-gas quality control. *Clin Chem* 1977; 23:493–503.

361. Abramson J, et al: Evaluation and comparison of commercial blood gas quality controls and tonometry. *Respir Care* 1980; 25:441:447.

362. Smith ER, Cissik JH, Reading PM: Influence of the Clark electrode blood-gas factor on calculation of pulmonary venous admixture. *CVP* June/July 1980; pp 23–29.

363. Oeseburg B, Kwant G: Inaccuracy of oxygen electrode systems. Reply by Brinklov MM, et al (letter). *Anesthesiology* 1979; 51:368–369.

364. Andersen PK, et al: Inaccuracy of oxygen electrodes at high blood oxygen tensions. *Anesthesiology* 1978; 49:61–62.

365. Holmes PL, et al: Evaluation of methods for calibration of O_2 and CO_2 electrodes. *Am J Clin Pathol* 1970; 54:566–569.

366. Hulands GH, Nunn JF, Paterson GM: Calibration of polarographic electrodes with glycerol/water mixtures. *Br J Anaesth* 1970; 42:9–14.

367. Winckers EK, Teunissen AJ, Van den Camp RA, et al: A comparative study of the electrode systems of three pH and blood gas apparatus. *J Clin Chem Clin Biochem* 1978; 16:175–185.

368. Fraser CG, Peake MJ: Problems associated with clinical chemistry quality control materials. *CRC Crit Rev Clin Lab Sci* 1980; 12:59–86.

369. McLear J, Ladenson JH: Temperature coefficient for pH of various control materials. *Clin Chem* 1979; 25:1981–1982.

370. Sullivan K, Dean WW: Multiple sample blood gas quality control system offering temperature independence and ease of use. *Clin Chem* 1980; 26:997.

371. Remington RD, Schork MA: *Statistics With Applications to the Biological and Health Sciences.* Englewood Cliffs, NJ, Prentice-Hall Inc, 1970.

372. Westgard JO, Barry PL, Hunt MR: A multi-rule Shewhart chart for quality control in clinical chemistry. *Clin Chem* 1981; 27:493–501.

373. Moran RF: Assessment of quality control of blood gas/pH analyzer performance. *Respir Care* 1981; 26:538–546.

374. Westgard JO, Groth T: Assessment of the performance characteristics of an interactive computer simulation program. *Clin Chem* 1980; 26:999.

375. Evans JR: A comparison of two methods of quality control of pH, PCO_2 and PO_2 measurements. *Ann Clin Biochem* 1978; 15:168–171.

376. Komjathy ZL, et al: Stability and precision of a new ampouled quality-control system for pH and blood-gas measurements. *Clin Chem* 1976; 22:1399–1401.

377. Ladenson JH, et al: Use of tris buffers for quality control of blood pH. *Clin Chem* 1974; 20:1337–1340.

378. Maas AHJ, Veefkind AH, Van den Camp RAM, et al: Evaluation of ampouled tonometered buffer solutions as quality control system for pH, PCO_2 and PO_2 measurement. *Clin Chem* 1977; 23:1718–1725.

379. Noonan DC, Burnett RW: Quality control system for blood pH and gas measurements, with use of tonometered bicarbonate-chloride solution and duplicate samples of whole blood. *Clin Chem* 1974; 20:660.

380. Noonan DC, Komjathy ZL: Long-term reproducibility of a new pH/blood-gas quality-control system compared to two other procedures. *Clin Chem* 1976; 22:1817–1820.

381. Bird BD, Henderson FA: The use of serum as a control in acid-base determination. *Br J Anaesth* 1971; 43:592–594.

382. Steiner MC, Shapiro BA, Kavanaugh J, et al: A stable blood product for pH-blood gas quality control. *Clin Chem* 1978; 24:793–795.

383. Leary ET, Graham G, Kenny MA: Commercially available blood gas quality controls compared with tonometered blood. *Clin Chem* 1980; 26:1309–1316.

384. Louderback A, Szatkowski P, Matthews H: A new and stable whole blood pH/blood gas control employed for monitoring all measured and calculated parameters associated with pH/blood gas analyzers and oximeter instrumentation. *Clin Chem* 1977; 23:1141.

385. Weisbrot IM, Kambli VB, Gorton L: An evaluation of clinical laboratory performance of pH-blood gas analysis using whole blood tonometer specimens. *Am J Clin Pathol* 1974; 61:923–935.

386. Cormier AD, Legg KD, Feil MC: Emulsion-based gas controls with high oxygen capacity. *Clin Chem* 1980; 26:997.

387. Rej R, Graffunder B, Bretaudiere JR: Suitability of materials for internal and external quality control of pH and blood gas measurements, abstracted. *Clin Chem* 1980; 26:1014.

388. Lancaster RC: Spectrophotometric instrumentation, in Davidsohn I, Henry JB (eds): *Clinical Diagnosis by Laboratory Methods,* ed 14. WB Saunders Co, Philadelphia, 1969.

389. Evenson MA: Principles of instrumentation, in Henry JB (ed): *Diagnosis and Management by Laboratory Methods,* ed 16. Philadelphia, WB Saunders Co, 1979.

390. Willard HH, Merritt LL, Dean JA: *Instrumental Methods of Analysis.* New York, D Van Nostrand Co, 1965.

391. Caraway WT: Analytic procedures and instrumentation, in Tutz NW (ed): *Fundamentals of Clinical Chemistry*, ed 2. Philadelphia, WB Saunders Co, 1976.

392. Horicker BL: The absorption spectra of hemoglobin and its derivatives in the visible and near infra-red regions. *J Biol Chem* 1943; 148:173–183.

393. Severinghaus JW, Astrup PB: History of blood gas analysis: VI. Oximetry. *J Clin Monit* 1986; 2:270–288.

394. Brown LJ: A new instrument for the simultaneous measurement of total hemoglobin, % oxyhemoglobin, % carboxyhemoglobin, % methemoglobin, and oxygen content in whole blood. *IEEE Trans Biomed Eng* 1980; 27 (No. 3) 132–138.

395. Nilsson NJ: Oximetry. *Physiol Rev* 1960; 40:1–23.

396. Falholt W: Blood oxygen saturation determined spectrophometrically. *Scand J Clin Lab Invest* 1963; 15:67–72.

397. Ramiere A Jr, Jatlow P, Seligson D: New method for rapid determination of carboxyhemoglobin by use of double-wavelength spectrophotometry. *Clin Chem* 1974; 20:278–281.

398. Gordy E, Drabken DL: Spectrophotometric studies: XVI. Determination of the oxygen saturation of blood by a simplified technique applicable to standard equipment. *J Biol Chem* 1957; 227:285–299.

399. *Operator's Manual 482: Co-Oximeter*. Instrumentation Laboratory Inc, Catalogue No. 79482, 1987.

400. Sidi A, Rush WR, Paulus DA, et al: Effect of fluorescein, indocyanine green and methylene blue on the measurement of oxygen saturation by pulse oximetry. *Anesthesiology* 1986; 65 (No. 3A):A132.

401. Scheller MS, Unger RJ: The influence of intravenously administered dyes on pulse oximetry readings. *Anesthesiology* 1986; 65 (No. 3A):A161.

402. Barker SJ, Tremper KK: The effect of carbon monoxide inhalation on pulse oximetry and transcutaneous PO_2. *Anesthesiology* 1987; 66(5):677–679.

403. Tsao MV, Sethma SS, Sloan CH, et al: Spectrophometric determination of the oxygen saturation of whole blood. *J Biol Chem* 1955; 217:479–487.

404. Chapman KR, Rebuck AS: Oximetry, in Nochomovity ML, Cherniack NS (eds): *Noninvasive Respiratory Monitoring*. New York, Churchill Livingstone, Inc, vol. 3, 1986.

405. Flick MR, Block AJ: Continuous in-vivo measurement of arterial oxygen saturation by oximetry. *Heart Lung* 1977; 6 (No. 6):990–993.

406. Yoshiya I, Shimada H, Tanaka K: Spectrophometric monitoring of arterial oxygen saturation in the fingertip. *Med Biol Eng Comput* 1980; 18:27–32.

407. Shimada H, Yoshiya I, Oka N: Effects of multiple scattering and peripheral circulation on arterial oxygen saturation measured with a pulse-type oximeter. *Med Biol Eng Comput* 1984; 22:475–478.

408. Peterson J: The development of pulse oximetry. *Science* 1986; 232:G135–136.

409. *Service Manual: Ohmeda Biox 3700 Pulse Oximeter.* Ohmeda, 1986, Catalogue No. 1118–303, Boulder, Colorado.
410. Yelderman M, New W Jr: Evaluation of pulse oximetry. *Anesthesiology* 1983; 59:349–352.
411. Polanyi ML, Hehir RM: New reflection oximeter. *Rev Scien Instru* 1960; 31 (No. 4):401–403.
412. Polanyi ML, Hehir RM: In-vivo oximeter with fast dynamic response. *Rev Sci Instru* 1962; 33 (No. 10): 1050–1054.
413. Johnson CC, Palm D, Stewart DC, et al: A solid state fiberoptics oximeter. *J Assoc Advan Med Instrumentation* 1971; 5 (No. 2):77–83.
414. Cole JS, Martin WE, Cheung PW, et al: Clinical studies with a solid state fiberoptic oximeter. *Am J Cardiol* 1972; 29:383–388.
415. Taylor JB, Lown B, Polanyi M: In-vivo monitoring with a fiber optic catheter. *JAMA* 1972; 221:667–673.
416. Lubbers DW: Theoretical basis of the transcutaneous blood gas measurements. *Crit Care Med* 1981; 9:721–733.
417. Eberhard P, Mundt W, Schafer R: Cutaneous blood gas monitoring in the adult. *Crit Care Med* 1981; 9:702.
418. Beran AV, Tolle CD, Huxtable RF: Cutaneous blood flow and its relationship to transcutaneous O_2/CO_2 measurements. *Crit Care Med* 1981; 9:736.
419. *Radiometer Transcutaneous Blood Gas Systems: User's Handbook*, Copenhagen, Denmark, radiometer, 1981.
420. *Kontron Instruments Operating Manual: Cutaneous PO_2 Monitor 820.* Münchenstein, Switzerland, Kontron Ltd, 1984.
421. *Kontron Instruments Operating Manual: Microgas 7640.* Münchenstein, Switzerland, Kontron Ltd, 1986.
422. Hill DW: Methods of analysis in the gaseous and vapor phase, in Scurr C, Feldman S (eds): *Scientific Foundations of Anesthesia*, ed. 3. Chicago, Year Book Medical Publishers Inc, 1982.
423. Beebe C, Liston MD: The development and performance of a mono-beam, ratio, non-dispersive infra-red gas analyzer. *ISA Trans* 1963; 2:331.
424. *PB 253 Operator's Manual.* Catalog No. 223779, Puritan Bennett Corporation of Massachusetts, 1985.
425. *PB 252/253 Airway Gas Monitor Service Manual.* Catalog No. 223778, Puritan Bennett Corporation of Massachusetts, Marlborough, Massachusetts, 1985.
426. Hill DW, Dolan AM: Biochemical instrumentation in the intensive care unit, in Hill DW, Dolan AM, Lenihan J (eds): Intensive Care Instrumentation. New York, Grune & Stratton, 1976.
427. Rebuck AS, Chapman KR: Measurement and monitoring of exhaled carbon dioxide, in Nochomovity ML, Chermack NS (eds): *Noninvasive Respiratory Monitoring.* New York, Churchill Livingstone Inc, 1986, vol 3.
428. Severinghaus TW, Larson CP, Eger EI: Correction factors for infrared carbon dioxide pressure broadening by nitrogen, nitrous oxide and cyclopropane. *Anesthesiology* 1961; 22:429–432.

429. Sodal IE, Swanson GD: Mass spectrometer in patient monitoring, in Gravenstein JS, Newbower RS, Ream Am, et al (eds): *Essential Noninvasive Monitoring in Anesthesia*. New York, Grune & Stratton, 1980.

430. Watson JT: Introduction, in Watson JT (ed): *Mass Spectrometry*. New York, Raven Press, 1985.

431. Angoline G, Massa RF: Medical mass spectrometry in simultaneous measurement of respiratory and blood gases, in Frigerio A (ed): *Recent Developments in Mass Spectrometry in Biochemistry and Medicine*. New York, Plenum Press, 1978.

432. Saari LA, Seitz WR: pH sensor based on immobilized fluoresceinamine. *Anal Chem* 1982; 54:821–825.

433. Angel SM: Optrodes: Chemically selective fiber-optic sensors. *Spectroscopy* 1987; 2:38–46.

434. Seitz WR: Chemical sensors based on fiberoptics. *Anal Chem* 1984; 56:17A–34A.

435. Lubbers DW, Opitz N: Blood gas analysis with fluorescence dyes as an example of their usefulness as quantitative chemical sensors, in *Proceedings International Meeting on Chemical Sensors, Fukuoka, Japan*. Amsterdam, Elsevier, 1983, pp 609–619.

436. Shapiro BA, Cane RD, Chomka CM, Bandala LE: Preliminary evaluation of an intra-arterial blood gas system in dogs and humans. *Crit Care Med* in press.

Index